Compendium medicine

Pocket
Dermatology

Romée Snijders & Veerle Smit
Anouk Verbeeck & Dominique de Vries

Together for Healthcare

Want to know more about Compendium Medicine? Check out our website!

www.compendiummedicine.com

First edition, 2025

© 2023 Compendium Medicine
All rights reserved. Published by Compendium Medicine B.V. under license from Synopsis B.V. as copyright holder. No part of this publication may be reproduced, stored in a computerised database and/or published in any form or in any manner, whether electronic, mechanical, by photocopying, recording or any other means, now known or hereafter invented, without the prior written consent of the publisher.

Neither the publisher nor any authors, contributors, or other representatives of Compendium Medicine assume any liability for any injury and/or damage to persons and property, as a matter of products liability, negligence or otherwise, or from any use or operation of any methods, products, instructions, or ideas in this book. This is a comprehensive limitation of liability that applies to all damages of any kind, including (without limitation) compensatory; direct, indirect, or consequential damages; loss of data, income, or profit; loss of or damage to property and claims of third parties. Links to third-party websites are provided by the publisher in good faith and for information only. The publisher disclaims any responsibility for the materials contained in any third-party website referenced in this work.

This book contains information contained from authentic and highly regarded sources. Every effort has been made to trace copyright holders and obtain their permission for the use of copyright material. Reprinted material is quoted with permission, and sources are indicated. The publisher does not provide medical advice or guidance and this work is merely a reference tool. Healthcare professionals, and not the publisher, are solely responsible for the use of this work including all medical judgments, and for any resulting diagnosis and treatments.

With respect to any pharmaceutical product identified, readers are urged to check the most current information provided on procedures featured by the manufacturer of each product to be administered, to verify the recommended dose or formula, the method, and duration of administration and contraindications. It is the responsibility of practitioners, relying on their own experience and knowledge of their patients, to make diagnoses, determine dosages and the best treatment for each patient, and take all appropriate safety precautions. Compendium Medicine does not accept responsibility or legal liability for any errors in the text, or for the misuse or misapplication of material in this work.

ISBN 9789083374093
BISAC MED 017000
Thema MJK

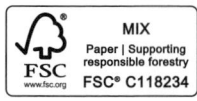

MIX
Paper | Supporting responsible forestry
FSC® C118234

Preface

Welcome to the *Compendium Community*!

'Together for Healthcare' – these three simple words encapsulate the spirit of our collective mission and underscore the essence of our work. In an era where the complexity of healthcare is becoming increasingly interconnected, collaboration is not merely an option but an imperative. Our books symbolise the effectiveness of collaboration, knowledge sharing, and a joint commitment to improve and interconnect healthcare.

We proudly present the first edition of our pocket *Dermatology*, with all the information you need at your fingertips. This comprehensive guide covers a wide range of skin conditions that will prove invaluable during your internship, residency, and in the outpatient clinic. You can explore chapters like dermatological examination, microscopy, and dermatological conditions with corresponding treatment strategies, including the most important rules regarding pharmacotherapy with a narrow therapeutic window.

The innovative *Compendium Method*©, designed for medical students and doctors, employs comprehensible illustrations for every medical condition, straightforward tables, icons, and useful mnemonics. It is visually appealing, to the point, and concise. We only focus on the essentials and make sure all the content is comprehensively presented.

Our strength lies in the diverse expertise of our close-knit medical team, consisting of students, doctors, and medical specialists. This collaborative approach ensures that our content is comprehensive and accurate.

We are committed to inclusivity and aim to make our texts and images a reflection of the diversity of patients our readers provide care to. We aspire for every (future) doctor and patient to find themselves reflected in our books. In this pocket, we focused on providing as many pictures of dermatological conditions on different skin types as possible. We aspire to offer the complete range; any contribution you can make is much appreciated!

We sincerely wish to express immense gratitude to our team of medical students and healthcare professionals. The outstanding result of their contributions is this extraordinary pocket - a pocket for everybody in healthcare.

Enjoy reading and enjoy working, and we hope to hear from you soon!

Amsterdam, June, 2025

Veerle Smit, MD & Romée Snijders, MD
Doctors and founders *Compendium Medicine*

Editorial staff

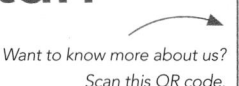

*Want to know more about us?
Scan this QR code.*

Editorial board

Romée J.A.L.M. Snijders, MD, PhD & Veerle L. Smit, MD

Chief editor

Gwendolyn Vuurberg, MD, PhD

Pocket editors

Current edition

Anouk Verbeeck, MD, Sexual Health Clinic, GGD Haaglanden, The Hague
Dominique de Vries, MD, PhD candidate, Amsterdam University Medical Center, Amsterdam

Previous edition

Carlijn Veldman, MD, University of Groningen, Groningen
Gwendolyn Vuurberg, MD, PhD, University of Amsterdam, Amsterdam

Authors

Current edition

Otte Borghouts, MD, Maastricht University, Maastricht
Dorina Kahedy, VU University, Amsterdam
Jay Yee, BSc, Erasmus University, Rotterdam

Previous edition

Linde Goijen, VU University, Amsterdam
Maud Vesseur, Maastricht University, Maastricht

Acknowledgements

Content quality assurance

The editorial board extends its sincere appreciation to the many contributions of doctors, specialists, and professors from around the world who played a pivotal role in crafting this pocket. We wish to express our thanks to the entire international team for their dedicated efforts and invaluable expertise. In particular, we are grateful to Vijay Dayalani who took the time to critically review the complete pocket. Special appreciation is also extended to the team of specialists who actively participated in shaping the previous edition.

Current edition

Deepak M.W. Balak, MD, PhD, Leiden University Medical Center, Leiden
Charlotte Burms, MD, Maastricht University Medical Center, Maastricht
Juan C. Galvis Martinez, MD, Medical Center Wetering Amsterdam, Amsterdam
Raidah Gangji, MD, Muhimbili University of Health and Allied Sciences and Kairuki University, Dar es Salaam
Vijay Dayalani, MD, Erasmus Medical Center, Rotterdam
Laurence V. Khoe, MD, Alrijne Hospital, Leiderdorp
Rutger C. Melchers, MD, PhD, Leiden University Medical Center, Leiden
Maryam Safaei, PharmD, Eastern Mediterranean University (EMU), Faculty of Pharmacy, Gazimağusa
Suzanne van Santen, MD, PhD, Leiden University Medical Center, Leiden
Pip Vlaanderen, MD, Maastricht University Medical Center, Maastricht
Prof. Henry J.C. de Vries, MD, PhD, Amsterdam University Medical Center, Amsterdam
Jim Zegelaar, MD, Flevoziekenhuis, Almere

Previous edition

Niloufar Ashtiani, MD, Dijklander Hospital, Hoorn
Deepak M.W. Balak, MD, Leiden University Medical Center, Leiden
CODING, Collective for Diversity and Inclusion in Dutch Medicine
Maria W.J.A. Dingen, MD, practice M.W.J.A. Dingen BVBA, Maasmechelen
Diversity Committee of the Dutch Society for Dermatology and Venereology
Yannick S. Elshot, MD, Amsterdam University Medical Center / Antoni van Leeuwenhoek, Amsterdam
Linde Goijen, MD, University Medical Center Groningen, Groningen
Colette L.M. van Hees, MD, Erasmus Medical Center, Rotterdam
Fabiënne Koekelkoren, MD, Erasmus Medical Center, Rotterdam
Priscilla A. Maria, MD, Amsterdam University Medical Center, Amsterdam
Leonie Meijerink - van 't Oost, MD, OLVG Hospital, Amsterdam
Jan R. Mekkes, MD, Amsterdam University Medical Center, Amsterdam
Ivo F. Nagtzaam, MD, Maastricht University Medical Center, Maastricht
Vidhya S. Narayan, MD, Amsterdam University Medical Center, Amsterdam
J. Marja Oldhoff, MD, University Medical Center Groningen, Groningen
Sanne G. Plug, MD, Leiden University Medical Center, Leiden
Lotte S. Spekhorst, MD, University Medical Center Utrecht, Utrecht
Prof. Henry J.C. de Vries, MD, Amsterdam University Medical Center, Amsterdam
Foppe H. Wiersma, MD, University Medical Center Utrecht, Utrecht
Jim E. Zeegelaar, MD, PhD, Flevoziekenhuis

Sounding board

Laura M. Barrantes Rodríguez, MD, University of Costa Rica, International Relations Manager Compendium Medicine
Fernando Dias Goncalves Lima, MD, PhD candidate, Amsterdam University Medical Center, Amsterdam
Josine Dolmans, MD, Maastricht University Medical Center, Maastricht
Emmilia Dowlatshahi, MD, PhD, OLVG Hospital, Amsterdam
Myrthe Moermans, MD, PhD candidate, Maastricht University Medical Center, Maastricht
Wouter O. van Seggelen, MD, OLVG Hospital, Amsterdam
Hitesh Suthar, MD, M. T. Agarwal Hospital, Mumbai
Fibyan bin Ishaq, Dhaka University, East West Medical College & Hospital (EWMCH), Dhaka

Editorial coordinators

Laura M. Barrantes Rodríguez, MD, junior editor
Pauline Blom, final editor
Vera den Boef, MSc, project manager
Melanie Goedegebure, product manager
Delano R. Sanches, MD, BSc, illustration manager

Illustrators

Yente S. Beentjes, MD, University Medical Center Utrecht, Utrecht
Dagmar Bouwer, Leiden University, Leiden
Susan Deelstra, University of Groningen, Groningen
Lotte Dupuis, Radboud University, Nijmegen
Gulizar Durak, University of Applied Sciences, Rotterdam
Astrid A.H. Feikema, Radboud University, Nijmegen
Iza Hogenelst, University of Applied Sciences, Amsterdam
Nicky Janssen, Maastricht University, Maastricht
Koen L.C. Ketelaars, MD, GP practice De Brink, Severum
Rosalie C. Krijl, MD, Ask Arbo Artsen, Zeist
Juliëtte M.E. Linskens, MD, Maastricht University, Maastricht
Laura Sanchez, MSc, KU Leuven, Leuven
Carlijn Sturm, BSc, Leiden University, Leiden

Language support

Bram van Breugelen, BSc, Radboud University, Nijmegen
Eva L. Brunner, MD, NSPOH, The Hague
Translation Agency Perfect
Mark Hannay, translator
Ruth Rose, editor

Graphic designers

Maria van Doorn, BASc
Ivana Kinkel

The Compendium Method© Manual

In *Compendium Medicine* we use the same concise, visual and schematic description of the various medical specialties. Everything is geared towards overview and structure, facilitating study and practice. We call this the *Compendium Method*©.

Fixed layout
All our medical specialties are presented in the same, recognisable way and each has its own colour and icon. The pockets have a fixed chapter structure. The table of contents of each pocket tells you exactly which topics are covered. The symbols in the corner of the page show what kind of information is being discussed.

- Anatomy
- Physiology
- Patient history
- Physical examination
- Diagnostics
- Treatment
- Differential diagnosis
- Conditions
- Clinical reasoning
- Appendices
- References
- Abbreviations
- Index

Illustrations
The figures provide at-a-glance insight into topics like anatomy or the typical patient. They are also intended for study and practice, such as checking whether you can identify the letters in a picture without looking at the caption.

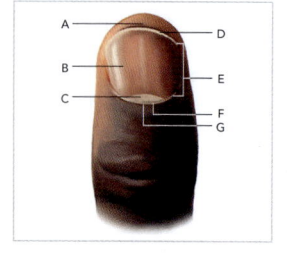

Figure 3 // Nail: external
A: Hyponychium **B:** Nail plate **C:** Lunula
D: Free margin **E:** Paronychium **F:** Cuticle
G: Eponychium

Conditions

Each condition in this pocket starts with a full-sentence definition followed by a telegram-style explanation. For each condition, the following icons (as applicable) are discussed. These visual cues that convey specific attributes or features of the condition are also useful when studying. You can cover the text and quiz yourself.

- (D) Definition
- (E) Epidemiology
- (Ae) Aetiology
- (R) Risk factors
- (Hx) Patient history
- (PE) Physical examination
  - (P) Place
  - (A) Arrangement
  - (S) Size
  - (S) Shape
  - (O) Outline
  - (N) Nuance/colour
  - (E) Efflorescence
- (Dx) Diagnostics
- (Tx) Treatment
  - 💬 General
  - 👁 Paramedical care
  - 💊 Pharmacological treatment
  - ✏️ Invasive, non-pharmacological treatment
- (P) Prognosis
- (!) Watch out/don´t forget

Tables

We use tables to arrange the information in a clear and structured manner, with columns representing different conditions and rows indicating features or characteristics. Centered formatting for matching features makes it easy to identify similarities and differences.

Diagrams

⟶ = positive/yes/+   ⟶ = negative/no/-

> Diagrams help you reason clinically, starting from a particular symptom, using the green and red arrows as signposts. Always remember that the full differential diagnosis may consist of additional diagnoses.

Icons & frames

Throughout this pocket you will find highlighted frames.

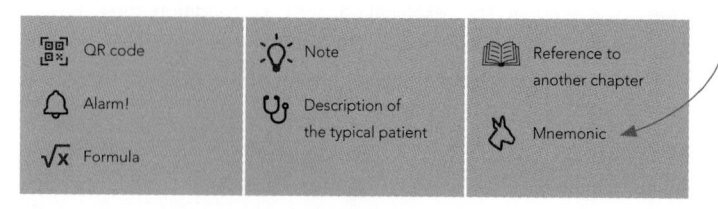

Fun fact: our founders are Dutch, and in the Netherlands, we refer to a mnemonic as a "donkey bridge". That's why the symbol for mnemonics in our books is a donkey.

QR code	Note	Reference to another chapter
Alarm!	Description of the typical patient	Mnemonic
Formula		

Punctuation marks

The punctuation in our books also focuses on overview and ensures that the subject matters are covered concisely and effectively.

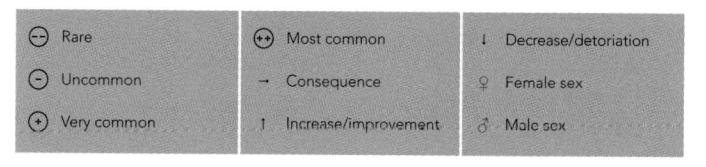

⊖ Rare	⊕ Most common	↓ Decrease/deterioration
⊖ Uncommon	→ Consequence	♀ Female sex
⊕ Very common	↑ Increase/improvement	♂ Male sex

Abbreviations

We make extensive use of abbreviations, medical terms and symbols for scientific units and quantities. Below are some examples of the abbreviations used in this pocket.

sec	second/seconds	d	day/days	min.	minimum
min	minute/minutes	wk	week/weeks	max.	maximum
h	hour/hours	mo	month/months	e.g.	for example
		y	year/years	L	litre/litres

Index
The pockets include a comprehensive and easy-to-use index. It contains all the topics covered in the books so you can quickly navigate and find the information you are looking for.

Appendices
In the pockets, you will find space for your notes, additional information, reminders, or insights. In addition, handy appendices have been added; these contain specific information that you would like to have at hand and are therefore located at the back of the pockets.

They/theirs
We realise that sex and gender identity are not binary and that there is more variation than just 'woman' or 'man'. For readability's sake (as well as for grammatical reasons) we have therefore chosen to use the pronouns 'they/theirs', regardless of sex or gender identity.

Warning
When studying this pocket, be mindful of the protocols within your own facility and adhere to the established guidelines. It is also essential to understand the circumstances under which you may or may not provide assistance in a given country, as this can potentially have legal consequences.

Want to know more about the Compendium Method©? Scan the QR code.

Table of contents
Dermatology

Anatomy	**18**
Skin	18
Adnexa	19
Hairs	19
Sebaceous glands	19
Sweat glands	19
Nails	20
Face	21
Aesthetic units	21
Relaxed skin tension lines	22
Danger zones	23
Venous system of the lower extremities	25
Physiology	**26**
Thermoregulation	26
Protective functions	26
Immunological function	26
Sensory function	27
Hair growth	27
Vitamin D3 production	27
Patient history	**28**
General	28
Malignancy risk factors	28
Course	29
Eliciting factors	29
Other	29
Past dermatological history	29
Chief complaint	29
Physical examination	**30**
PASS ONE©	30
Colour	31
Efflorescence	33
Dermoscopy	36
Wood's lamp	36
Skin type	36
Fitzpatrick Skin Type Classification	36
Colorimetric Scale Skin Tone Classification	38
Diagnostics	**40**
Skin biopsy and excision	40
Immunofluorescence biopsy	42
Histopathological and immunohistochemical testing	42
Duplex ultrasound	43
Allergy testing	44
Epicutaneous test (patch test)	44
Skin prick test	44
Serology	44
Radioallergosorbent test	44
Phadiatop test	45
Microscopy	45
Microbiological testing	45
Parasitic diagnostics	45
Mycological test	45
Infections and arthropods	45
Gram staining	46
Serological testing	46
General	46
Proctological examination	47
High-resolution anoscopy	47
Anal swab	47
Treatment	**48**

Pharmacological treatment	48		Keratolytics	66
Analgesics	48		Retinoids	67
Opioids	48		General	67
Ointments and creams	50		Topical retinoids	67
Non-medicated therapy	50		Oral retinoids	67
Creams	50		Topical fluorouracil	68
Ointments	50		Dimethyl fumarate	68
Immunosuppressive drugs	51		Invasive, non-pharmacological treatment	70
Corticosteroids	51		Cryotherapy	70
General	51		Electrocoagulation	70
Local corticosteroids	51		Excision biopsy melanoma	70
Intralesional corticosteroids	51		Therapeutic lipoma excision	72
Other anti-inflammatory and immunosuppressive drugs	52		Knot-tying and suturing techniques	73
			Suturing	73
Biologicals	54		Knot-tying	78
TNF-alpha blockers	54		Suture removal	78
Interleukin inhibitors	55		Mohs micrographic surgery	78
Janus kinase inhibitors	58		Wound treatment	78
Antibacterial therapy	60		Treatment of varicose veins	79
General	60		Compression therapy	79
Groups of antibiotics	60		Sclerotherapy (injecting varicose veins)	79
Antibiotic resistance and switch therapy	63		Endovenous techniques (cauterisation from within the vein)	79
Topical antibiotics	65		Muller procedure (ambulatory phlebectomy)	79
Other	65		Stripping and crossectomy	79
Antiviral therapy	65		PUVA/UVA/UVB	79
Antiparasitic therapy	65		Photodynamic therapy	80
Antimycotics	66			
Hydroxychloroquine	66			
Antihistamines	66			

Table of contents
Dermatology

Laser therapy	80
Differential diagnosis	**82**
Pruritus (itching)	82
Pruritus with primary skin lesions	82
Pruritus without primary skin lesions	82
Erythema	83
Generalised erythema (erythroderma)	83
Local erythema	84
Generalised erythema in children	84
Facial pustules	85
Hair loss	85
Suspicious skin lesions	85
Conditions	**86**
Pustular dermatoses	**86**
Acneiform dermatoses	86
Acne vulgaris	86
Comedonal acne	88
Papulopustular acne	88
Acne conglobata	89
Acne keloidalis nuchae	89
Perioral dermatitis	91
Hidradenitis suppurativa	92
Rosacea	94
Erythematotelangiectatic rosacea	95
Papulopustular rosacea	95
Pyodermas	96
Folliculitis	96
Pseudofolliculitis barbae	97
Furuncle and carbuncle	99
Impetigo vulgaris	100
Palmoplantar pustulosis	101
Bullous dermatoses	**102**
Bullous pemphigoid	102
Dermatitis herpetiformis	103
Bullous impetigo	105
Pemphigus vulgaris	106
Toxic epidermal necrolysis	107
Nodular dermatoses	**109**
Erythema nodosum	109
Prurigo nodularis	110
Papulomatous dermatoses	**111**
Granuloma annulare	111
Lichen planus	112
Keratosis pilaris	114
Eczematous dermatoses	**115**
Constitutional dermatitis	115
Acrovesicular eczema	116
Allergic contact dermatitis	118
Irritant contact dermatitis	119
Intertriginous dermatitis	121
Nummular dermatitis	122
Seborrhoeic dermatitis	123
Lichen simplex chronicus	125
Prurigo	**126**
Xerosis cutis	126
Notalgia paresthetica	127
Erythematous dermatoses	**128**
Acute urticaria and angioedema	128

Erythema chronicum migrans	129	Lipoma	151
Erythema multiforme minor	130	Seborrhoeic keratosis	152
Erythema multiforme major	131	Dermatosis papulosa nigra	153
Polymorphous light eruption	132	Benign lichenoid keratosis	153
Lichen sclerosus	134	Neurofibroma	154
Infectious exanthem	135	**Premalignant skin lesions**	**155**
Cutaneous adverse drug reactions	136	Actinic keratosis	155
		Bowen's disease	157
Erythematosquamous dermatoses	**137**	**Malignant skin tumours**	**158**
Pityriasis rosea	137	Basal cell carcinoma	158
Psoriasis vulgaris	138	Squamous cell carcinoma	160
Guttate psoriasis	141	Melanoma	161
Scalp psoriasis	141	Lentigo maligna	163
Psoriasis inversa	141	Cutaneous t-cell lymphoma	164
Cutaneous lupus erythematosus	142	**Naevi**	**166**
Acute cutaneous lupus erythematosus	142	Acquired melanocytic naevus	166
		Becker naevus	168
Subacute cutaneous lupus erythematosus	142	Halo naevus	168
		Naevus sebaceous	169
Chronic cutaneous lupus erythematosus	142	Naevus spilus	169
		Spitz naevus	169
Pityriasis lichenoides	144	**Pigmentation disorders**	**170**
Pityriasis lichenoides chronica	144	Café-au-lait macule	170
		Solar lentigo	171
Pityriasis lichenoides et varioliformis acuta	144	Lentigo simplex	172
		Melasma	173
Skin tumours	**146**	Pityriasis versicolor	174
Benign skin tumours	146	Vitiligo	175
Epidermoid cyst	146	Postinflammatory hyperpigmentation	176
Dermatofibroma	147		
Keloid	148	Pityriasis alba	177
Keratoacanthoma	149	Acanthosis nigricans	178

Table of contents
Dermatology

Erythema dyschromicum perstans	179
Progressive macular hypomelanosis	180
Cutaneous amyloidosis	181
Macular cutaneous amyloidosis	182
Lichen amyloidosis	182
Pressure ulcers	**183**
Pressure ulcers	183
Lymphology	**186**
Lymphoedema	186
Vascular conditions	**187**
Venous skin conditions	187
Chronic venous insufficiency	187
C2 varicose veins	189
Venous leg ulcer	190
Arterial skin conditions	**192**
Arterial leg ulcer (Fontaine IV)	192
Pernio	193
Cherry angioma	195
Pyogenic granuloma	195
Sexually transmitted infections	**197**
Chlamydia	197
Gonorrhoea	198
Genital herpes	199
Condylomata acuminata	200
Pediculosis capitis	201
Pediculosis pubis (phthiriasis pubis)	202
Scabies	203
Syphilis	204
Trichomoniasis	207
Lymphogranuloma venereum	208
Human immunodeficiency virus infection and acquired immunodeficiency syndrome	209
Human papilloma virus induced malignancies/pre-malignancies	212
Anal intraepithelial neoplasia	213
Bacterial infections	**215**
Cellulitis	215
Erysipelas	215
Erythrasma	216
Necrotising fasciitis	217
Viral infections	**218**
Oral herpes	218
Herpes zoster	219
Molluscum contagiosum	220
Verruca vulgaris	221
Kaposi sarcoma (KS)	223
Classic KS (Sporadic)	224
Iatrogenic KS (Immuno-compromised)	224
Endemic KS (African)	225
Aids Associated KS	225
Dermatomycoses	**226**
Onychomycosis	226
Tinea capitis	227
Tinea corporis	228
Tinea pedis	229
Trichosis	**230**
Alopecia areata	230

Androgenetic alopecia	232	**Clinical reasoning**	**254**
Cicatricial alopecia	233	Allergic reactions	254
Lichen planopilaris	234	Suspicious skin lesion	255
Frontal fibrosing alopecia	234	**Appendices**	**256**
Dissecting cellulitis of the scalp	235	Appendix 1: Medication dosage	256
Folliculitis decalvans	235	**References**	**261**
Telogen effluvium	236	**Illustrations & figures**	**262**
Hirsutism	237	**Epilogue**	**265**
Central Centrifugal Cicatricial alopecia	238	**About us**	**268**
Traction alopecia	239	**Compendium Compass©**	**270**
Hyperhidrosis	240	**Abbreviations**	**272**
Paediatrics	**241**	**Index**	**275**
Measles (morbilli)	**242**		
Scarlett fever (scarlatina)	242		
Rubella (German measles or three-day measles)	242		
Erythema infectiosum (5th disease)	243		
Exanthema subitum (6th disease, roseola infantum)	243		
Chickenpox (varicella)	243		
Haemangioma (strawberry naevus)	246		
Diaper dermatitis	248		
Congenital dermal melanocytosis	249		
Naevus flammeus	249		
Seborrhoeic dermatitis of the head (cradle cap)	251		
Neonatal acne	252		

Anatomy

Skin

The skin is the largest organ of the body and consists of several layers (see Figure 1). The superficial layer of the skin (epidermis) consists of keratinised squamous cell epithelium. Melanocytes in the basal layer of the epidermis produce pigment called melanin. There are two types of melanin (eumelanin and pheomelanin), with their amount and mutual ratio determining the pigmentation of the skin. Below the epidermis lies a highly vascular layer of connective tissue (dermis), which is home to the adnexa of the skin. The epidermis and dermis are connected by the basal membrane, and together make up the cutis. The dermis supplies the avascular epidermis with oxygen and nutrients (see Table 1). Below the dermis is a layer of loose adipose and connective tissue (subcutis/hypodermis, subcutaneous connective tissue).

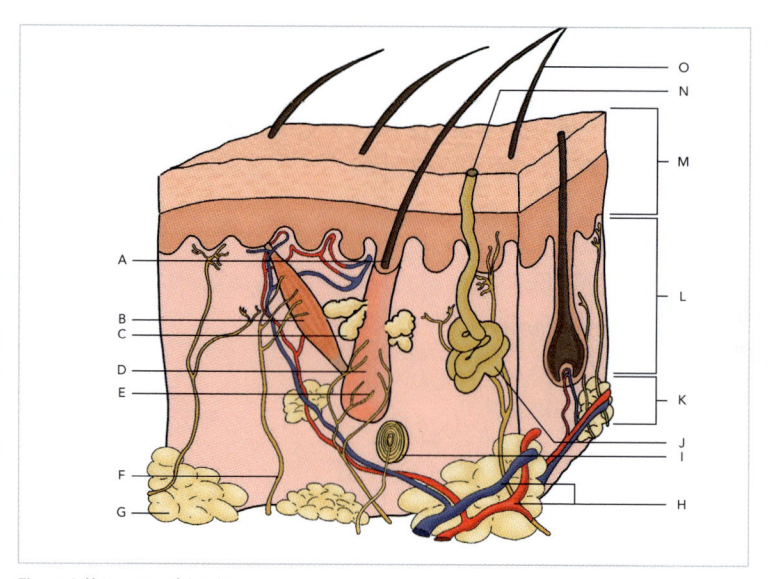

Figure 1 // Anatomy of the skin
A: Hair follicle **B:** Arrector pili muscle **C:** Sebaceous (oil) gland **D:** Hair root **E:** Hair follicle receptor **F:** Sensory nerve fiber **G:** Adipose tissue **H:** Cutaneous vascular plexus **I:** Pacinian corpuscle **J:** Eccrine sweat gland **K:** Hypodermis **L:** Dermis **M:** Epidermis **N:** Pore of sweat gland duct **O:** Hair shaft

SKIN LAYER	CHARACTERISTICS
Epidermis (A)	Keratinised squamous cell epithelium, melanocytes, Merkel cells, Langerhans cells, avascular
Dermis (D)	Connective tissue, adnexa, highly vascular
Subcutis (F)	Fat cells

Table 1 // Characteristics of skin layers

Adnexa

The skin contains the following structures: hair, sebaceous glands, sweat glands, and nails. Together, these structures are known as the adnexa or appendages.

Hairs

Hair consists of a root and a shaft, growing from a hair follicle located in the dermis. A hair follicle consists of a hair papilla with capillaries, a nerve, a sebaceous gland, and the arrector pili muscle, the little muscle that causes hair to stand on end. This muscle is surrounded by stem cells from which new hair follicles can grow.

Sebaceous glands

Sebaceous glands develop from hair follicles, and the ducts through which these glands secrete sebum usually run through the same follicles (see Figure 1). Free sebaceous glands have ducts that lead directly to the surface of the epidermis. They are found e.g. in the areola, the tip of the penis, the vermillion border, and the perianal region (see Figure 2). Sebum keeps the skin moist and has antimicrobial properties.

Sweat glands

There are two types of sweat glands: eccrine and apocrine. Eccrine glands are the more common type and are localised on the palms of the hands, soles of the feet, scalp, and armpits. These glands produce sweat in hot weather and during stressful, emotional experiences. The apocrine sweat glands are activated during puberty, secreting sweat in response to hormonal factors. The moisture-producing part of a sweat gland is located in the lower part of the dermis and in the subcutis. Sweat ducts run through the dermis, making several coils and opening to the skin's surface (see Figures 1 and 2).

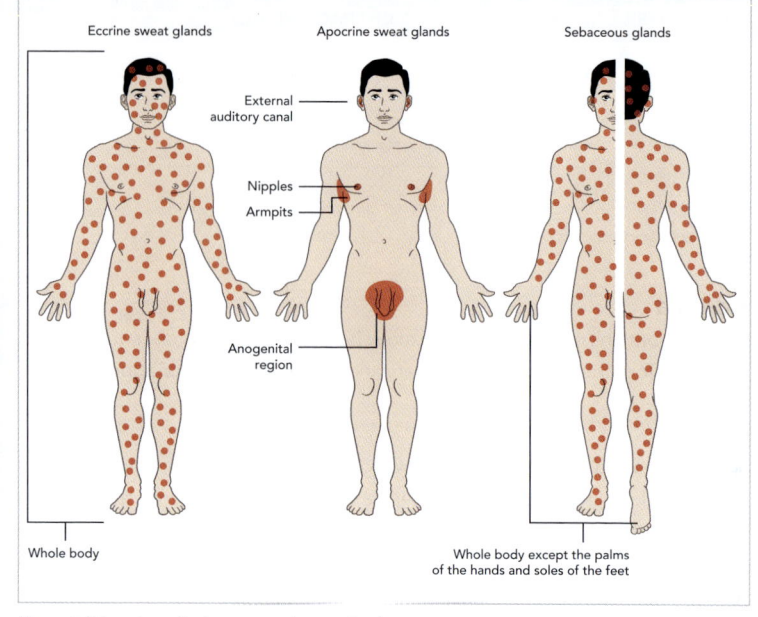

Figure 2 // Locations of sebaceous and sweat glands

Nails

Nails are keratinised plates that grow from the nail matrix, with the nail root as the most proximal part. The nail grows distally over the nail bed, which consists of a thickened layer of epidermis (stratum corneum) (see Figures 3 and 4).

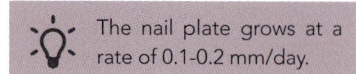

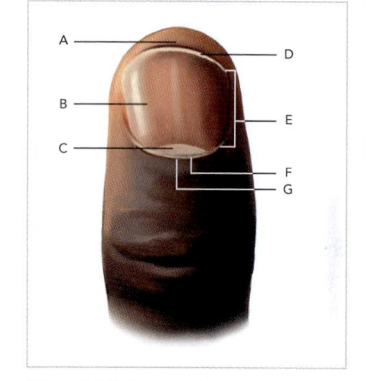

> The nail plate grows at a rate of 0.1-0.2 mm/day.

Figure 3 // Nail: external
A: Hyponychium **B:** Nail plate **C:** Lunula **D:** Free margin **E:** Paronychium **F:** Cuticle **G:** Eponychium

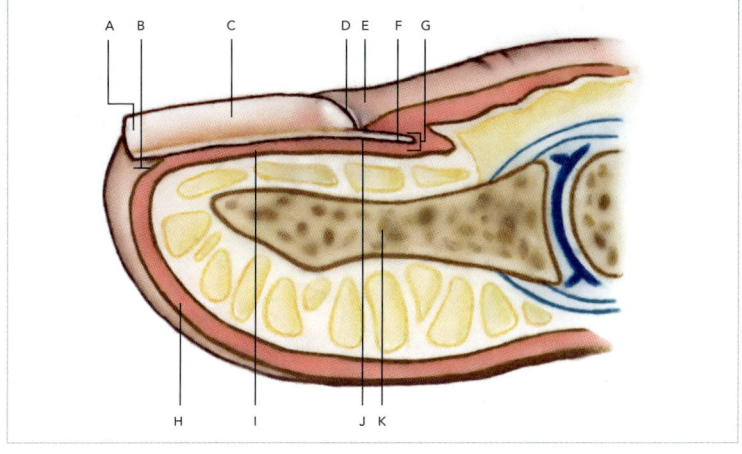

Figure 4 // Nail: internal
A: Free margin **B:** Hyponychium **C:** Nail plate **D:** Cuticle **E:** Eponychium **F:** Nail root **G:** Nail fold (dorsal and ventral matrix) **H:** Cutis **I:** Nail bed **J:** Nail matrix **K:** Distal phalanx

Face

Aesthetic units

The face can be divided into nine 'aesthetic units', each with smaller subunits (see Figure 5). The central units (nose, lips, eyelids) are distinguished from the peripheral units (cheeks, forehead, chin). These units are used to guide incisions for procedures, as incisions made at the interface of several units are less likely to create deformities and produce better functional and aesthetic results. A scar in the furrow adjacent to the ala of the nose (interface between units B3 and D1) is less noticeable than a scar that runs across the ala (unit B3).

> It is very important to distinguish central from peripheral aesthetic units, as the principles of facial reconstruction apply more to the former than the latter. For instance, asymmetry in central units is more noticeable.

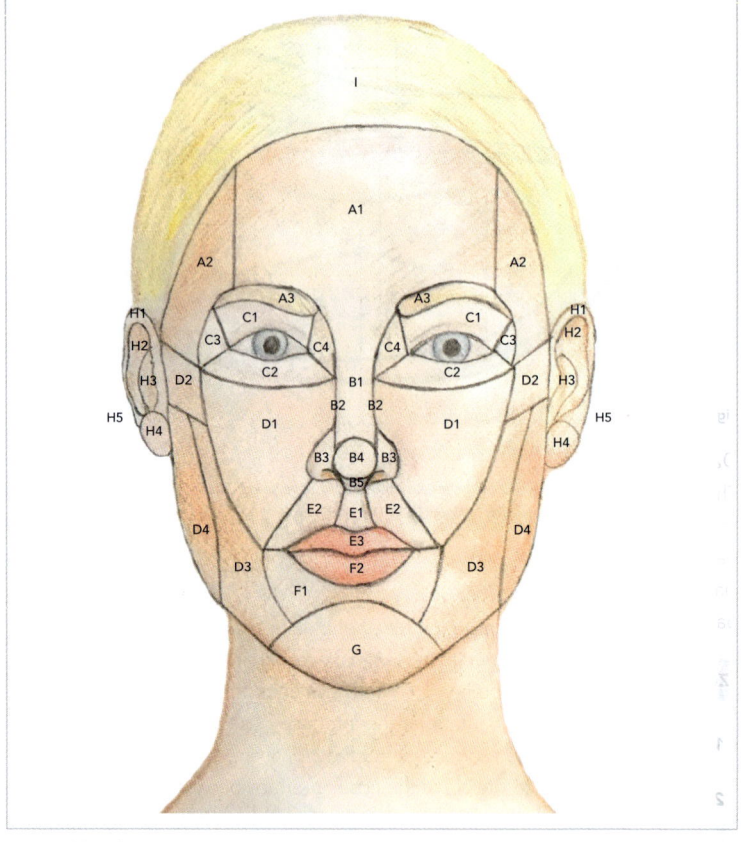

Figure 5 // Aesthetic units
A: Forehead **B:** Nose **C:** Periorbital **D:** Cheeks **E:** Upper lip **F:** Lower lip **G:** Chin **H:** Ears **I:** Scalp

Relaxed skin tension lines (RSTL)

RSTL are imaginary lines across the skin that run perpendicular to the directional pull of the underlying muscles. Closing skin defects along the RSTL produces more aesthetically satisfying scars by taking advantage of the elasticity of the skin. See Figure 6 for the RSTL of the face.

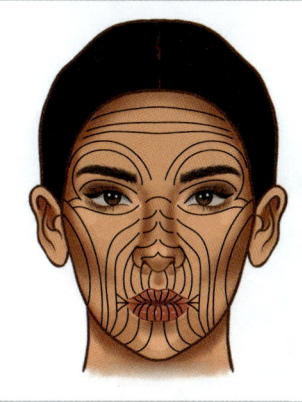

Figure 6 // Relaxed skin tension lines of the face

Danger zones

There are seven different 'danger zones' in the face (see Figure 7). It is important to pay attention to these danger zones when performing facial dissection. The danger zones are the most common areas in which damage to the peripheral facial nerves occurs. Damage to these nerves can cause permanent numbness or paralysis of facial muscles (see Table 2).

ZONE	NERVE	SYMPTOMS OF NERVE PALSY
1 (S)	Greater auricular nerve	Numbness of the lower two-thirds of the ear, the surrounding part of the cheek, and the neck
2 (M)	Temporal branch of the facial nerve	Paralysis of the eyebrow
3 (M)	Marginal mandibular branch of the facial nerve	Paralysis of the lower lip
4 (M)	Zygomatic and buccal branches of the facial nerve	Paralysis of the upper lip and cheek
5 (S)	Supraorbital nerve, supratrochlear nerve	Numbness of the forehead, upper eyelid, bridge of the nose, and skull
6 (S)	Infraorbital nerve	Numbness of the nasal sidewalls, cheek, upper lip, and lower eyelid
7 (M)	Mental nerve	Numbness of the chin and part of the lower lip

Table 2 // Danger zones in the face
(M), motor nerve branch; (S), sensitive nerve branch

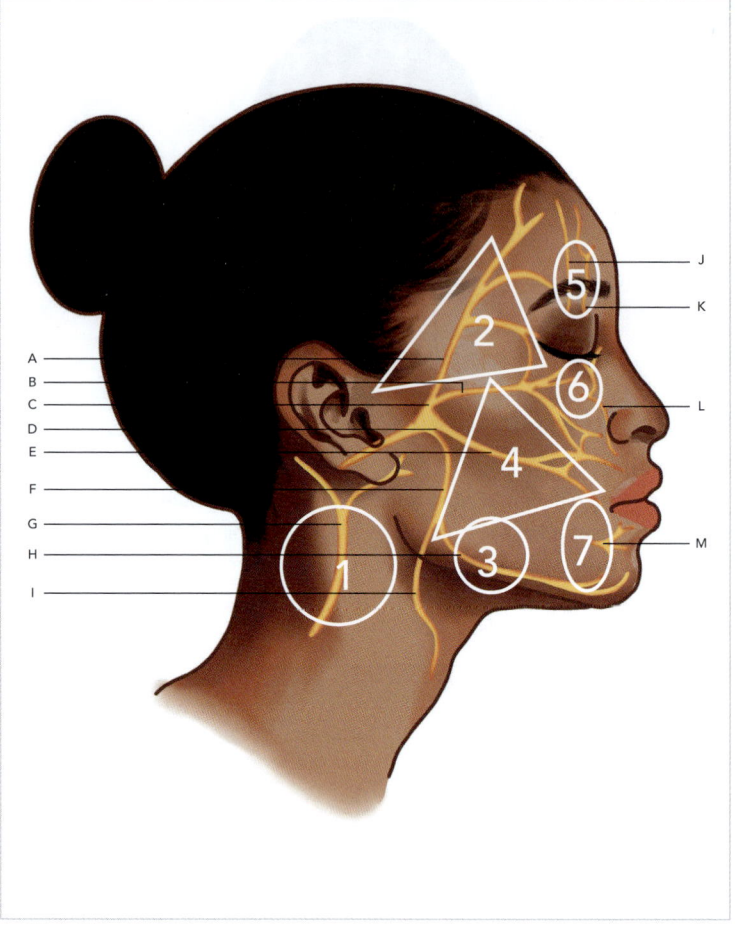

Figure 7 // Danger zones in the face

A: Temporal branch of the facial nerve **B:** Zygomatic branch of the facial nerve **C:** Temporal branch of the facial nerve **D:** Cervical branch of the facial nerve **E:** Buccal branch of the facial nerve **F:** Sub-branch of the facial nerve **G:** Greater auricular nerve **H:** Marginal mandibular branch of the facial nerve **I:** Cervical branch of the facial nerve **J:** Supraorbital nerve of the trigeminal nerve **K:** Supratrochlear nerve of the trigeminal nerve **L:** Infraorbital nerve of the trigeminal nerve **M:** Mental nerve of the trigeminal nerve

Venous system of the lower extremities

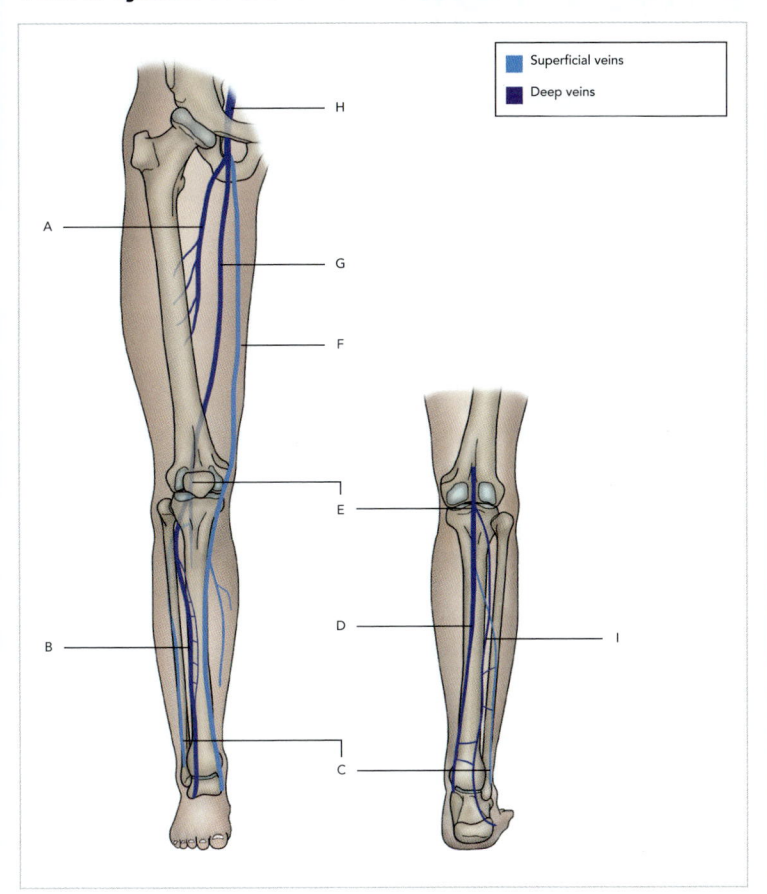

Figure 8 // Venous system of the lower extremities
A: Deep femoral vein **B:** Anterior tibial vein **C:** Small saphenous vein **D:** Posterior tibial vein **E:** Popliteal vein
F: Great saphenous vein **G:** Femoral vein **H:** External iliac vein **I:** Fibular veins

Physiology

Thermoregulation

The skin maintains a constant body temperature by regulating temperature reduction and retention. Temperature reduction is promoted by increasing skin perfusion (vasodilation) and stimulating sweat secretion, while retention is achieved by decreasing skin perfusion (vasoconstriction) and reducing sweat secretion.

> 💡 The main function of sweating is to cool the skin.

Protective functions

The skin, as the body's largest organ, has several protective functions:

- The skin serves as a barrier between the organism and the outside world. With the help of the stratum corneum, it prevents moisture loss and maintains a stable internal environment.
- The skin possesses several protective mechanisms against potentially pathogenic microorganisms. An intact stratum corneum, which regenerates rapidly, is an important line of defence against microorganisms. Antimicrobial peptides such as defensins and cathelicidins can kill various microorganisms, while the free fatty acids present on the skin also have an antibacterial effect. Finally, the skin flora prevents other microorganisms from colonising the skin surface.
- The presence of dermal and subcutaneous collagen and elastin means that the skin can be stretched and indented, preventing mechanical damage.
- The skin provides protection against the harmful effects of UV radiation. Epidermal melanin and the protein barrier in the stratum corneum both protect the body by absorbing UV radiation, reducing damage to cellular components such as deoxyribonucleic acid (DNA). Increased melanin production causes the skin to tan. Melanin is stored in melanosomes, which are found in adjacent basal keratinocytes. Exposure to the sun also thickens the stratum corneum. Skin tans due to an increase in the number of both melanocytes and melanosomes.
- The skin secretes sweat to prevent the body from overheating. It also functions as an insulating layer that retains heat in the cold.

Immunological function

The immune system detects and eliminates foreign bodies and microorganisms. The body has an innate and an acquired immune system. Dendritic cells are part of the adaptive (or acquired) immune system and are called Langerhans cells when found in the skin. Langerhans cells have a gatekeeper function in the epidermis and are capable of phagocytosing foreign particles. After phagocytosis, dendritic cells migrate through the lymphatic vessels to the lymph nodes, where they present antigens to T lymphocytes.

Sensory function
Nerve endings are distributed in the skin and are responsible for perceiving sensations such as heat, cold, pain, itching, pressure, vibration, and touch. Merkel cells also play a role in this process.

Hair growth
Hair growth is a cycle consisting of three phases: the anagen phase (growth phase, four to six years, 80% of all hair), the catagen phase (transition phase, fourteen days), and the telogen phase (resting phase, three to four months). Hair is shed after the telogen phase (see Figure 9).

Vitamin D3 production
See Figure 10 for an overview of vitamin D3 production.

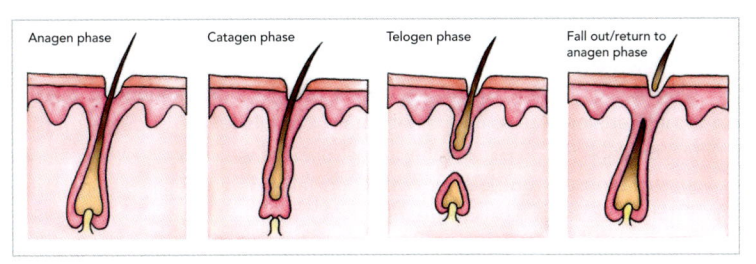

Figure 9 // Cycle of hair growth

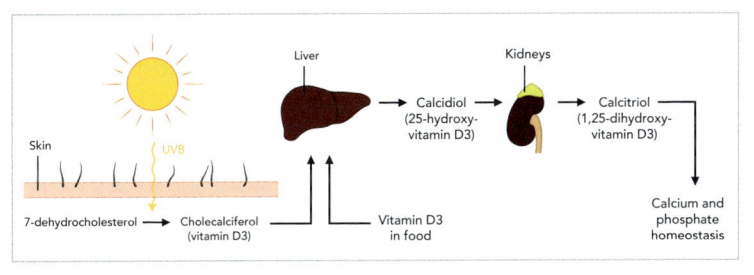

Figure 10 // Vitamin D3 production

Patient history

Introduction	Patient history	Concluding
· Introduce yourself · Check personal details · Assess the patient: acute or non-acute, determine reason for consultation and/or chief complaint, non-verbal communication	· General patient history · History of presenting complaint/current illness · History of relevant system (full review of systems if necessary)	· Summarise your findings · Patient's remarks and/or questions · Explain physical examination and/or indicated diagnostics

Consider psychosocial variables such as language barriers, cultural differences between patients and physicians, financial backgrounds, and addiction, which may impact disease progression.

Diagram 1 // Patient history

General
While taking the dermatological history, it is important to enquire about the chief complaint, as well as the course and possible cause of the symptoms. Many skin pathologies can be diagnosed at first glance - a quick look is enough to give fair diagnostic certainty. Assessing the patient's risk profile for developing a particular skin condition can help make the correct diagnosis (e.g. family history of skin cancer, sun exposure, outdoor job, etc.). See Table 3 for specific history-taking for common dermatological symptoms.

General patient history
Medical history, medication use (exact dosage, frequency, last dose, administration form), history of substance use (smoking, alcohol, drugs), allergies (latex, plasters, medication, contrast agents), family history, psychosocial history, travel history, social history (home situation, work, study, social support), vaccinations, ill individuals in immediate vicinity.

Malignancy risk factors
Always enquire about the following risk factors if skin cancer is suspected: sun exposure, rapid burning, little pigmentation after sun exposure, visit to the tropics, tanning bed use, use of sunscreen, past sunburn, blisters from sunburn, pos-

itive medical history (PMHx) (melanoma, basal cell carcinoma (BCC), squamous cell carcinoma (SCC)), smoking, immunodeficiency (e.g. use of immunosuppressive medications), work (frequently outdoors).

Course
Pathogenesis, duration of symptoms, growth, colour change, shape change, recurrence, quiet spells, location, and spread.

Eliciting factors
Work, stress, hobbies, light and sunlight, contact with chemicals, treatment to date, effect of treatment, relatives with similar condition, baths/showers, soap/cosmetic use (e.g. new detergent, fabric softener), trauma, contact with animals.

Other
Itching, scratching, pain, bleeding, scaling, burning.

Past dermatological history
Skin cancer, atopy (asthma, hay fever, eczema/dermatitis), other skin diseases.

Chief complaint
Influence on daily life, psychological impact (e.g. due to shame), patient expectations.

SUSPECTED DIAGNOSIS	HISTORY
Skin cancer	Growth, colour change, itching, bleeding, pain, enquire about risk factors
Eczema	Location, course, psychological impact, dry skin, FHx (atopy, asthma, dermatitis, hay fever), evidence of food allergy in children, external factors such as bathing/showering, soap use, work, contact with metals, symptoms consistent with venous insufficiency
Psoriasis	Location, course, itching, pain, therapy to date, past trauma, effect of sunlight, joint pain, psychological impact
Acne	Location, course, oral contraception, factors exacerbating/relieving symptoms, medication use, overweight, menstrual disorders, virilising features (hirsutism, excessive male-pattern hair, voice drop, clitoral enlargement), psychological impact
Sexually transmitted infection (STI)	Symptoms, course, multiple sexual partners, unprotected intercourse, partner with similar symptoms, partner with known STI, type of intercourse, discharge, itching, fever, dysuria, pollakisuria, contact bleeding, intermenstrual bleeding, swelling, pain, stool (blood, mucus)

Table 3 // History-taking for several common dermatological symptoms

Physical examination

The next chapter provides a systematic guide to performing a general physical examination. Emphasis is placed on the importance of clear communication and patient comfort throughout the examination. The most important aspects of the dermatological examination are presented.

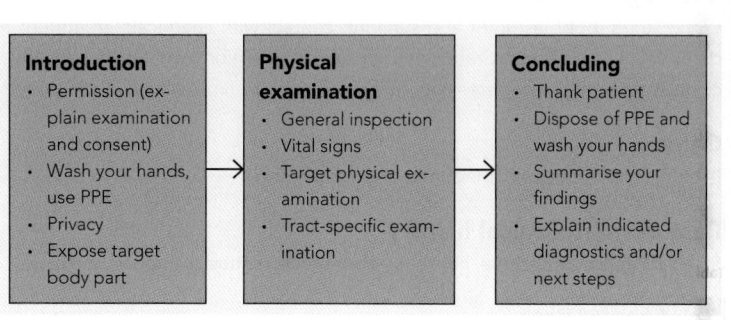

Introduction	Physical examination	Concluding
• Permission (explain examination and consent) • Wash your hands, use PPE • Privacy • Expose target body part	• General inspection • Vital signs • Target physical examination • Tract-specific examination	• Thank patient • Dispose of PPE and wash your hands • Summarise your findings • Explain indicated diagnostics and/or next steps

Diagram 2 // Physical examination
PPE, personal protective equipment

PASS ONE©

The PASS ONE© method is used to describe the morphology of dermatological pathology. It is an acronym, as explained in Table 4.

ACRONYM	DESCRIPTION	EXAMPLE
P **Place**	Location of the lesion	• Volar wrist, scalp, etc. • Symmetry
A **Arrangement**	How the lesions are distributed across the body and arranged with respect to each other (see Figure 12)	• Solitary (1 lesion), grouped/herpetiform (in clusters), discrete (separated), contiguous, diffuse (widespread), disseminated/dispersed (evenly distributed across body), reticular (net-like), coalescent, follicular • Extent: solitary (1 single lesion), circumscribed, regional (larger area), segmental (dermatome), generalised (large area of skin), universal (across the skin)

Table 4A // PASS ONE© method

ACRONYM	DESCRIPTION	EXAMPLE
(S) **Size**	Number and size of lesions, extent of lesions	• Number: several, multiple, dozens, hundreds • Size: in cm or mm, common descriptors include miliar (1-2 mm), lenticular (3-10 mm), and nummular (1-3 cm)
(S) **Shape**	Shape of the lesion, two-dimensional and three-dimensional (see Figures 13 and 14)	Round, oval, linear, polycyclic, jagged, etc.
(O) **Outline**	Border of the lesion	Descriptors include very well-defined, well-defined, moderately well-defined, ill-defined, and irregular
(N) **Nuance/ colour**	Nuance and colour of the lesion	Hyperpigmented, hypopigmented or depigmented skin, brown, yellow, blue, green, red, orange-red, black, white, purple
(E) **Efflorescence**	Efflorescence of the lesion (see Figure 15)	See Table 5

Table 4B // PASS ONE© method

> 🔔 Conditions according to PASS ONE© may manifest differently on different skin types, e.g. redness may appear as dark or bluish discoloration on darker skin types. This is mentioned where applicable. See Figure 11 for an example of how psoriasis can present differently in different skin types.

> 💡 Lenticular and nummular are terms used to describe both size (3-10 mm and 1-3 cm respectively) and shape (round).

Colour

When describing colour, we use the terms 'redness' and 'erythema'. Erythema is redness resulting from vasodilation that blanches when under pressure. Redness may be harder to spot on darker skin than on lighter skin. How redness presents varies per condition and skin type: it may manifest as hyperpigmentation or greying. It is a sign of inflammation, but it is also important to watch out for signs of infection, such as warmth, pain, and swelling.

> 💡 PASS ONE© is a clinical method used to describe skin lesions. In this section, PASS ONE© is used to categorise the conditions, based on their common presentation.

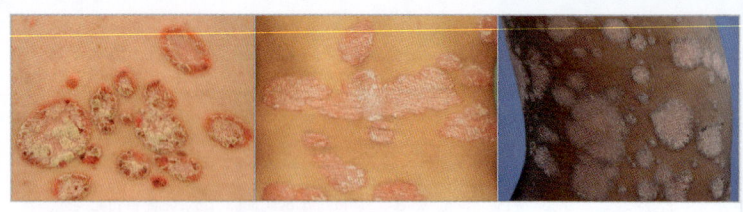

Figure 11 // Presentation of psoriasis in different skin types

- Dermatological inspection gives information about the skin condition, giving rise to a differential diagnosis.
- Palpating the lesions may provide more information, for example help differentiate between types of efflorescence.
- Commonly missed locations during dermatological exams are mucous membranes, nails, scalp, skin between the fingers, under the soles of the feet, behind the ears, and the anogenital region.

Are the lesions symmetrical? Asymmetry may be indicative of an exogenous cause, such as infection or trauma.

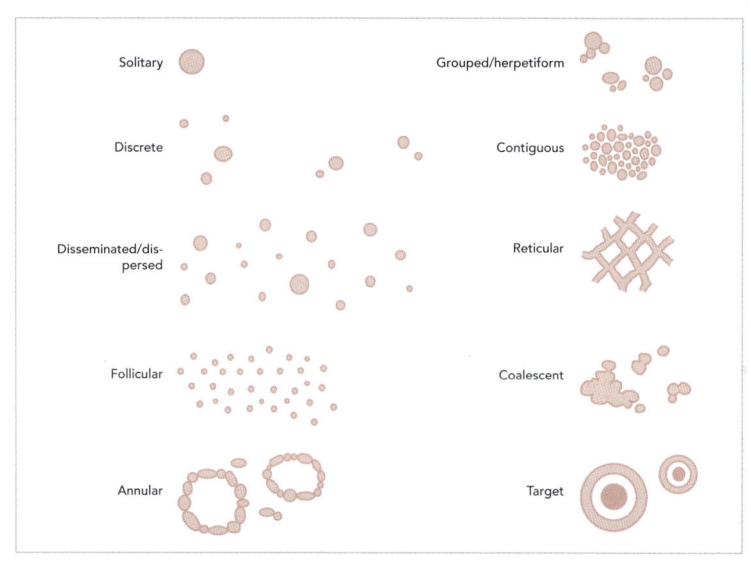

Solitary	Grouped/herpetiform
Discrete	Contiguous
Disseminated/dispersed	Reticular
Follicular	Coalescent
Annular	Target

Figure 12 // PASS ONE© arrangement

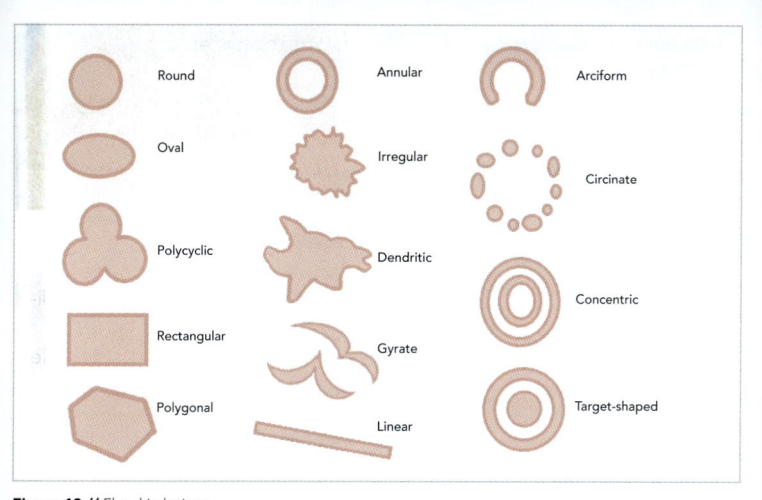

Figure 13 // Flat skin lesions

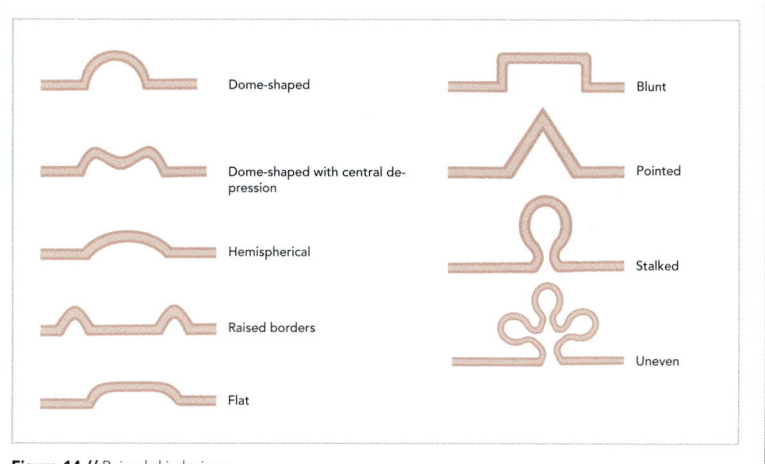

Figure 14 // Raised skin lesions

Efflorescence

Efflorescence classifies skin pathology by its primary morphology, helping practitioners describe skin lesions. This facilitates clear communication and diagnosing patients. See Table 5 and Figure 15 for the most common efflorescences.

EFFLORES-CENCE	SYNONYM	DESCRIPTION
Primary		
Macule	Spot	Flat, diffuse or demarcated colour change without elevation or depression: non-palpable
Papule	Papule	Solid, circumscribed lesion <1 cm
Plaque	Plaque	Persistent, flat, raised lesion, ≥1 cm
Nodule	Small lump	Firm, circumscribed lesion, in or under the skin, <1cm
Large nodule	Large lump	Identical to nodule, but ≥1 cm
Urtica	Wheal/hive	Migratory, flat, and raised lesions secondary to dermal oedema
Vesicle	Blister	Cavity filled with clear fluid or blood, no proper wall under the epidermis, <1 cm
Bulla	Blister	Cavity filled with clear fluid or blood, no proper wall under the epidermis, ≥1 cm
Pustule	Abscess or pustule	Cavity in the skin, filled with pus or purulent fluid, may be sterile, <1 cm, no proper wall
Secondary		
Crusta	Crust	Dried blood, exudate, or pus
Squama	Scale	• Abnormal scaling (detached keratinocytes) • Various forms: pityriasis (fine, powdery scales), keratotic (calloused, friable), psoriasiform (plate-like, white, silvery), ichthyosiform (diamond-shaped, resembling fish scales), collarettes, craquelure (cracked, like a paint or varnish coating), seborrhoeic (yellowish, oily)
Erosion	Loss of the epidermis	Superficial, non-bleeding skin defect
Excoriation	Scratch mark	Epidermal and dermal tissue damage caused by scratching
Ulcer	Ulcer or wound	Epidermal and dermal defect that may penetrate down to the subcutis

Table 5 // Most common efflorescences

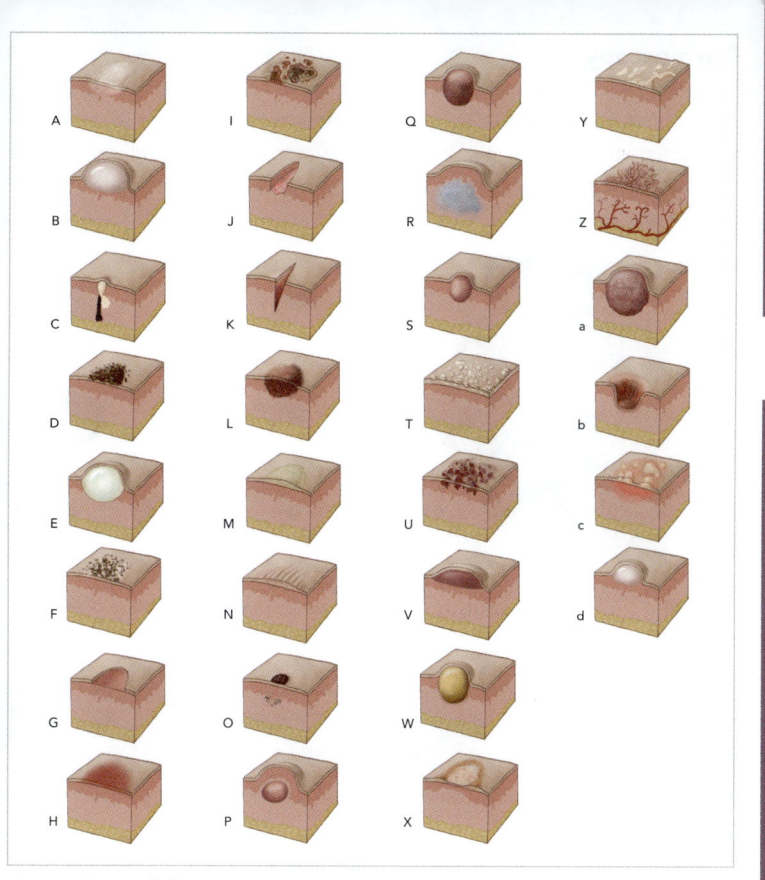

Figure 15 // Types of efflorescence and common skin pathology

A: Atrophy **B:** Bulla **C:** Comedo **D:** Crusta **E:** Cyst **F:** Dyschromia **G:** Erosion **H:** Erythema **I:** Erythematosquamous disease **J:** Excoriation **K:** Fissure/rhagade **L:** Haematoma **M:** Hyperkeratosis **N:** Lichenification **O:** Macule **P:** Nodule **Q:** Large nodule **R:** Oedema **S:** Papula **T:** Parakeratosis **U:** Purpura **V:** Plaque **W:** Pustule **X:** Sclerosis **Y:** Squama **Z:** Telangiectasias **a:** Tumour **b:** Ulcer **c:** Hive **d:** Vesicle

> Erythema or purpura? Use a glass slide to apply pressure to the lesion. Erythema blanches to pressure.

> Erythematosquamous efflorescence is a common hybrid type in which the skin is both red and scaly.

Dermoscopy

Dermoscopy is a diagnostic tool used to complement the physical exam (see Figure 16). A dermatoscope is a portable instrument with a ten times magnification factor and a built-in light. It makes it easier to distinguish between benign and malignant pigmented lesions and can also be used to accurately measure the size of a lesion.

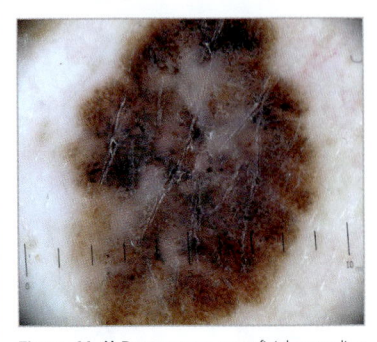

Figure 16 // Dermoscopy: superficial spreading melanoma

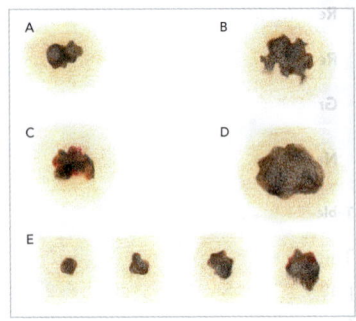

Figure 17 // ABCDE rule
A: Asymmetry **B:** Border **C:** Colour **D:** Differential and diameter **E:** Evolution

> Stolz's **ABCDE** rule of dermoscopy is used to assess pigmented lesions. ABCDE is short for **a**symmetry, **b**order, **c**olour, **d**ifferential structures, **d**iameter, and **e**volution – be alert for sudden changes to a birthmark! (see Figure 17)

Wood's lamp

A Wood's lamp is a portable UVA light source used as a diagnostic tool for e.g. mycoses (tinea capitis) and erythrasma, which appear fluorescent (see Table 6). It is also used in diagnosing vitiligo. (see Table 6).

Skin type
Fitzpatrick skin type classification

> The Fitzpatrick classification is often mistakenly used to classify skin tones. However, it is designed to assess the risk of skin cancer. To refer to different skin tones, the Colorimetric scale is used (see Table 8).

COLOUR OF FLUORESCENCE	PATHOGENS
Green	*Trichophyton schoenleinii, Microsporum audouinii, Microsporum canis*
Yellowish brown	*Malassezia furfur* (pseudohyphae of *Pityrosporum orbiculare* (pityriasis versicolor))
Red, bright orange	*Corynebacterium minutissimum* (erythrasma)
Red in a follicular pattern	Progressive macular hypomelanosis
Greenish yellow	Hair stumps infected with favus (*Trichophyton schoenleinii*)
No fluorescence	Other *Trichophyton* species show endothrix growth (inside the hair) and no fluorescence

Table 6 // Fluorescence and corresponding pathogens

This classification is based on the skin's response to UV light exposure. The Fitzpatrick classification of sun-reactive skin types categorises people based not only on whether they sunburn and their erythematous reaction, but also on whether they tan and their tanning reaction. Additionally, the classification considers features such as eye colour and the presence or absence of freckles, as these characteristics can also influence an individual's susceptibility to sun damage and skin reactions (see Figure 18 and Table 7).

FITZPATRICK TYPE	SKIN COLOUR	RESPONSE TO SUN EXPOSURE
Type I	Very fair, pale white	Always burns, never tans
Type II	Fair white	Usually burns, tans with difficulty
Type III	Light-to-medium beige	Sometimes mild burn, gradually tans
Type IV	Olive, moderate brown	Rarely burns, tans easily
Type V	Dark brown	Very rarely burns, tans very easily
Type VI	Deeply pigmented dark brown	Never burns, always tans

Table 7 // Fitzpatrick Skin Type Classification

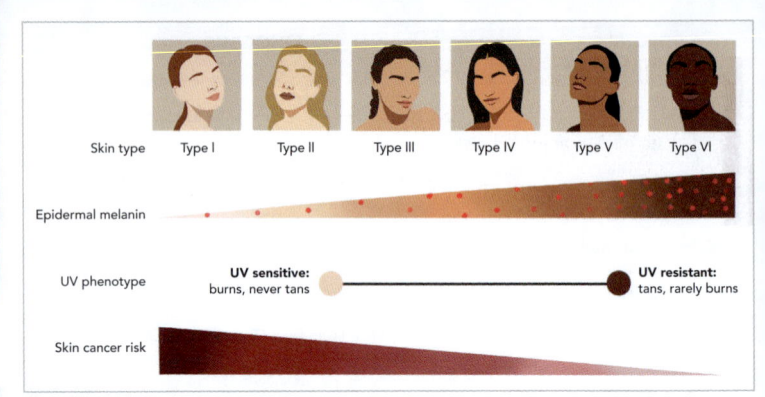

Figure 18 // Skin type classification according to Fitzpatrick

Colorimetric scale skin tone classification

The colorimetric scale classifies skin colour independently of ethnic background. It enables quick classification of skin tones, facilitating accurate skin cancer risk assessment and improved management of cosmetic procedures. Colour is defined by the visible light spectrum. Neither white nor black are visible on this spectrum, which is why these two colours are not included in this classification (see Table 8).

COLORIMETRIC SCALE	TYPE AND NAME	SKIN COLOUR
Type 0A	Pale skin	
Type 0	Fair skin	
Type 1	Very light beige	
Type 2	Light brown	
Type 3	Medium brown	
Type 4	Dark brown	
Type 5	Very dark brown	

Table 8 // Colorimetric scale, skin types and names, and skin colour

These chapters deal specifically with dermatological issues. See the pocket *Acute Medicine* for more information on an extended general patient history, physical exam, and diagnostics.

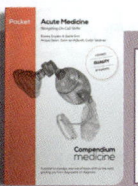

Diagnostics

Skin biopsy and excision

A skin biopsy is the removal of a piece of skin for histopathological examination (see Figure 19). Skin biopsies are widely used within dermatology for diagnostic purposes. Indications for a skin biopsy include suspected malignancy, bullous dermatoses, hair disorders, atypical presentation of a skin lesion and poor response to therapy. There are several ways to take a biopsy. Three-millimetre punch biopsies are most common, but shave biopsies are also used for superficial lesions. Excisions are used to remove raised lesions, such as dermatofibromas. To avoid sample error (e.g. progression of melanoma in another part of the lesion) suspicious pigmented lesions should be excised in total, rather than examining a small sample through a punch biopsy. For pigmented lesions, include the lesion's edge and adjacent healthy skin for comparison.

> It may be helpful to photograph the suspicious skin pathology in advance so that it can be reassessed retrospectively.

The procedure for performing a skin biopsy is as follows:
1. Lay out the materials for the procedure
2. Mark the location of the biopsy
3. Disinfect the skin
4. For superficial lesions, inject small quantities of lidocaine superficially under the skin. For deeper lesions, inject lidocaine subcutaneously. Subcutaneous injections of lidocaine take effect after about 5-10 min.
5. Once the lidocaine has taken effect - this can be tested by pricking the skin with a needle - pull the skin taut using the thumb and index finger of your non-dominant hand
6. Apply the biopsy puncher to the skin with the dominant hand and rotate the biopsy probe in one direction, applying light pressure. The puncher should reach the subcutis, as signalled by a noticeable drop in resistance.
7. Using forceps, gently grasp the specimen and pull it up slightly. Avoid injuring the patient with the biopsy forceps.
8. Using scissors, cut the specimen at the base
9. Place the specimen in the formalin jar

10 Apply pressure to the wound with gauze. Complete the request form for the pathology department. Secondary closure is used for wounds <4 mm. Primary closure methods can be used for wounds >4 mm.

11 Tell the patient to take paracetamol for any pain and that infection, and scarring are very rare

> Mark the skin pathology prior to anaesthetising the skin, as the pathology may become less visible after the injection.

Punch biopsy - detail

Punch biopsy - execution

Excisional biopsy

Shave biopsy

Anaesthetising the skin

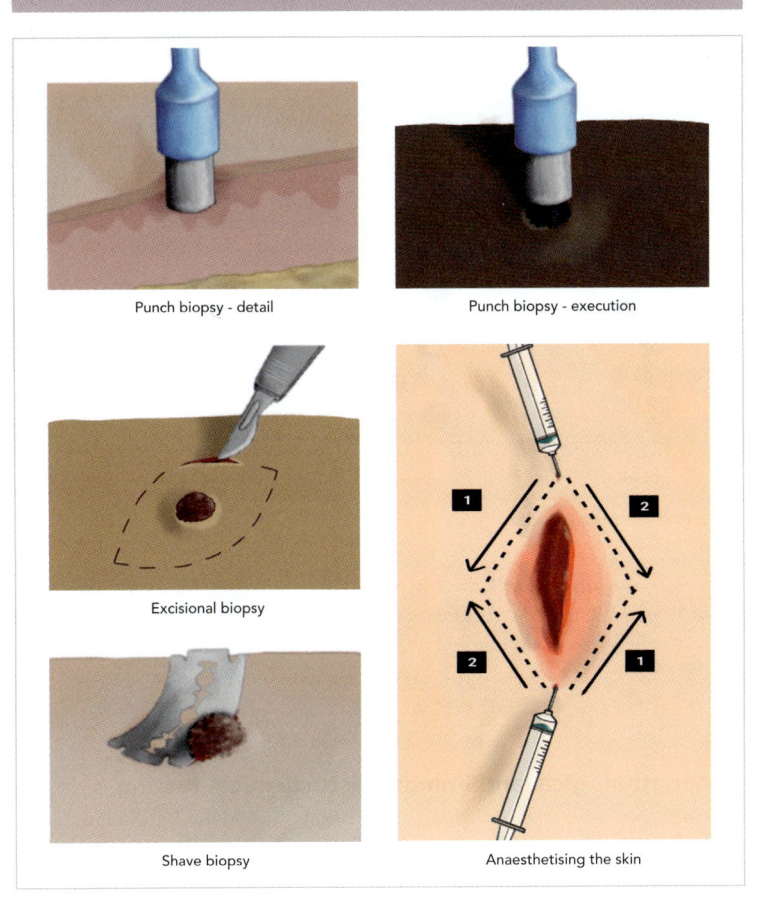

Figure 19 // Skin biopsies

Immunofluorescence (IF) biopsy

Immunofluorescence is a technique used to detect specific proteins and antibodies in tissues. It involves binding an antibody to a fluorescent (light-emitting) substance (e.g. fluorescein and rhodamine). There are two immunofluorescence techniques (see Figure 20).

Indications for immunofluorescence include diagnosis of autoimmune diseases (e.g. subacute cutaneous lupus (SCLE)), detection of vasculitis (e.g. small vessel vasculitis), blistering diseases (e.g. bulleus pemphigoid). Immunofluorescence can also be used to visualise cell division.

> Fluorescence microscope: uses excitation light (e.g. UV light) to fluoresce (illuminate) a particular substance. Different wavelengths (and therefore colours) can be used to distinguish between different substances.

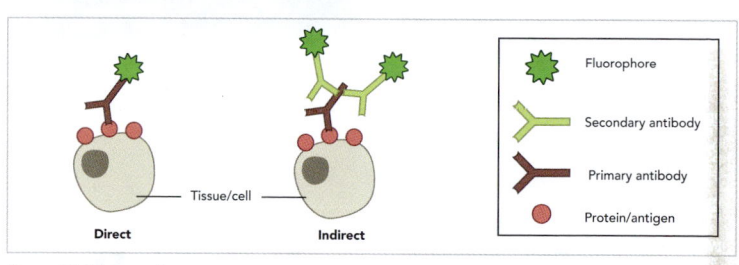

Figure 20 // Immunofluorescence

> Haematoxylin and eosin staining (H&E staining) is a gold standard in histology. The alkaline haematoxylin stains the nucleus of the cell, giving it a deep purple-bluish colour. The eosin, an acidic dye, stains the cytoplasm red or pink (depending on the quantity and density of the structures to be stained).

Histopathological and immunohistochemical testing

After a biopsy, H&E staining is frequently used to distinguish between different cell and tissue types and to reveal structural changes at the cellular level. This method provides essential information that helps refine the diagnosis.

> The colours of the histology stains can be remembered as follows:
> - Haematoxylin = alkaline = purple-bluish
> - Eosin = acid = red or pink

Duplex ultrasound

Duplex ultrasounds, or duplex Dopplers, combine Doppler with ultrasound. Depending on the velocity and direction of the blood, a frequency difference can be measured between the transmitted and the received frequency of the sound wave (Doppler shift). In a duplex ultrasound, the Doppler shift (vertical axis) is plotted against time (horizontal axis). Frequency shifts within the audible spectrum can also be played through a speaker (see Figure 21). Here the pitch is proportional to the velocity of the blood. Duplex ultrasound is used to find/exclude vascular stenosis and is therefore also used for detecting and ruling out deep vein thrombosis (DVT). Another common dermatological indication is assessing varicose veins (valve function, great saphenous vein (GSV), small saphenous vein (SSV)).

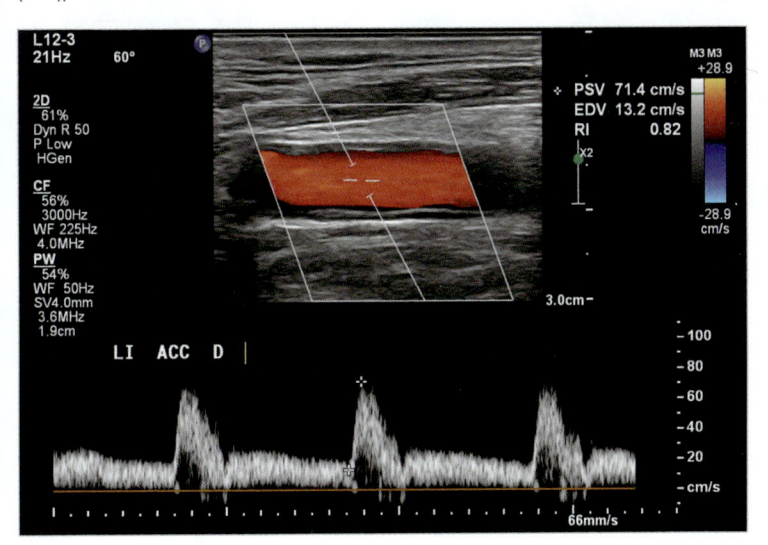

Figure 21 // Normal duplex ultrasound of the left common carotid artery. Increase in velocity of blood flow will turn yellow/white in a stenosis. The graph pattern below the ultrasound image resembling a sawtooth indicates peak systolic velocity (PSV) and the end diastolic velocity (EDV). The horizontal axis indicates time and the vertical axis indicates velocity of blood flow in cm/s.

Allergy testing
Epicutaneous test (patch test)

Epicutaneous patch testing consists of taping patches directly to the skin of patients with a suspected contact dermatitis (see Figure 22). The patches are applied on day 1 and are removed on day 3. The results are evaluated on day 4 or 5. Based on the patient's history, the treating physician decides which substances to test; this can include products the patient brings in. The patient should not shower between day 1 (application of patches) and day 3 (removal of patches). The test is positive if the material causes an inflammatory reaction, leading to redness, swelling, sores, and/or bumps (see Figure 23). A reaction on the first day is usually due to irritation and not to contact allergies (type IV hypersensitivity reaction).

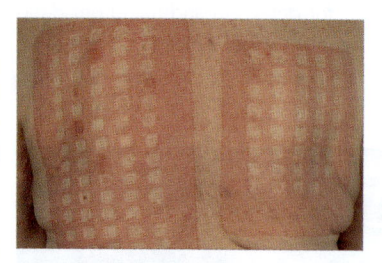

Figure 22 // Epicutaneous test

Figure 23 // Contact dermatitis

Skin prick test

The skin prick test consists of applying a small amount of allergen extract percutaneously on the volar side of the forearm or sometimes on the back. The standard panel of inhalation allergens consists of house dust mites, grass, tree and weed pollen, cat and dog epithelium, and fungi. Skin prick tests always involve a negative (buffer solution) and a positive (often histamine) control.

Serology
Radioallergosorbent test (RAST)

The RAST is a serological blood test designed primarily to evaluate food and respiratory allergies (e.g. hay fever, dust mite allergy). The patient's blood is added to the suspected allergen in a test tube. If the serum contains antibodies (IgE) against the allergen, these antibodies will bind to the allergen. After washing away the unbound IgE antibodies, radiolabeled anti-human IgE antibodies are added to the tube, which then bind to the IgE bound to the allergen. The radioactivity measured in the test tube is proportional to the quantity of serum IgE immunoglobulins against the allergen.

Phadiatop test

The Phadiatop test is a general screening for the presence of IgE immunoglobulins in the blood against inhalant and/or food allergens. Inhalant allergies virtually always involve IgE immunoglobulins. When allergies are the suspected cause of the symptoms, the Phadiatop test is used to demonstrate atopy (predisposition to allergy) and sensitisation (sensitivity) to a combination of allergens. A positive result indicates that the patient is sensitive to common inhalant and food allergens, which are, however, not always clinically relevant. Positive results can also be broken down into the following common allergens: grass, weed and tree pollen, dust mites, cat and dog epithelium, and fungi. The RAST can then be used to narrow down the diagnosis.

> Increased levels of IgE immunoglobulins can also be caused by viral, bacterial and parasitic infections, and Kahler's disease (multiple myeloma).

Microscopy
Microbiological testing
Parasitic diagnostics

Microscopy can be used as a method to detect scabies mites in clinical practice (potassium hydroxide (KOH) preparation).

Mycological test

Mycological tests are usually performed with a heated KOH preparation of skin scales, nails, or hair. The KOH preparation test is used to confirm the presence of a fungal skin infection. KOH dissolves cell walls and keratin, but not fungal hyphae. In addition to revealing fungi and yeasts (dermatophytes, *Candida*, and *Malassezia*), KOH preparations can also be used to detect *Corynebacteria* (erythrasma and trichomycosis), and *Demodex* (demodicosis).

Infections and arthropods

Microscopy is a widely used method for observing bacteria. Cultures are performed first. Bacteria can be identified by using methylene blue staining. Gram staining distinguishes between Gram-positive and Gram-negative bacteria.

Ziehl-Neelsen or auramine staining stains Mycobacteria. Arthropods are identified by examining the specimen brought in by the patient or found on the patient during physical examination with the naked eye, under a magnifying glass, or under a microscope.

Gram staining

Gram staining is a commonly used method to distinguish two classes of bacteria by their cell wall: a thick peptidoglycan layer (Gram-positive bacteria) and a thin peptidoglycan layer (Gram-negative bacteria). Gram staining is performed as follows:

1. A patient specimen is prepared on a slide
2. The patient specimen is fixed on the slide (one minute in alcohol or several passes through a flame)
3. The preparation is stained in crystal violet dye and then in iodine, forming a crystal violet-iodine complex
4. Next, the preparation is rinsed with alcohol, causing Gram-negative bacteria to decolourise. Gram-positive bacteria retain the crystal violet-iodine complex and turn purple (see Figure 24).
5. The preparation is counterstained in aqueous fuchsin, causing the decolourised Gram-negative bacteria to turn pink

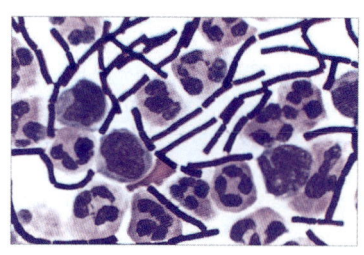

Figure 24 // Gram-positive bacilli between polymorphonuclear leukocytes (PMNLs, granulocytes)

> The distinction between Gram-positive and Gram-negative bacteria can be remembered using the **4 Ps**: **p**rokaryote, Gram-**p**ositive, **p**eptidoglycan, and **p**urple.

Serological testing
General

Serological testing can be used to detect antibodies and autoantibodies indicating infection and autoimmune diseases. A venipuncture is performed, after which the clotted blood is separated from the serum. An antibody titre test is then performed to determine the concentration of antibodies in the serum. Indi-

cations for serological testing are:
- Immune status testing, e.g. in autoimmune diseases (incl. systemic lupus erythematosus (SLE)), or infections by microorganisms (incl. syphilis serology testing)
- Hypersensitivity testing (e.g. RAST)

Serological tests include the complement binding assay, immunofluorescence, and enzyme-linked immunosorbent assay (ELISA). Serological diagnostics are increasingly being replaced by molecular diagnostics, which produce significantly faster results.

Proctological examination

A proctological examination involves using a proctoscope, which is a short tube inserted into the anal canal to visualise the anal canal and mucous membrane from the inside (see Figure 25).

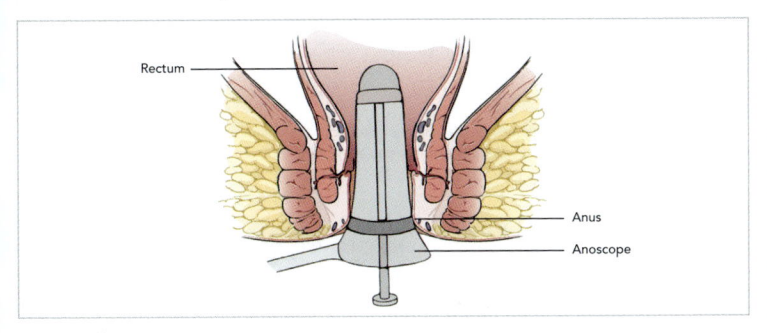

Figure 25 // Anoscopy

High-resolution anoscopy (HRA)

HRA is a technique used to examine the anal canal for the presence of malignant/premalignant lesions. This method involves applying acetic acid and Lugol's iodine, and using a camera with high magnification to enhance the visualisation of the area of interest. HRA is used to identify malignant/premalignant anal lesions and to obtain histological specimens if needed.

Anal swab

Anal swabs can be used for cytopathological examination and high-risk HPV testing. Some centres use anal swabs for screening, as a pre-selection method for HRA. Other centres screen directly using HRA.

Treatment
Pharmacological treatment

Analgesics

MEDICATION		MECHANISM OF ACTION	ADVERSE EFFECTS
	Paracetamol	Analgesic and antipyretic properties via unknown mechanism	Mild adverse effects profile: risk of liver damage at high doses (>150 mg/kg) and in cases of alcoholism and pre-existing liver damage
NSAIDS	Diclofenac	Classic non-selective inhibitors of the COX enzyme with analgesic, antipyretic, and anti-inflammatory properties	• GI: risk of peptic ulcer • Renal: peripheral oedema, acute/chronic renal insufficiency esp. in patients on RAS inhibitors, diuretics, pre-existing renal insufficiency, heart failure, dehydration, sepsis • Cardiovascular: potential ↑ risk esp. with COX-2 inhibitors and diclofenac, incl. risk of heart failure
	Ibuprofen		
	Naproxen		
	Aspirin		
	Celecoxib	Selective COX-2 inhibitor with fewer renal and GI adverse effects	

Table 9 // Analgesics
COX, cyclooxygenase; GI, gastrointestinal; NSAID, non-steroidal anti-inflammatory drug; PMHx, past medical history; PPI, proton pump inhibitor; OAC, oral anticoagulation; RAS, renin-angiotensin system; SSRI, selective serotonin reuptake inhibitor

Opioids

MEDICATION		MECHANISM OF ACTION
OPIOIDS	Codeine	• Opioid receptor agonist: 　- μ receptor: analgesia (main effect) 　- κ and δ receptor: spinal and peripheral analgesia • Fentanyl is more potent than morphine and can be administered transdermally ($t_{1/2}$ 17h), via IV ($t_{1/2el}$ 6-8h), and nasally ($t_{1/2}$ 3-4h) • Codeine is a prodrug of morphine that has unpredictable variability in conversion to morphine (10x less potent) • Tramadol and buprenorphine are partial agonists. Tramadol also has an SNRI mechanism of action.
	Tramadol	
	Morphine	
	Oxycodone	
	Fentanyl	

Table 10 // Opioids
SNRI, serotonin-norepinephrine reuptake inhibitors; TCA, tricyclic antidepressant; COPD, chronic obstructive pulmonary disease

> To prevent constipation, always prescribe **opioids** with a **laxative**: e.g. docusate sodium/calcium, bisacodyl, macrogol, lactulose, magnesium sulfate/citrate/hydroxide, methylnatrexone, naloxegol, or enema.

Legend

- 💡 = Additional information
- 🟢 = Indication for prescribing medication
- ⇔ = Interaction with drugs or high-risk groups
- ✖ = Indication for stopping with medication
- 🔺 = Intoxication management

NOTES
⇔ Administer lower dose in cases of alcoholism, chronic malnutrition, hepatic insufficiency, or dehydration   🔺 N-acetylcysteine (cysteine derivative) as an antidote
🟢 Prescribe PPI in patients aged >70, peptic ulcer in PMHx, or age >60 with DM, heart failure or use of corticosteroids, SSRIs, OAC, or acetylsalicylic acid   🟢 At low doses of ascal/carbasalate calcium: PPI in patients aged >80, >60 with ulcer in PMHx, or >70 using corticosteroids, OAC, SSRIs, or clopidogrel

ADVERSE EFFECTS	NOTES
· Central nervous system (CNS): respiratory depression (esp. high-risk in COPD), miosis, delirium, sedation, dependence · Pulmonary: bronchoconstriction · GI: motility ↓ (constipation, nausea and vomiting)	⇔ Risk of constipation ↑ due to immobility, poor water and fibre intake, and use of anticholinergics, antidepressants, and diuretics ↑ 🟢 So do not forget to prescribe a laxative when starting an opioid ⇔ Risk of respiratory depression and sedation ↑ with alcohol and CNS depressants (anaesthetics, anxiolytics, TCA, hypnotics, and sedatives) ⇔ Tramadol combined with SSRIs produces ↑ risk of serotonin syndrome 🔺 Naloxone (competitive antagonist) as an antidote for opioid-induced adverse effects 💡 Consider opioid rotation in case of adverse effects or poor effect

STEP 1	Start with paracetamol and add an NSAID if pain relief is insufficient. Diclofenac is 1st choice for colic pain. Consider selective COX-2 inhibitors with CIs for classic NSAIDs.
STEP 2	Add a weak-acting opioid (tramadol) or substitute the non-opioid. Codeine is still used primarily as an antitussive and not for additive pain relief.
STEP 3	Combine a strong oral or transdermal opioid (morphine, fentanyl, oxycodone) with a non-opioid. Fentanyl patches provide relief for nausea, vomiting and small bowel obstruction.
STEP 4	Opt for subcutaneous or IV route

Table 11 // Treatment of nociceptive pain (World Health Organization (WHO) analgesic ladder)

Ointments and creams

OINTMENT	CREAM
Oil-based topical treatment	Water-based topical treatment to which a small amount of grease has been added

Table 12 // Ointments and creams

Non-medicated therapy

Non-medicated therapy consists of applying non-medicated ointments, creams, balms, lotions, shake lotions, etc. These products are designed to return the skin to its normal condition, e.g. an oily ointment for dry skin, a cream or lotion for wet skin. Non-medicated products do not contain active ingredients but do help cure skin disease.

Creams

Non-medicated creams are emulsions of water and fats with an added emulsifier. The outer layer of these creams consists of water, with the inner layer containing a small amount of fat. They have a neutral effect on dry and wet skin. Examples: Cetomacrogol cream or Lanette cream, with or without Vaseline®.

Ointments

Non-medicated ointments have a more viscous consistency than creams. Ointments can be subdivided into:
- Ointments: emulsions of water and fats that are greasier to the touch and often thicker than creams (see Table 12). Example: cooling ointment and hydrous ointment.
- High-fat ointments: generally anhydrous preparations composed largely of paraffin and petroleum jelly
- Emulsifying ointments: usually high-fat ointments that adhere to moist skin due to their relatively high emulsifier content and can be washed off with water. Example: Cetomacrogol and lanolin ointments.

Depending on the percentage of Vaseline®, ointments cover dry skin, causing it to lose less water through evaporation. As a result, the skin is rehydrated from the dermis up. Hydrous or cooling 'ointments' also have a cooling effect because the water phase evaporates immediately after application, leaving only the fatty components on the skin.

> Wool wax allergies (wool alcohols, lanolin) are a contraindication (CI) to many non-medicated products (e.g. shampoo, certain cosmetics and skin care products, shaving foam/soap).

Immunosuppressive drugs
Corticosteroids
General

Corticosteroids can be split into glucocorticoids and mineralocorticoids (see Table 13). Mineralocorticoids regulate electrolyte balance. Glucocorticosteroids have an anti-inflammatory effect and are used in dermatological treatment as systemic therapy, or through local or intralesional application. Adverse effects are less commonly observed with local or intralesional applications due to the lower dosage and lack of systemic effects.

Local corticosteroids

Local corticosteroids are anti-inflammatory ointments, creams, or lotions that can be applied on the skin. Local corticosteroids help calm inflamed skin by inhibiting immune cells and slowing down cell division. This reduces redness and itching, with minimal systemic side effects. There are different classes of topical corticosteroids, classified by strength.

Examples per class:
- Class I: Hydrocortisone acetate (hydrocortisone)
- Class II: Triamcinolone acetonide (triamcinolone)
- Class II-III: Hydrocortisone-17-butyrate (Locoid)
- Class III: Desoximetasone (Ibaril)
- Class III-IV: Betamethasone dipropionate (Diprosone)
- Class IV: Clobetasol-17-propionate (Dermovate)

Intralesional corticosteroids

This approach involves injecting corticosteroid medication directly into the affected skin area. Triamcinolone acetonide is most commonly used for this purpose, although dexamethasone, betamethasone, or methylprednisolone acetate can be used as well. Triamcinolone preparations are available as micronised suspensions. This enhances the delivery of small corticosteroid crystals to the treatment site, leading to a reduction in the total administered dose. This approach helps limit side effects. Furthermore, the corticosteroid crystals are retained in the tissues and slowly released in the course of several weeks.

	MEDICATION	INDICATIONS	MECHANISM OF ACTION
GLUCOCORTICOSTEROIDS	**Corticosteroids general**	• Chronic inflammatory skin conditions (e.g. dermatitis, psoriasis) • Hidradenitis suppurativa (HS)	Anti-inflammatory effect: • Stimulating protein degradation → inhibition formation of granulation tissue • Stabilisation of lysosomal membrane of leukocytes • Vasoconstrictive effect and antagonise vasodilation → inflammatory exudate and local oedema ↓ Immunosuppressive (anti-allergic) action: cell migration ↓ and inhibition of phagocytic activity of leukocytes and monocytes → activity and volume of the lymphatic system ↓ and suppression of humoral immunity (only at very high doses)
	Prednisolone, prednisone		
	Dexamethasone		

Table 13 // Overview of corticosteroids

Other anti-inflammatory and immunosuppressive drugs

	MEDICATION	INDICATIONS	MECHANISM OF ACTION
CALCINEURIN INHIBITOR	**Ciclosporin**	• Psoriasis • Atopic dermatitis • Alopecia areata • Lichen planus	Binding to specific cytoplasmic immunophilin, Ca^{2+}, and calmodulin → inhibition/suppression of calcineurin's phosphatase activity → prevention of dephosphorylation → disruption of the nuclear factor of activated T-cells' signalling pathway → decreased interleukin-2 (IL-2) production → reduced T-cell activation and release of inflammatory cytokines
	Tacrolimus	Topical tacrolimus is often used for inflammatory skin disorders, e.g. vitiligo, psoriasis, alopecia areata, contact dermatitis, and lichen planus	Binding to specific cytoplasmic immunophilin, Ca^{2+}, and calmodulin → inhibition/suppression of calcineurin's phosphatase activity → prevention of dephosphorylation → disruption of the nuclear factor of activated T-cells' signalling pathway → decreased interleukin-2 (IL-2) production → reduced T-cell activation and release of inflammatory cytokines

Table 14A // Anti-inflammatory and immunosuppressive drugs

ADVERSE EFFECTS	NOTES
- Sodium and fluid retention, heart failure in susceptible patients, potassium loss, hypokalaemic alkalosis, hypertension, calcium excretion ↑ - GI symptoms: peptic ulcer, nausea, oesophagitis, pancreatitis, GI bleeding, perforation - Delayed wound healing, thin skin, acne, petechiae and ecchymosis, facial erythema, rosacea-like dermatitis - Erythrocytosis and agranulocytosis, moderate leucocytosis, lymphopenia and eosinopenia, thromboembolism - Intracranial hypertension with papilloedema - Hirsutism, Cushing's syndrome, adrenal insufficiency, manifestation of latent DM - Weight ↑, mood changes, insomnia, depression - Susceptibility to infection ↑, masking of clinical signs, impaired immune response - Steroid myopathy (atrophy and weakness), osteoporosis, avascular necrosis (AVN) of esp. femoral/humeral head, tendon rupture (esp. of the Achilles tendon), tendinitis	✖ CI: - Ventricular and duodenal ulcer - Acute infectious processes, esp. viral infections and systemic fungal infections - Parasitic infections, tropical worm infections

ADVERSE EFFECTS	NOTES
- GI symptoms: nausea, abdominal pain - Reversible nephrotoxicity in short term treatment - Hypertension	● Significant efficacy in severe cases of psoriasis, atopic dermatitis, alopecia areata, urticaria, lichen planus, and other inflammatory skin conditions 💡 Patients often experience a reduction in symptoms such as itching, redness, and flaking, hence an improved quality of life
Local redness, warmth, pain, increased skin sensitivity, skin tingling, or skin irritation after alcohol consumption	💡 Only minimally absorbed through the skin → less adverse effects ⇔ Tacrolimus may heighten the risk of sunburn, so it is advisable to regularly apply sunblock to sun-exposed areas that have been treated 💡 Apart from potential skin irritation or a burning sensation, the safety profile of tacrolimus is comparable to that of corticosteroids

	MEDICATION	INDICATIONS	MECHANISM OF ACTION
PDE4 INHIBITOR	**Apremilast** (Otezla®)	• Psoriatic arthritis, plaque psoriasis • Oral ulcers associated with Behçet's disease	Specifically inhibits phosphodiesterase 4 (PDE4) → prevents degradation of cyclic adenosine monophosphate (cAMP) to AMP in inflammatory cells → modulates expression of pro-inflammatory and anti-inflammatory mediators
IMMUNOSUPPRESSIVE DRUGS, OTHER	**Methotrexate**	• Chronic inflammatory skin conditions (e.g. psoriasis, systemic lupus erythematosus (SLE), dermatomyositis) • Severe atopic dermatitis • Alopecia areata, sarcoidosis, mycosis fungoides	Inhibits the enzyme 5-aminoimidazole-4-carbox-amide-1-β-D-ribofuranoside (AICAR) transformylase → interfering with adenosine and guanine metabolism → adenosine accumulation → inflammation → and suppression of T-cell and B-cell activity

Table 14B // Anti-inflammatory and immunosuppressive drugs

Biologicals

Biologicals or biologics are artificial proteins that are identical to proteins produced naturally in the body. Most biologicals used as medication are antibodies directed against a naturally produced protein, often one that plays a role in maintaining inflammation. By binding to this protein, the artificial antibody inhibits inflammation (see Table 15).

TNF-alpha blockers

These agents belong to the group of second-line antipsoriatics, as they inhibit chronic inflammation in psoriasis. The same agents can be used to treat e.g. hidradenitis suppurativa.

TNF-alpha blockers bind specifically to tumour necrosis factor alpha (TNF-alpha, an important cytokine in the pathogenesis of inflammatory diseases), thus blocking the interaction of TNF-alpha with TNF receptors on the cell surface. This inhibits the biological activity of TNF, therefore preventing a TNF-mediated cellular response. The effect is inhibition of the inflammatory process and reduced proliferation of keratinocytes.

ADVERSE EFFECTS	NOTES
• GI symptoms: diarrhoea, nausea • Headache • Upper respiratory tract infections	⊗ CI: patients with severe renal insufficiency, pregnancy and lactation ⚡ Apremilast is an oral, systemic PDE4 inhibitor that plays a critical role in modulating inflammatory pathways ● Reduction of inflammation → skin clearance and relief from joint pain, stiffness, and swelling ● A non-biologic treatment option, offering an alternative for patients who may not respond to or tolerate biologic therapies
• GI symptoms ⊖: nausea, vomiting, mucosal ulcers, loss of appetite • Hepatotoxicity (mild elevation of aminotransferases) ⊕: liver steatosis, fibrosis, or cirrhosis ⊖ • Risk of toxicity if prescribed in high dose: bone marrow suppression (aplastic anaemia, low white blood cell (WBC) count), alopecia, fatigue, fever, infections, pancreatitis, GI bleeding, lymphoproliferative disorders, renal failure	● Lowers chronic inflammation → can reduce pain and prevent injuries to tissues affected by autoimmune conditions ⚡ Avoided as first-line therapy for mild dermatological conditions due to its potential for serious side effects (e.g. hepatotoxicity, myelosuppression) ⚡ Always prescribe folic acid alongside methotrexate, to reduce side effects ⚡ Concomitant use of probenecid, trimethoprim-sulfamethoxazole, and salicylates can result in toxic concentrations of MTX. ⊗ Teratogenicity, patients with abnormal liver function tests

Interleukin (IL) inhibitors

IL inhibitors target cytokines involved in differentiation and activation of T cells, and are commonly used for the treatment of moderate-to-severe plaque psoriasis, psoriatic arthritis (IL-12, IL-17, and IL-23), and atopic dermatitis (IL-4/IL-13 inhibitors).

> Clinical notes
> - Infections: biologicals suppress parts of the immune system, making patients more susceptible to infections, particularly opportunistic infections like tuberculosis (TB) and fungal infections. Screening for TB (with a chest X-ray) before starting treatment is mandatory.
> - Vaccination: patients should receive appropriate vaccinations before initiating biologicals, esp. live vaccines, which cannot be given during therapy.
> - Monitoring: routine monitoring for infections, liver function, and other potential adverse effects is critical. Each biological may require different screening or monitoring protocols.

	MEDICATION	INDICATIONS	MECHANISM OF ACTION
TNF-ALPHA BLOCKERS	**Etanercept** (e.g. Enbrel®)	Psoriasis, psoriatic arthritis	Targets TNF-alpha
	Infliximab (e.g. Remicade®, Remsima®, Inflectra®, Flixabi®, Zessly®)	Psoriasis, psoriatic arthritis	
	Adalimumab (e.g. Humira®, Hulio®, Hyrimoz®, Amgevita®, Imraldi®)	Psoriasis (adults), psoriatic arthritis, hidradenitis suppurativa	
IL INHIBITORS	**Ustekinumab** (Stelara®)	Plaque psoriasis in patients who do not tolerate or respond to ciclosporin or methotrexate and PUVA	Targets IL-12, IL-23
	Guselkumab (Tremfya®)	Plaque psoriasis	Targets IL-23
	Tildrakizumab (Ilumya®)	Psoriasis	
	Risankizumab (Skyrizi®)		
	Secukinumab (Cosentyx®)	Psoriasis (adults), psoriatic arthritis	Targets IL-17A
	Ixekizumab (Taltz®)	Psoriasis, psoriatic arthritis	
	Brodalumab (Siliq®)	Psoriasis	Targets IL-17R

Table 15A // Biologicals

ADVERSE EFFECTS	NOTES
• Headache • Allergic reactions, pruritus, rash, urticaria	✖ CI: active infections, sepsis
Infections, fever	
• GI symptoms: stomachache, nausea, diarrhoea, constipation • Dizziness, vertigo • Hypoesthesia	✖ CI: active TB, sepsis, opportunistic infections, moderate-to-severe heart failure (NYHA III-IV)
• Respiratory tract infections, conjunctivitis • Headache, migraine, dizziness • Tachycardia • GI symptoms: stomachache, nausea, vomiting • Muscle aches, hypoesthesia • Anaemia, thrombocytopenia, leukocytosis • Hypersensitivity, alopecia	
• GI symptoms: nausea, vomiting, diarrhoea • Upper respiratory tract infections • Dizziness, headache, fatigue, muscle aches • Erythema	✖ CI: active infections
• Upper respiratory tract infections • Diarrhoea • Headache	
• GI symptoms: nausea, vomiting, diarrhoea • Upper respiratory tract infections • Headache • Antibody formation against the drug	
• Upper respiratory tract infections • Headache, fatigue • Tinea infections, pruritus, dermatitis • Antibody formation against the drug	✖ CI: active TB
• GI symptoms: nausea, diarrhoea • Upper respiratory tract infections, oral herpes infections • Urticaria • Headache, fatigue	
• Upper respiratory tract infections • Nausea • Tinea infections, mucocutaneous herpes simplex infections	
• GI symptoms: nausea, diarrhoea • Upper respiratory tract infections, tinea infections (e.g. tinea pedis) • Headache, fatigue, muscle ache	✖ CI: active Crohn's disease, active TB

	MEDICATION	INDICATIONS	MECHANISM OF ACTION
IL INHIBITORS	**Dupilumab** (Dupixent®)	Atopic dermatitis, prurigo nodularis	Targets IL-4R
	Omalizumab (Xolair®)	Chronic spontaneous urticaria	Targets IgE

Table 15B // Biologicals

Janus kinase (JAK) inhibitors

JAK inhibitors are a class of small-molecule drugs that modulate the activity of the JAK-STAT (Signal Transducer and Activator of Transcription) signaling pathway, which plays a pivotal role in immune regulation and inflammation. JAK inhibitors have shown beneficial effects in dermatological conditions such as atopic

	MEDICATION	INDICATIONS	MECHANISM OF ACTION
JAK INHIBITORS	**Tofacitinib** (Xeljanz®)	Psoriatic arthritis	Inhibition of JAK enzymes → prevent activation of downstream signalling molecules that lead to inflammation. These typically include cytokines (e.g. IL-4, IL-13, and IL-31 in atopic dermatitis, IL-12, IL-23 in psoriasis, and IFN-γ and IL-15 in vitiligo and alopecia).
	Ruxolitinib (Jakavi®)	Atopic dermatitis, graft-versus-host disease	
	Abrocitinib (cibinqo)	Atopic dermatitis	
	Upadacitinib (Rinvoq®)	Atopic dermatitis, psoriatic arthritis	
	Baricitinib (Olumiant®)	Atopic dermatitis, alopecia areata	

Table 16 // JAK inhibitors

ADVERSE EFFECTS	NOTES
Conjunctivitis, oral herpes infection, eosinophilia	☼ CI: none
Fever (in children), headache, upper respiratory tract infections	

dermatitis, alopecia areata, psoriatic arthritis, and vitiligo. Some JAK inhibitors are tofacitinib, baricitinib, and upadacitinib. JAK inhibitors have shown promising results in connective tissue diseases like dermatomyositis and cutaneous lupus erythematosus, where they target type-I interferons and thereby reduce inflammation and improve symptoms (see Table 16).

ADVERSE EFFECTS	NOTES
• GI symptoms: stomachache, vomiting, diarrhoea • Pneumonia, herpes zoster, urinary tract infections • Anaemia, lymphopenia • Headache • Hypertension	✖ CI: active TB, sepsis, severe liver insufficiency (Child-Pugh score 10-15), pregnancy and lactation
• CMV infections, sepsis, urinary tract infection • Anaemia, thrombocytopenia, neutropenia • Hypertension • Nausea	✖ CI: pregnancy and lactation
• Nausea, vomiting • Herpes zoster infection • Headache, dizziness	✖ CI: active infections (e.g. TB), severe liver function disorders, pregnancy and lactation
• GI symptoms: stomachache, nausea • Upper respiratory tract infections, herpes zoster, pneumonia • Neutropenia, anaemia • Urticaria • Headache, vertigo	✖ CI: active TB, severe liver function disorders, pregnancy and lactation
• Upper respiratory tract infections • Herpes zoster infection • Headache • Hypercholesterolemia, thrombocytosis • Rash • GI-tract symptoms: stomachache, nausea	✖ CI: pregnancy and lactation

Antibacterial therapy

General

Antibiotics (AB) are medications used to fight bacterial infections. It is important that they are used purposefully and moderately. AB can kill bacteria (bactericidal action) or stop bacteria from multiplying, allowing the body to clear the microorganism itself (bacteriostatic action).

Groups of antibiotics

Bacteria can be roughly divided into Gram-positive and Gram-negative cocci or bacilli based on Gram staining. Gram-positive bacteria have a thicker cell wall than Gram-negative bacteria, which have only a thin cell wall with a lipopolysaccharide outer membrane. Bacteria can also be further subdivided as aerobic and anaerobic. Table 17 classifies the most common bacterial strains. AB act on various processes taking place in these bacteria. Table 18 lists different groups of AB used for cutaneous infections. Table 13 lists different groups of AB of which adverse effects include cutaneous manifestations.

ANTIBIOTIC	BACTERIAL ACTION	ANTIMICROBIAL ACTION
Penicillins • Penicillinase-resistant (flucloxacillin) • Broad-spectrum (amoxicillin, piperacillin) • Penicillin G	Bactericidal	• Esp. with Gram-positive pathogens • Flucloxacillin: also active against beta-lactamase-producing pathogens, e.g. *Staphylococcus aureus* • Broad spectrum: also effective against Gram-negative bacteria (piperacillin also against *Pseudomonas*) • Addition of clavulanic acid + amoxicillin makes beta-lactamase-producing bacteria treatable
Cephalosporins • 1st: cefazolin • 2nd: cefuroxime • 3rd: ceftazidime, cefotaxime		• 1st generation: narrow spectrum, esp. effective against Gram-positive bacteria • 2nd generation: more effective against Gram-negative bacteria due to beta-lactamase insensitivity • 3rd generation: broader spectrum, esp. effective against Gram-negative bacteria
Macrolides Azithromycin, clarithromycin	Bacteriostatic, with some species bactericidal	• Like narrow-spectrum penicillins but with a broader spectrum (*Staphylococcus aureus, Mycoplasma, Legionella, Mycobacterium avium*) • For penicillin resistance or hypersensitivity

Table 18A // AB used for cutaneous infections; CYP, cytochrome P450

GRAM STAINING	MORPHOLOGY	GENUS
Gram-positive	Cocci	*Staphylococcus, Streptococcus, Enterococcus*
	Bacilli	*Clostridium, Corynebacterium, Cutibacterium*
Gram-negative	Cocci	*Neisseria, Bordetella, Rickettsiae*
	Bacilli	*Escherichia (E. coli), Campylobacter, Proteus, Haemophilus, Salmonella, Shigella, Yersinia, Pseudomonas*

Table 17 // Classification of bacteria

> Generally speaking, Gram-positive bacteria are cocci and Gram-negative bacteria are bacilli (exceptions are listed in Table 17).

> When antibiotics are prescribed for their anti-inflammatory properties, they are often used for the long term. An example is doxycycline to manage rosacea.

ADVERSE EFFECTS	INTERACTIONS AND RISK GROUPS
GI symptoms (nausea, abdominal pain, diarrhoea), toxicoderma (7-8% with amoxicillin, see Figure 26), hypersensitivity (1%), anaphylactic shock (0.01-0.04%), amoxicillin + EBV: generalised rash	There is cross-sensitivity between penicillins. Cross-sensitivity with cephalosporins is much less common.
GI (nausea, abdominal pain, diarrhoea), bone marrow depression (thrombocytopenia, leukopenia, granulocytopenia), haemolytic anaemia	· Cross-sensitivity with penicillins (limited) · Avoid simultaneous parenteral administration with calcium-containing solution → precipitation
GI symptoms (nausea, abdominal pain, diarrhoea), hypersensitivity	· Potent inhibition of CYP3A4 (increased risk of adverse effects with statins (myopathy and rhabdomyolysis), warfarin and digoxin) · Risk of QT prolongation ↑

ANTIBIOTIC	BACTERIAL ACTION	ANTIMICROBIAL ACTION
Tetracyclines Doxycycline, tetracycline	Bacteriostatic, with some species bactericidal	• Very broad spectrum, incl. *Mycoplasma*, *Rickettsiae*, *Chlamydia*, *Borrelia*, spirochetes, and protozoa • Doxycycline is the 1st choice to treat Lyme disease
Aminoglycosides Gentamicin (IV)	Bactericidal	• Mainly active against aerobic Gram-negative rods, as well as various Gram-positive organisms • Synergy with beta-lactam AB

Table 18B // AB used for cutaneous infections

ANTIBIOTIC	BACTERIAL ACTION	ANTIMICROBIAL ACTION
Carbapenems Meropenem	Bactericidal	Esp. against highly resistant Gram-negative bacteria, e.g. ESBL (extended spectrum beta-lactamase) because of its very broad spectrum. SPACE bugs: Serratial Proteus/Pseudomonas, Citrobacter, Enterobacter
Quinolones Ciprofloxacin, levofloxacin		• Broad spectrum, esp. effective against Gram-negative bacteria (enterocolic), as well as *H. influenzae*, *Campylobacter*, and *Pseudomonas* • Ciprofloxacin is the 1st choice for treating complicated UTIs

Table 19 // Groups of AB whose adverse effects include cutaneous manifestations

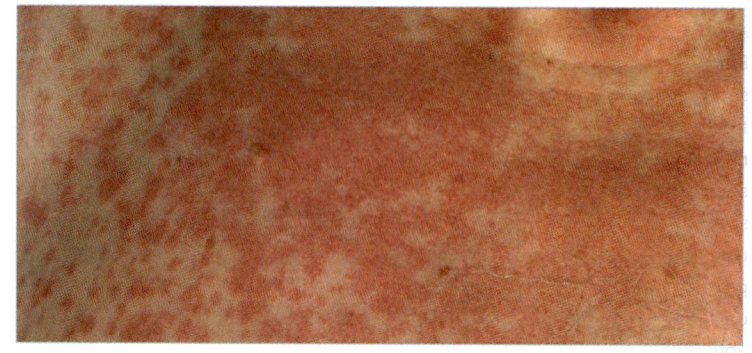

Figure 26 // Toxicoderma: reaction of the skin, mucous membranes, and appendages caused by drugs

ADVERSE EFFECTS	INTERACTIONS AND RISK GROUPS
Photosensitivity (photodermatitis, photo-onlycholysis, hyperpigmentation), calcium chelation (dental discolouration, dental hypoplasia, delayed osteogenesis)	• Chelation of metal ions • Dental discolouration/osteogenesis ↓: avoid in pregnant women from 16 wk and in children up to age 8 • Potentiates effect of oral anticoagulants
Dose-dependent: ototoxicity (irreversible vertigo, ataxia, deafness), reversible nephrotoxicity	• Ototoxicity: loop diuretics • Nephrotoxicity: renal insufficiency, nephrotoxic medication • Teratogenic • Therapeutic drug monitoring necessary due to narrow therapeutic index

ADVERSE EFFECTS	INTERACTIONS AND RISK GROUPS
GI symptoms (nausea, abdominal pain, diarrhoea), thrombocytaemia, hives, severe skin reactions ⊖ e.g. SJS, TEN, erythema multiforme	Concomitant use of bacteriostatic AB → bactericidal effect of carbapenems ↓
GI symptoms (nausea, abdominal pain, diarrhoea), hypersensitivity, neurotoxicity, hives, rash, itching, angioedema ⊖	Complex formation with calcium, magnesium, zinc, iron → strong decrease in absorption (be careful with antacids, milk, iron supplements)

Antibiotic resistance and switch therapy

Prudent AB use is essential in minimising the risk of antibiotic resistance. As soon as the pathogen and sensitivity pattern are known, an initial broad-spectrum therapy should make way for a narrower, more targeted therapy. While narrow-spectrum AB act against fewer species of bacteria than their broad-spectrum counterparts, they do reduce the risk of antibiotic resistance. Narrow-spectrum antibacterial agents are also gentler on the functional intestinal flora and have fewer adverse effects. When an admitted patient shows clinical improvement, switch from IV to oral antibiotic therapy (ABx) after 2-3 days, or 3-4 days for severe infections. The patient must be haemodynamically stable and able to swallow. This is known as switch therapy, a more patient-friendly, less labour-intensive option for the nursing staff which also leads to considerable

cost savings. If a patient does not improve after several days on AB, consider the following causes:
- Resistance
- The infection is viral or is caused by a different bacteria
- It is a febrile, non-infectious inflammation caused e.g. by an autoimmune disease, malignancy, or drug-induced fever
- The antibiotic agent cannot reach the focus of infection, e.g. due to an abscess, empyema, sequestrum, foreign body (prosthesis, infusion, catheter), poorly vascularised tissue (DM, peripheral vascular disease) or due to its location per se (brain, bone, heart valve)

Antibiotic resistance is caused by roughly four different biochemical mechanisms:
- The bacteria produce an enzyme that inactivates the AB: main examples are the production of beta-lactamase in beta-lactam AB and the production of acetyltransferase in aminoglycosides
- The AB-sensitive target molecule changes, as with aminoglycosides, erythromycin, and penicillin: one example is a mutation in the ribosomal protein to which aminoglycoside normally binds
- Increased AB efflux, as with tetracyclines
- The development of alternative pathways using other enzymes, as with the sulfonamides and trimethoprim

> Consider the following factors when selecting an AB:
> - Effective against the suspected pathogen
> - Reaches the focus of infection
> - Minimises the emergence of resistant microorganisms
> - No more toxic than an equivalent agent
> - Preferred mode of administration
> - No more expensive than an equivalent agent

> See *Appendix 1* for medication dosage of corticosteroids, methotrexate, and fumarates.

> Switching from IV to oral ABx is possible if:
> - Symptoms are improving
> - Vital signs are normal
> - Temperature is <37.8°C/100°F for >8h
> - Labs: WBC ↓ and C-reactive protein (CRP) ↓
> - A suitable oral option is available
> - The patient is capable of swallowing
> - Follow-up at home is possible

Topical antibiotics

Topical AB are highly effective for delivering medication directly to the affected area, maximising the presence of the drugs at the site of infection. Additional benefits of using topical AB include minimal drug usage and cost-effectiveness.

Topical AB are commonly indicated for the treatment of minor skin infections like impetigo, and to prevent infections in minor cuts, scrapes, and burns. Commonly used topical AB include fusidic acid, mupirocin, and silver sulfadiazine.

Other
Antiviral therapy

Antivirals interfere with viral replication cycles. Viruses have different replication cycles and are therefore treated differently. Antivirals are effective only if the virus replicates and should therefore be given as soon as possible after the start of the infection. Antiviral resistance can develop rapidly due to the high mutation rate during virus replication, possibly necessitating a combination of multiple antiviral drugs. HSV I and II can be treated with antivirals such as valaciclovir, famciclovir, and aciclovir.

Antiparasitic therapy

When deciding on antiparasitic therapy, consider the type of parasitic infection (helminthiasis, protozoan infection, arthropod infection), the complexity of life cycles, and differences in parasite metabolisms. Key is to choose an agent that acts on host-parasite differences such as drug uptake, folate metabolism, polyamine uptake, trypanothione-dependent reduction mechanisms, cytoskeleton proteins (tubulin), neurotransmitters, intracellular calcium levels, and oxidative phosphorylation. Some AB have antiprotozoal activity (e.g. metronidazole, tetracycline).

Antimycotics

Compared to the vast array of antibacterial agents, the arsenal of antifungal agents is rather sparse. This is because it's more difficult to create selective toxicity against eukaryotes than against prokaryotes. Antifungal agents have several points of action, including inhibition of cell membrane synthesis (azoles), interference with cell wall synthesis (echinocandins), inhibition of cell membrane function (polyenes), and inhibition of nucleic acid synthesis.

As with AB, resistance to antifungal agents is becoming increasingly common, particularly because of their use in animal husbandry and agriculture (the 'one world, one health' principle).

Hydroxychloroquine

Hydroxychloroquine (HCQ) is a 4-aminoquinoline oral antimalarial drug with immunomodulatory properties, widely used in dermatology for the treatment of e.g. lupus erythematosus, porphyria cutanea tarda, dermatomyositis, cutaneous sarcoidosis, disseminated granuloma annulare, and lichen planus (see Table 20).

Antihistamines

Antihistamines are administered orally or intramuscularly in the symptomatic treatment of allergic conditions mediated by histamine release, including urticaria (hives); atopic dermatitis; other skin diseases based on direct allergies, esp. pruritus, insect bites; medication allergies; food allergies, angioedema; and anaphylactic shock (only in combination with epinephrine and corticosteroids). Antihistamines are also used to treat hay fever and allergic rhinitis. The effect of these drugs is a decrease in the symptoms of allergic diseases, resulting from the release of histamine.

Keratolytics

This group of agents remove the upper layer of skin (epidermis) in a process known as keratolysis. Keratolytics are used for e.g. dry and flaky skin, acne, ichthyosis, corns, calluses, hyperkeratosis, and warts. They act directly on the adhesive intercellular junctions (desmosomes) to prevent adhesion between keratinocytes. Their hygroscopic and keratolytic properties also reduce the density of the stratum corneum, thus impairing comedone formation and size.

Retinoids

General

Retinoids are a group of compounds that are derived from vitamin A or share structural and functional similarities with it. Vitamin A is also known as retinol, and its metabolites consist of retinaldehyde/retinal and retinoic acid. This fat-soluble organic substance and its metabolites play roles in immune function, reproduction, vision, cellular communication, and differentiation. Vitamin A is obtained through the human diet in two forms, preformed vitamin A (retinol) and provitamin A (carotenoids), and both forms are stored in the liver. Vitamin A is stored and converted into retinyl esters in the skin by keratinocytes and activates retinoid receptors to influence the development of cells.

Retinoids impact the proliferation and differentiation of cells. Cytosolic binding proteins and nuclear hormone receptors are responsible for regulating retinoids' biological effects. Retinoids normalise abnormal desquamation by increasing the turnover of follicular epithelial cells and accelerating the shedding of corneocytes.

Topical retinoids

Topical retinoids like tretinoin have proven to be extremely effective in the treatment of acne vulgaris and various other skin conditions, including disorders of keratinisation and sun-damaged skin. These topical treatments can cause side effects such as dryness and irritation at the site of application, as well as photosensitivity. The use of topical retinoids offers several advantages compared to oral retinoids, including localised treatment with reduced systemic exposure, making them a preferred option for managing dermatological conditions while minimising potential systemic side effects.

Oral retinoids

Oral retinoids (e.g. isotretinoin) have shown significant efficacy in the treatment of severe acne, psoriasis, disorders of keratinisation, gram-negative folliculitis, ichthyosis, acne rosacea, and hidradenitis suppurativa. Patients using oral retinoids can experience side effects, such as dry skin/lips/eyes, muscle pains, headaches, and changes in the liver function tests. Due to its known teratogenicity it is vital that patients do not become pregnant while using retinoids until one month after ceasing the retinoid therapy. Patients undergoing oral retinoid therapy must be closely monitored due to these potential adverse effects.

Topical fluorouracil

Topical fluorouracil (5%), also known as 5-fluorouracil or 5-FU, belongs to a class of chemotherapy drugs and is an FDA-approved therapy for the management of actinic keratoses and superficial basal cell carcinomas (see Figure 27 and Table 20).

Dimethyl fumarate

Dimethyl fumarate (DMF) is an oral immunomodulatory agent originally approved for the treatment of multiple sclerosis (MS), which has also gained use in dermatology for the treatment of moderate-to-severe psoriasis. It is effective in reducing the hyperproliferation of skin cells and inflammation associated with the disease (see Table 20).

MEDICATION	INDICATIONS	MECHANISM OF ACTION
Fluorouracil 5% (5-FU) (topical)	Actinic or solar keratoses, superficial basal cell carcinomas	• 5-FU is converted into fluorodeoxyuridine monophosphate (FdUMP) upon entering cells → FdUMP complex formation with thymidylate synthase → inhibition of deoxythymidine monophosphate (dTMP) production → imbalance in intracellular nucleotides and depletion of DNA replication and repair → generation of double-stranded DNA breaks → cell death of rapidly proliferating cells • 5-FU has a selective cytotoxic effect on actinic skin lesions, without damaging normal skin, potentially due to selective inhibition of thymidylate synthase • Other mechanisms by which 5-FU may exert its effects include interference with RNA processing and increased p53 expression
Hydroxychloroquine (Plaquenil®)	Lupus erythematosus, porphyria cutanea tarda, dermatomyositis, cutaneous sarcoidosis, disseminated granuloma annulare, lichen planus	• Antiproliferative, anti-inflammatory, immunomodulatory, and photoprotective effects • Accumulation in immune cells → increase in vacuolar pH → disruption of antigen presentation → reduced immune overactivity • HCQ is believed to downregulate the arachidonic acid pathway → production of pro-inflammatory molecules ↓ and protection against oxidative damage ↓
Dimethylfumarate (DMF)	Psoriasis	• Activating the nuclear factor (erythroid-derived 2)-like 2 (Nrf2) pathway → oxidative stress ↓ • Elevating intracellular glutathione (GSH) levels → shifting immune responses from T helper cell 1/17 (pro-inflammatory) to T helper cell 2 (anti-inflammatory) → inhibiting the production of inflammatory cytokines • Inhibiting NF-κB activity → cytokine production ↓ and inflammation in T cells and other immune cells ↓

Table 20 // Other medications used in dermatological treatment

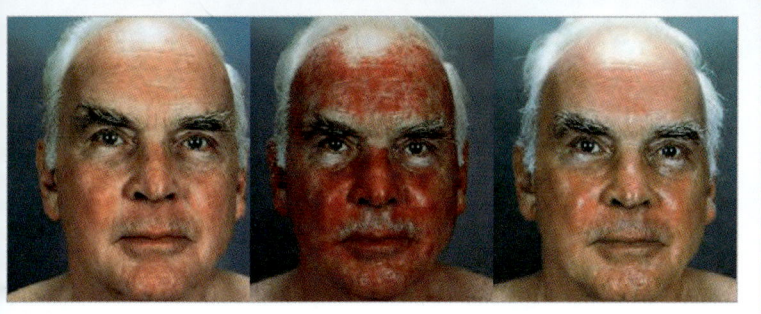

Figure 27 // Example of skin reaction before (left), during (middle), and after (right) topical treatment with fluorouracil

ADVERSE EFFECTS	NOTES
Localised skin irritation (ulceration or local infection), pruritus, pain, crusting, dermatitis	✗ CI: pregnancy (associated with ventricular septum defects and an risk ↑ of miscarriage), highest risks of teratogenicity during the 1st trimester
• GI symptoms (e.g. nausea, vomiting, anorexia, diarrhoea) • Headache, blurred vision • Skin rash • Prolonged use may rarely lead to retinopathy, necessitating regular ophthalmological testing	✗ CI: patients with retinal disease ⇔ Caution in patients with known prolonged QT intervals, reduced liver function, myasthenia gravis, porphyria, or G6PD deficiency
• GI symptoms (e.g. nausea, diarrhoea, abdominal pain) • Flushing • Long-term use requires monitoring due to potential risks like lymphopenia, liver enzyme elevation, and rare cases of progressive multifocal leukoencephalopathy	✗ CI: patients with severe infections, liver dysfunction, or hypersensitivity to the drug

✎ Invasive, non-pharmacological treatment

Cryotherapy
Cryotherapy is the use of liquid nitrogen to freeze benign or malignant skin conditions. Lesions are frozen with a nitrogen spray held a few mm to >1 cm from the lesion, depending on the size of the lesion. This produces an 'ice disk' that should remain frozen for 10-20 seconds. After the disk defrosts, the procedure is often repeated. Cryotherapy is indicated for e.g. warts, actinic keratosis, Bowen's disease, and superficial BCCs. The skin usually heals within one to three weeks, with the blister/crust falling off spontaneously. The most common adverse effect is hypopigmentation.

Electrocoagulation
Electrocoagulation is a technique that uses electrical current to heat and coagulate tissue. It is indicated for e.g. cutting tissue and stopping bleeding during interventions with minimal carbonisation. Additionally, electrocoagulation is commonly used to remove small skin lesions, such as skin tags, condylomata, and spider angiomas (spider naevi).

Excision biopsy melanoma
Suspected melanoma is also called atypical naevus/mole. Procedure for excision of atypical naevi:

1. Lay out the materials for the procedure
2. Using a surgical marker, draw an elliptical shape around the excision site. Align the incision with the direction of the locally draining lymph node, using a 3:1 length-to-width ratio, approx. 30° angles, and a 2 mm margin, while also factoring in the course of the skin lines (see Figure 28).
3. Disinfect the area centrifugally with gauze and disinfectant
4. Anaesthesia: field block with lidocaine; test sensitivity and inject more if area is still sensitive, then wait several minutes before making the first incision
5. Cover the area with a surgical drape with a hole
6. Using a scalpel, cut straight down to the subcutis while pulling the skin taut with the thumb and index finger of your non-dominant hand. Use surgical forceps to lift the flap of skin.
7. Remove the flap
8. Suturing: cutaneous and possibly subcutaneous
9. Dress the wound with gauze and consider applying pressure dressing to

stop the bleeding

10. Tell the patient to keep the wound dry for one day, come back if they notice signs of infection (redness, heat, swelling, pain, loss of function), and to have the sutures removed after 7-10 days

A therapeutic re-excision is performed if the diagnostic excision reveals the presence of melanoma. Therapeutic re-excision is performed by the dermatologist, with a margin of 10-20 mm depending on the Breslow depth. Patients who qualify for a sentinel node procedure will be referred to a surgeon due to possible satellite lesions. Satellite lesions are more likely at greater Breslow depths.

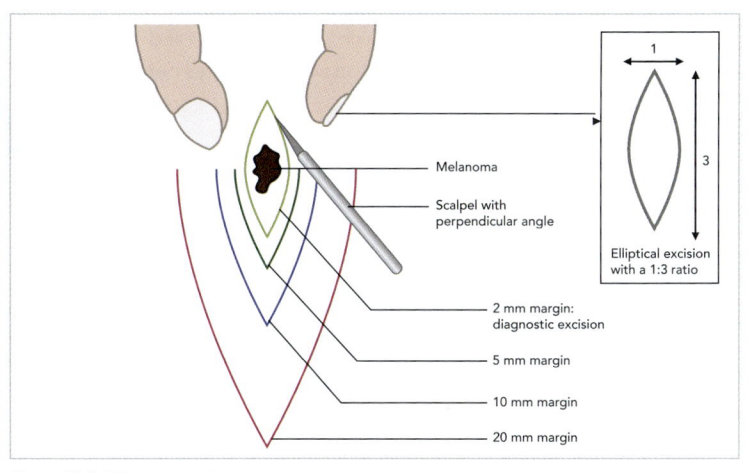

Figure 28 // Melanoma excision

Excision margins:
- Diagnostic, atypical naevus/melanoma: 2 mm
- Therapeutic, superficial, low-risk nodular (BCC): 3 mm (superficial with preference for applying fluorouracil or imiquimod over surgery)
- Therapeutic, spiky, micronodular BCC: 5 mm
- Therapeutic, primary low-risk squamous cell carcinoma (SCC): 5 mm
- Therapeutic, melanoma in situ: 5 mm
- Therapeutic, high-risk or recurrent SCC: 10 mm
- Therapeutic, Breslow ≤2 mm: 10 mm
- Therapeutic, Breslow >2 mm: 20 mm

> For therapeutic excisions the same procedure can be used as for diagnostic excisions, but a therapeutic excision requires greater excision margins.

Therapeutic lipoma excision

Lipoma excision consists of removing a subcutaneous lump of fatty tissue (see Figure 29). Indications for lipoma excision include aesthetic preference, lipoma size >5 cm, and/or pain. The procedure for lipoma excision is as follows:

1. Using a surgical marker, draw the incision line on the skin, factoring in skin lines and length
2. Disinfect the area centrifugally with gauze and disinfectant
3. Anaesthesia: field block with lidocaine. Test sensitivity and inject more lidocaine if the area is still sensitive. Wait several minutes before making the first incision.
4. Cover the area with a surgical drape with a hole
5. Make an incision along the marked line with a scalpel
6. Free the lipoma using pressure and traction of the fingers and gauze and continue with scissors if necessary
7. Cut through any residual structures
8. Stop any bleeding
9. Suturing: cutaneous and possibly subcutaneous
10. Dress the wound with gauze and consider applying pressure dressing to stop the bleeding
11. Tell the patient to keep the wound dry for one day, come back if they notice signs of infection (redness, heat, swelling, pain, loss of function), and to have the sutures removed (after 7-14 days, dependig on the location)

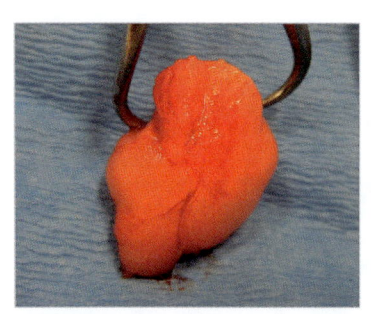

Figure 29 // Removed lipoma with a clear smooth structure

> Referral to a general surgeon is indicated for growing lipomas attached to e.g. a muscle or tendon. These lipomas are no longer mobile relative to their substrate upon palpation. Typical locations are the neck or upper back (nuchal lipoma).

> If the lipoma does not resemble normal adipose tissue, request histopathological testing.

Knot-tying and suturing techniques
Suturing

Inspect the wound and determine which suturing technique to use (see Table 21). Deep wounds are often closed with subcutaneous sutures to reduce tension on the skin. The thickness of a suture gauge depends on the different tissue types, and always consists of a variable x and 0, separated by a hyphen (x-0). The higher the value of x, the thinner the wire. Anaesthetise the skin with lidocaine (10 mg/ml = 1%) prior to suturing with the chosen technique. Adrenaline can be used in acral areas as well (e.g. nose tip, nipple, penis, fingers, toes, earlobe).

In addition to selecting an appropriate thread and suturing technique, practitioners need to handle the equipment properly. Holding the forceps and needle holders as a knife and fork makes it easier to move the wrists (fine movements). Use the needle holder to grasp the needle at $3/4$ down from the tip (see Figure 30). As a general rule for suturing, always insert the needle at a 90° angle to the skin, to keep the opening as small as possible and point the wound edges more towards each other; the two sides of the suture should mirror each other, i.e. the entrance and exit must be equidistant from the wound edge.

> All sutures ending in '-yl' are soluble.

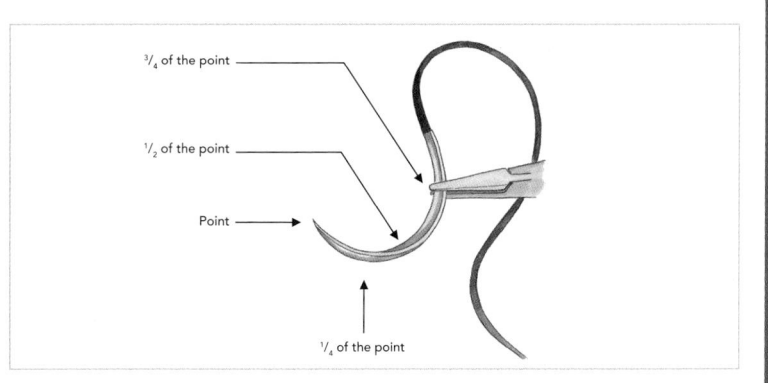

- $3/4$ of the point
- $1/2$ of the point
- Point
- $1/4$ of the point

Figure 30 // Proper handling of needle and needle holder

CHARACTERISTICS	INTERRUPTED MATTRESS SUTURE	DONATI SUTURE
Wound	Most widely used suture, suitable for virtually any wound (see Figure 31)	Suitable for deep wounds, receding wound edges, or inverted wound edges (see Figure 32)
Technique	1. Insert the needle, making sure the depth of the wound and the distance between the sutures are equal on both sides 2. Make sure the edges lie together, without pulling the skin too taut 3. Tie a knot in the suture, making sure that the knot is not over the wound edge and that all knots are on the same side	1. Insert the needle at a greater distance from the wound and deeper than in a mattress suture 2. Next, reinsert the needle closer to the wound edge and more superficially, so that the needle comes out on the same side as the first suture 3. See mattress suture
Advantages	Easy to place, strong, least likely to affect blood circulation	Well-approximated wound edges, more tension can be applied to wound
Disadvantages	• Takes longer to place than running suture • More likely to produce a 'railroad track' scar	Time-consuming
Preferred suture material	Non-resorbable monofilament	

Table 21 // Suturing techniques

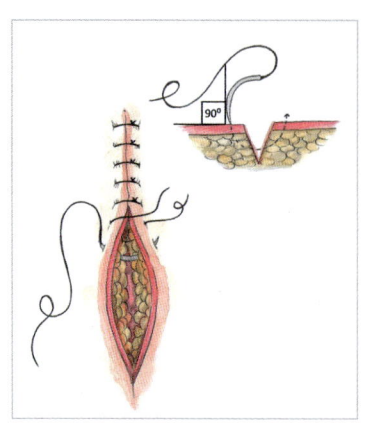

Figure 31 // Interrupted, mattress suture

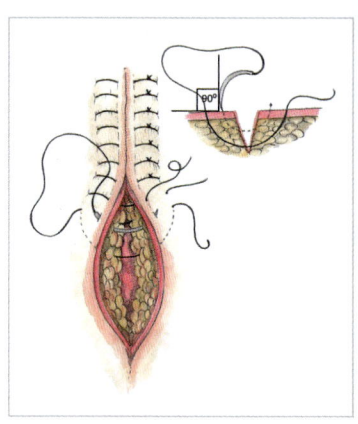

Figure 32 // Donati suture

RUNNING MATTRESS SUTURE	RUNNING INTRACUTANEOUS SUTURE
Suitable for wound edges that are not under tension. Often combined with subcutaneous sutures. This suture is widely used in skin grafts (see Figure 33).	Intracutaneous sutures are the preferred choice for wounds that require optimal cosmetic results (esp. in the face), but they can only be placed if the wound edges are under minimal tension (see Figure 34)
1. See mattress suture, tie a knot as with the mattress suture but without cutting the thread 2. Repeat the mattress suture technique to the end of the wound, without tying knots 3. See mattress suture	First tie a knot in the end of the suture thread 1. Starting above the apex of the wound, take a bite to the inside of the apex 2. Now insert the needle perpendicularly into the wound edge opposite the exit and make a horizontal turn below the skin until the needle exits the skin at the same side of the wound 3. Repeat this technique until you reach the other apex 4. Insert the needle from the distal wound apex to just above the wound, like the initial insertion, and pull the thread until the wound edges are well approximated 5. Knot the end of the thread to the outer edge of the wound
Less scarring thanks to fewer knots, easy and time-efficient	Only a knot at the wound apexes → better cosmetic result
Greater chance of dehiscence if suture breaks	• More time-consuming technique • Avoid if risk of wound infection is very high
Non-resorbable monofilament	Resorbable monofilament

Figure 33 // Running mattress suture

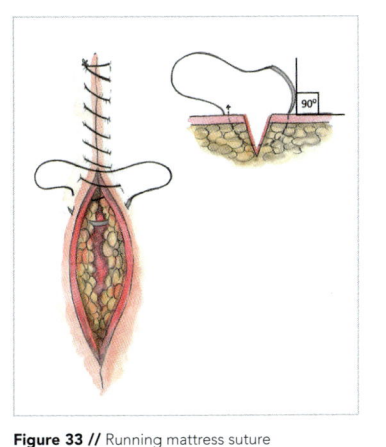

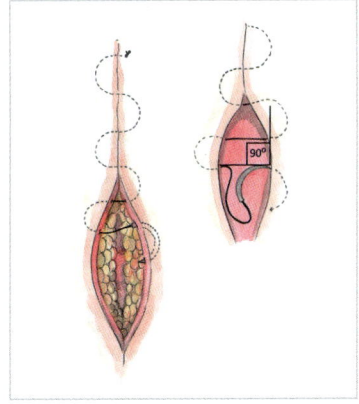

Figure 34 // Running intracutaneous suture

LOCAL FLAP	EXPLANATION	VISUALISATION
Advancement flap	• Advancement flaps are a type of sliding flap in which tissue is slid directly to an adjacent defect. Advancement flaps are generally made by deepening the defect, after which the skin is stretched out slightly to cover the defect. Advancement flaps can be designed with or without Burow's triangles. • Tissue is advanced unidirectionally. Examples are H, V-Y or Y-V plasty.	Incision, Lesion, Elevated skin flap, Excision of Burow's triangle (to prevent dog ear), Scar pattern
H plasty	• Incisions are made in the skin next to the defect, moving medially and laterally towards the defect • This creates an H-shaped scar	Incision, Lesion, Elevated skin flap, Excision of Burow's triangle (to prevent dog ear), Scar pattern
V-Y plasty	• Type of tissue displacement in which a triangular flap is raised and advanced over the subcutaneous fat • Y-V plasty is based on the same principle but produces broader width gains than V-Y plasty	Lesion, Incision, A, B, C, Elevated skin flap, Scar pattern
Rotation flap	• The defect is deepened and the donor skin is rotated around a fixed point to close the defect. The donor site is then closed primarily if possible. • The tissue is moved with a rotating motion	Incision, Elevated skin flap, Lesion, Scar pattern
Transposition flap	• A donor flap is moved to the defect. The flap can be of any shape. • The tissue is moved with a more or less rotating motion • Examples are Z-plasty, rhomboid flaps, nasolabial flaps, and bilobal flaps	Burrow's triangle, Lesion, Incision, Scar pattern

Table 22A // Most commonly used local flaps

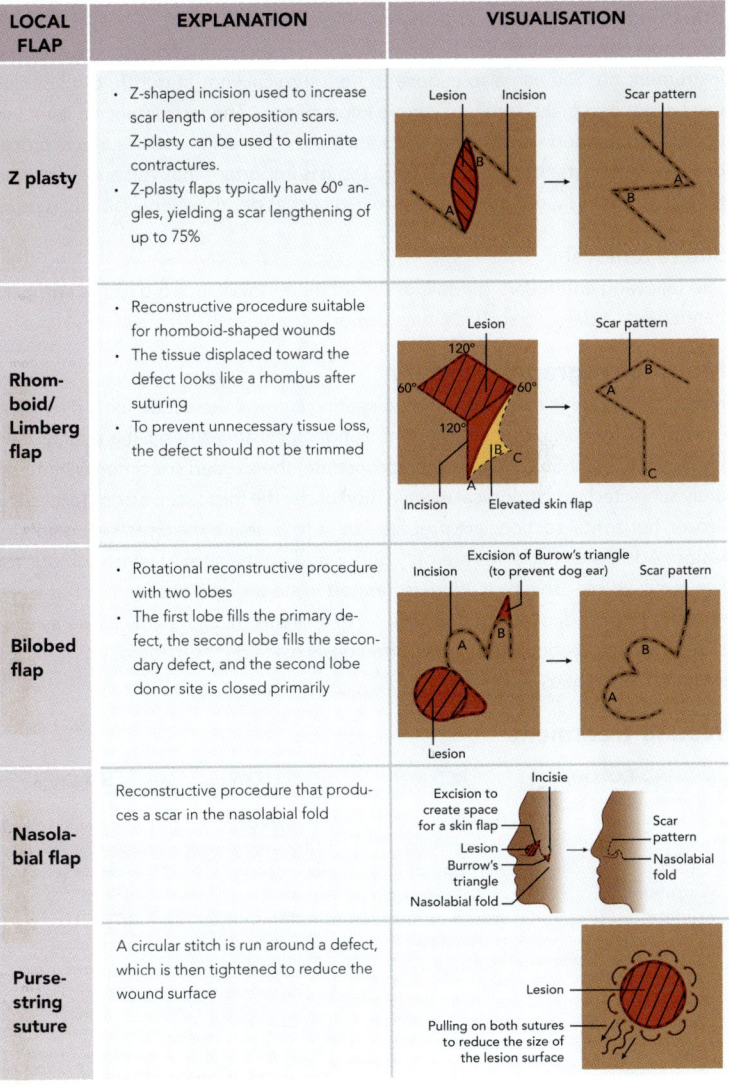

LOCAL FLAP	EXPLANATION	VISUALISATION
Z plasty	• Z-shaped incision used to increase scar length or reposition scars. Z-plasty can be used to eliminate contractures. • Z-plasty flaps typically have 60° angles, yielding a scar lengthening of up to 75%	Lesion, Incision → Scar pattern
Rhomboid/ Limberg flap	• Reconstructive procedure suitable for rhomboid-shaped wounds • The tissue displaced toward the defect looks like a rhombus after suturing • To prevent unnecessary tissue loss, the defect should not be trimmed	Lesion, 120°, 60°, Incision, Elevated skin flap → Scar pattern
Bilobed flap	• Rotational reconstructive procedure with two lobes • The first lobe fills the primary defect, the second lobe fills the secondary defect, and the second lobe donor site is closed primarily	Incision, Excision of Burow's triangle (to prevent dog ear), Lesion → Scar pattern
Nasolabial flap	Reconstructive procedure that produces a scar in the nasolabial fold	Incisie, Excision to create space for a skin flap, Lesion, Burrow's triangle, Nasolabial fold → Scar pattern, Nasolabial fold
Purse-string suture	A circular stitch is run around a defect, which is then tightened to reduce the wound surface	Lesion, Pulling on both sutures to reduce the size of the lesion surface

Table 22B // Most commonly used local flaps

Knot-tying

Flat knots can be made with a one-hand technique, two-hand technique, or the instrument tie. You can also choose to tie a surgical knot at depth, but visibility can be poor so make sure you can tie knots blindly. The instrument tie is mainly used when suturing skin. Manual knots are more commonly used in surgical procedures and subcutaneous sutures. Here too it is important that you are able to tie these knots blindly, as you may have to tie knots at depth, where visibility is poor.

Suture removal

The following criteria are guidelines for suture removal: face 5 days, head/neck/hands/arms 7 days, torso 10-14 days, lower extremities 10-18 days.

Mohs micrographic surgery

Mohs micrographic surgery is a tissue-sparing surgical technique for the removal of high-risk local skin cancer, performed under local anaesthesia. It is mainly used for facial BCCs or SCCs. During this procedure, the excised specimen is immediately subjected to histological examination under the microscope prior to surgery. Frozen horizontal sections are prepared so as to examine the cross-section of the lesion. Additional excisions are only performed on the sites at which tumour tissue is still visible. This procedure is iterated in stages until the tumour has been radically removed, allowing the surgeon to spare as much healthy tissue as possible. Reconstruction of the defect often takes place on the same day. For reconstruction techniques, see Table 22.

Wound treatment

WOUND/COLOUR	RED	YELLOW	BLACK
Wet/abundant exudate	• Hydrofibre • Foam dressing • Wet gauze dressing 3x/d or soaked in antiseptic solution • Hydrocolloid • Paraffin gauze	• Wet gauze dressing 3x/d or soaked in antiseptic solution • Alginate • Hydrofibre • Foam dressing • Hydrocolloid • Surgical debridement	• Wet gauze dressing 3x/d or soaked in antiseptic solution • Alginate • Hydrogel • Hydrocolloid • Surgical necrosectomy
Dry/little exudate	• Hydrogel • Hydrocolloid • Paraffin gauze • Wet gauze dressing 3x/d or soaked in antiseptic solution	• Hydrogel • Hydrocolloid • Wet gauze dressing 3x/d or soaked in antiseptic solution • Surgical debridement	• Dry dressing • Surgical necrosectomy

Table 23 // Wound treatment

Treatment of varicose veins
Compression therapy
Compression therapy consists of using elastic stockings to help manage insufficiency of the deep or superficial venous system, e.g. the GSV or its branches. It is also used to treat heavy legs without indications for surgical intervention.

Sclerotherapy (injecting varicose veins)
Sclerotherapy consists of injecting varicose veins with an irritating solution to provoke an inflammatory reaction in the vascular wall. A compression bandage is then applied to close the vessel. The technique can also be performed with foamed solution, especially for larger varicose veins – this is called foam sclerotherapy. It may be unsuitable for spider (thread) veins, as these veins are smaller than the needles used for the procedure. Very small varicose veins can be treated with external laser therapy.

Endovenous techniques (cauterisation from within the vein)
Endovenous cauterisation is used to close the GSV and small saphenous vein (SSV) from within, using either radio waves or the heat (VNUS closure). Both methods damage the interior of the vein, causing it to close. Other methods for damaging the vein are laser beams, electricity, and freezing, all of which use duplex ultrasound for guidance.

Muller procedure (ambulatory phlebectomy)
The Muller procedure consists of making small incisions next to the vein under local anaesthesia before extracting the vein with small hooks. Following this procedure, a compression bandage is applied for two weeks. Ambulatory phlebectomy is indicated for large, superficial branches of saphenous veins.

Stripping and crossectomy
Stripping is the surgical removal of varicose veins by a vascular surgeon. It is used for particularly tortuous trunk veins or large, superficial varicose veins. Crossectomy involves locating the GSV junction with the femoral vein through an incision in the groin, clearing and transecting the junction, and ligating branches with sutures. When treating the SSV, the incision is made in the hollow of the knee.

PUVA/UVA/UVB
Exposure to sunlight, and ultraviolet (UV) radiation in particular, can have a beneficial effect on skin pathology. UV radiation has an inhibitory effect on rapid cell

proliferation, stimulation of proteolytic enzymes, and modulation of cells in an inflammatory concentrate.

UV radiation can be split into three bands: UVA (315-400 nm), UVB (280-315 nm) and UVC (100-280 nm). UVA penetrates deeper into the skin (down to the dermis or subcutis) than UVB (down to the epidermis) because of its longer wavelength. UVA and psoralens plus ultraviolet A (PUVA) are types of phototherapy in which the patient is exposed to UVA light in a booth. In PUVA therapy, the patient is given a psoralen tablet first to enhance the skin's sensitivity to UVA light. Bath-water PUVA is a variation in which the patient soaks their hands or feet in a psoralen bath before the treatment. UVA1 dosimetry is categorised into low (10-29 J/cm^2), medium (30-69 J/cm^2), and high (>60 J/cm^2) dosage regimens. The mechanism of action is based on the generation of oxygen radicals by UVA, which causes lymphocytes, monocytes, and eosinophils to go into apoptosis. Main indications for UVA1 phototherapy are severe atopic dermatitis, scleroderma, urticaria pigmentosa, and mycosis.

UVB is a type of phototherapy in which the patient is exposed to UVB in a booth. The mechanism of action relies on UVB-induced damage to DNA leading to activation of transcription factors, cytokine secretion, immunosuppression, and apoptosis. The dose is gradually increased depending on the skin type. This treatment is used mainly for psoriasis, but is also suitable for atopic dermatitis, vitiligo, and pruritus. UVB therapy is not appropriate for deeper skin pathologies, which are easier to reach with UVA or PUVA.

Photodynamic therapy (PDT)

PDT consists of administering a local photosensitiser before exposing the skin to light, activating the agent and damaging the skin. Indications include superficial premalignant and malignant skin pathology such as actinic keratosis, Bowen's disease, and superficial BCCs.

Laser therapy

Laser therapy uses light energy, which can induce changes in the skin when absorbed in sufficient amounts. The type of treatment depends on the condition being treated. Lasers deliver monochromatic, coherent, collimated, high-intensity beams of light. Depending on the indication, different types of laser therapy can be chosen.

- Vascular lasers emit radiation that is selectively absorbed by oxyhemoglobin and deoxyhemoglobin, causing a targeted increase in temperature within the blood vessels. This heat is transferred to the vascular wall, leading to coagulation and necrosis at temperatures above 60°C/104°F. These lasers are primarily used for treating vascular lesions. Common vascular lasers are the Pulsed Dye Laser (PDL), with varying wavelengths (e.g. 577 nm) and the Neodymium Aluminium Garnet laser (Nd:YAG, 1064 nm).
- Fractional lasers use many narrow beams to create small columns of necrosis in the skin, surrounded by intact tissue. This technique ensures quicker healing and minimal side effects. There are over a hundred different fractional lasers, categorised into ablative and non-ablative types, used primarily for cosmetic treatments like rejuvenation, pigmentation issues, wrinkle removal, and acne scars.
- Intense Pulsed Light (IPL) is not a laser, but a device that emits electromagnetic radiation via a xenon lamp. Unlike lasers, which emit a single wavelength, IPL emits a spectrum of wavelengths (~500-1200 nm). The ability to switch filters allows for the same device to be used for various treatments, such as vascular lesions, pigmentation issues, and hair removal.
- Pigment lasers target melanin or external pigments (e.g., iron, drug-induced pigmentation, tattoos) through selective absorption. These lasers use very short pulse durations tailored to the size of pigment particles (melanosomes). Examples are the Q-switched Ruby laser (694 nm), Q-switched Alexandrite laser (755 nm), and Q-switched Nd laser.
- Ablative lasers remove tissue using electromagnetic radiation absorbed by water in the tissue, with very short pulse durations achieving temperatures above 300°C/572°F. Effects include ablation, coagulation, collagen necrosis, thermal damage, and collagen contraction. Initially developed for cosmetic treatments such as wrinkle removal and acne scars, common systems include the carbon dioxide (CO_2) laser (10,600 nm), and the Erbium Yttrium Aluminium Garnet laser (Er:YAG laser).
- Hair removal lasers use the presence of melanin in the hair shaft, infundibulum, and matrix to selectively destroy hair follicles. Common lasers are the long-pulse Alexandrite laser (755 nm), diode laser (800/810 nm), and long-pulse Nd laser (1064 nm). The long-pulse Nd laser allows for safe treatment of individuals with skin types V and VI.

Differential diagnosis

> This section lists several examples of diagnoses to consider for specific complaints. The differential diagnosis (DDx) shown here are examples only.

Pruritus (itching)
Pruritus with primary skin lesions
- Dermatitis
  - Constitutional dermatitis
  - Contact dermatitis
  - Statis dermatitis
  - Nummular dermatitis
- Hives
- Xerosis cutis (dry skin)
- Dermatomycosis
- Epizoonoses
  - Scabies
  - Insect bites
- Folliculitis
- Psoriasis
- Pemphigoid
  - Bullous
  - Non-bullous
- Adverse drug reaction (calcium antagonists, ACE inhibitors, hydrochlorothiazide, and opioids)
- Lichen simplex chronicus
- Lichen ruber planus
- Dermatitis herpetiformis
- Varicella

Pruritus without primary skin lesions
- Neurological
  - Multiple sclerosis (MS)
- Psychogenic

- Adverse drug reactions (toxicoderma)
- Gynaecological
  - Pregnancy
  - Postmenopausal
- Xerosis cutis
- Parasitic infections
- Systemic causes
  - Liver disease with cholestasis
  - Chronic renal insufficiency
  - Diabetes mellitus (DM)
  - Hyperparathyroidism, hyperthyroidism, and hypothyroidism
  - Gout
  - AIDS
- Haematological
  - Anaemia/iron deficiency
  - Polycythaemia vera
  - Malignancy
  - Leukaemia
  - Lymphomas (Hodgkin, non-Hodgkin)
  - Multiple myeloma
  - Tumours (Grawitz tumour, breast or gastric cancer)

> In pruritus without primary skin lesions, secondary skin lesions may develop over time, e.g. lichenification, papules, excoriations

Erythema
Generalised erythema (erythroderma)
- Solar erythema
- Toxicoderma
- Psoriasis
- Dermatitis
  - Atopic
  - Seborrhoeic
- Hives
- Dermatomyositis
- Lichen planus
- Paraneoplastic
  - Carcinoma
  - Adenocarcinomas
  - Flushes secondary to carcinoid syndrome/pheochromocytoma

- Secondary syphilis
- Erythema multiforme
- SLE
- Malignant reticulosis
- Idiopathic (red man syndrome)
- Sezary syndrome
- Ichthyosis

Local erythema
- Hives
- Intertrigo/diaper rash
- Insect bite
- Blushing
- Facial erythema
- Palmar erythema
- Erysipelas
- Cellulitis
- Erythema nodosum
- Rosacea
- Contact dermatitis
- Raynaud's phenomenon
- Butterfly erythema secondary to SLE
- Solar erythema (sunburn)
- Naevus flammeus (port-wine stain)
- Erythema migrans (Lyme disease)

Generalised erythema in children
- Hives
- Nonspecific viral exanthems
- Febrile erythema of unknown origin
- Staphylococcal scalded skin syndrome (SSSS)
- Infectious diseases
  - Erythema infectiosum (5th disease)
  - Exanthema subitum (6th disease)
  - Mononucleosis infectiosa (Pfeiffer's disease)
  - Enterovirus infections (ECHO and coxsackie virus)
  - Morbilli (measles)
  - Rubella
  - Scarlet fever

Facial pustules
- Acne
  - Acne vulgaris (pimples)
  - Acne conglobata
  - Steroid acne
  - Acne keloidalis
  - Other forms of acne
- Herpes virus
  - Herpes zoster (shingles)
  - Herpes simplex (HSV)
- Impetigo
- Rosacea
- Perioral/periocular dermatitis
- Folliculitis
  - Folliculitis barbae
- Furuncle/carbuncle
- Senile comedones
- Keratosis pilaris

Hair loss
- Androgenetic alopecia
- Telogen effluvium
- Post-pregnancy
- Anagen effluvium
- Alopecia areata
- Trauma/trichotillomania
- Medication

Suspicious skin lesions
- Actinic keratosis
- Basal cell carcinoma
- Bowen's disease
- Squamous cell carcinoma (SCC)
  - Keratoacanthoma
- Cutaneous horn
- Dysplastic naevus
- Lentigo maligna
  - Melanoma

Conditions

Pustular dermatoses

Acneiform dermatoses

Acne vulgaris
- (D) Acne vulgaris is a multifactorial condition of the sebaceous glands and hair follicles that presents primarily in the teenage years, characterised by a combination of papules, pustules, comedones, and nodules (see Figure 35).
- (E) Prevalence ↑ with age ↓, estimated prevalence 35-90% in adolescents
- (Ae) Combination of increased sebum excretion (e.g. due to hormonal changes in puberty), hyperkeratosis of the follicular duct, and *Propionibacterium acnes* colonisation
- (R) Adolescents and young adults
- (Hx) Pimples arising during puberty, oily skin
- (PE)
  - (P) Face, chest, upper back, shoulders
  - (A) Bound to the sebaceous gland complex, grouped
  - (S) Several to dozens, 1-5 mm
  - (S) Round
  - (O) Moderately well-demarcated
  - (N) Red, yellow-white pustules, black (open) and white (closed) comedones
  - (E) Comedones, papules, pustules, nodules, scarring
- (Dx) No added value
- (Tx) 💊 Gradually increasing doses of:
  - Mild acne: benzoyl peroxide alone or in combination with topical retinoids (tretinoin, adapalene, tazarotene) or topical ABx (e.g. erythromycin 1% solution or clindamycin 2% gel)
  - Moderate-to-severe acne: combination therapy using bezoyl peroxide or topical retinoids, and topical/systemic ABx (e.g. doxycycline, minocycline for 3-4 mo)
  - Primarily comedonal acne: topical retinoids alone or in combination with topical or oral ABx (e.g. doxycyline, minocyline, erythromycin 1% solution)
  - Primarily papulopustular acne: topical retinoid (preferred option adapalene) in combination with benzoyl peroxide, topical dapsone 5% gel

- Post-inflammatory hyperpigmentation: azelaic acid
- Treatment-resistant acne or acne producing physical scarring: oral isotretinoin, with routine pregnancy tests and monitoring of liver function tests, serum cholesterol, and triglycerides, as well as signs of inflammatory bowel disease or depressive symptoms

- Exacerbations and remissions occur, acne disappears before age 25 in 85% of patients
- Complete remission after isotretinoin (±70% cure rate after 1 course and ±95% after 2 courses)
- There may be recurrences despite complete remission
- There are many other variants of acne besides acne vulgaris, such as acne conglobata (see Figure 38), acne tarda, comedonal acne (see Table 24), acne fulminans, acne excorie (see Table 24)
- Severity can be assessed based on number and type of lesions, anatomical sites, and presence of scarring
- Rule out an underlying polycystic ovary syndrome (PCOS) when acne presents in women <12y or >20y, or when there are other symptoms such as hirsutism and menstrual cycle alterations
- Skin of colour is more prone to post-inflammatory hyperpigmentation, so consider initiating systemic treatment at an earlier stage
- Think of pityrosporum folliculitis when there are many small, itchy pustules (forehead, chest)
- Rule out any medicinal underlying cause

> Acne scars often have a typical crater-like appearance and are also known as ice-pick scars (see Figure 39).

> Comedones are a sine qua non for acne vulgaris, as the absence of comedones may also point towards papulopustular rosacea.

> Isotretinoin is highly teratogenic. Pregnancy is an absolute contraindication and use in patients of childbearing age is recommended only with a negative pregnancy test and appropriate contraception.

	COMEDONAL ACNE	**PAPULOPUSTULAR ACNE**
D	Comedonal acne is a form of acne vulgaris that is primarily characterised by open and closed comedones.	Papulopustular acne is a form of acne vulgaris that is primarily characterised by papulopustules (see Figure 36).
E	See Acne vulgaris	
Ae	Micronodules, formed by stimulation of sebaceous glands by circulating androgens, dysbiosis of the pilosebaceous follicle microbiome, and cellular immune responses, are converted into closed comedones by gradual accumulation of keratinous material, and sebum converts into microcomedones. Through continuous distension, the follicular orifice expands, resulting in the formation of an open comedo.	*C. acnes* and its antagonising cellular immune responses contribute to the development of inflammatory pustules and papules
R	Adolescents and young adults, use of comedogenic products	Adolescents and young adults
Hx	Pimples arising during puberty, oily skin, primarily comedones	Pimples arising during puberty, oily skin, primarily papules and pustules
PE	(P) Face, chest, upper back, shoulders (A) Bound to the sebaceous gland complex, grouped (S) Several to dozens, 1-5 mm (S) Round (O) Moderately well-demarcated (N) Black (open) and white (closed) comedones (E) Primarily comedones	(P) Face, chest, upper back, shoulders (A) Bound to the sebaceous gland complex, grouped (S) Several to dozens, 1-5 mm (S) Round, dome-shaped (O) Moderately well-demarcated (N) Red, yellow-white pustules (E) Primarily papules and pustules
Dx	Clinical diagnosis, consider additional testing in patients with signs of hyperandrogenism	
Tx	🖉 Topical retinoids alone or in combination with topical or oral AB	🖉 Topical retinoids (preferred option adapalene) in combination with benzoyl peroxide, topical dapsone 5% gel

Table 24A // Common subtypes of acne

ACNE CONGLOBATA	ACNE KELOIDALIS NUCHAE
Acne conglobata is a severe form of nodular acne vulgaris that often presents with sinus tracts and severe scarring (see Figure 38).	Acne keloidalis nuchae is a common, chronic disorder characterised by inflammation and scarring of the hair follicles and development of keloid-like papules and plaques (see Figure 37).
See Acne vulgaris	
Follicular hyperkeratinisation, hormonally-induced sebum production, and inflammation (e.g. by *Cutibacterium acnes* (formerly *Propionibacterium acnes*))	Might be triggered by chronic irritation or occlusion of the follicles due to shaving, easily ingrowing hair in tightly curled hair patterns, trauma, friction, heat, or due to infection, autoimmunity, increased sensitivity to androgens, seborrhea, medications (e.g. ciclosporin)
♂>♀, anabolic steroids, FHx of acne conglobata	More common in individuals with darker skin, esp. people of African-American descent, ♂:♀ = 20:1
Larger interconnecting comedones, cysts, nodules merging to sinus tracts, scarring	Papules, pustules primarily on neck
(P) Back, chest, and buttocks, but can also appear on the face (A) Multiple, grouped (S) Several, variable in size (S) Dome-shaped (O) Moderately well-demarcated (N) Red, yellow-white (pustules, comedones) (E) Papulopustules, interconnecting comedones, cysts, nodules merging to sinus tracts, scarring	(P) Posterior scalp and neck (A) Multiple, grouped, follicle bound (S) Several to dozens, variable in size (S) Round, dome-shaped (O) Moderately well-demarcated (N) Red or pink (papules), yellow-whitish (pustules), brown or dark brown in darker skin types (E) Firm papules and sometimes pustules, and keloidal scarring plaques
Clinical diagnosis, consider additional testing in patients with signs of hyperandrogenism	

💊 • Oral isotretinoin
• Systemic glucocorticoids may sometimes be required before or during isotretinoin therapy
	💊 • Inflammatory lesions:
	    - Combination therapy of topical high-potency corticosteroid, antibacterial agents (e.g. benzoyl peroxide), and/or topical retinoid
	    - Oral doxycycline for severe inflammatory papules
	    - Oral isotretinoin for refractory cases
	• Keloidal lesions:
	    - Intralesional corticosteroid injections or surgical excision

	COMEDONAL ACNE	PAPULOPUSTULAR ACNE
P	• Exacerbations and remissions occur, acne disappears before age 25 in 85% of patients • There may be recurrences despite complete remission	
!	• Severity can be assessed based on number and type of lesions, anatomical sites, and presence of scarring • Skin of colour is more prone to post-inflammatory hyperpigmentation, so consider initiating systemic treatment at an earlier stage	

Table 24B // Common subtypes of acne

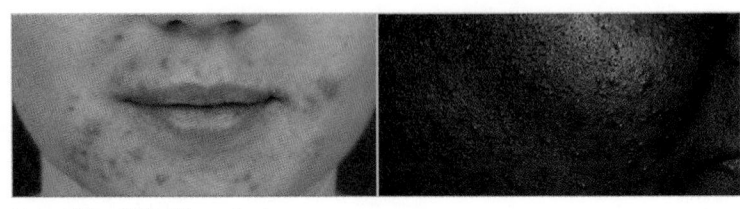

Figure 35A and 35B // Acne vulgaris

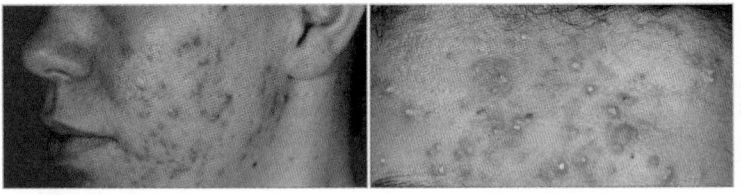

Figure 36 // Papulopustular acne

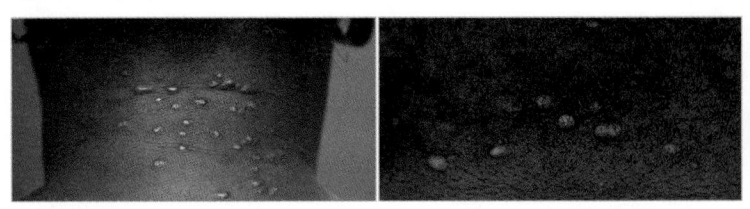

Figure 37 // Acne keloidalis nuchae

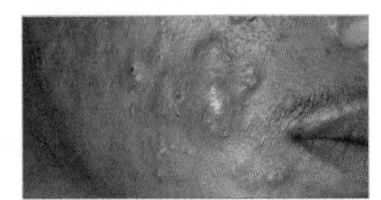

Figure 38 // Acne conglobata

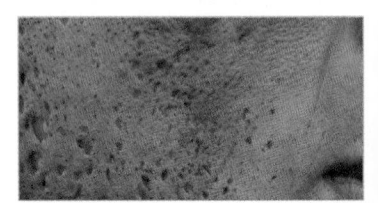

Figure 39 // Acne vulgaris: ice-pick scars

ACNE CONGLOBATA	ACNE KELOIDALIS NUCHAE

- Exacerbations and remissions occur, acne disappears before age 25 in 85% of patients
- There may be recurrences despite complete remission

- Severity can be assessed based on number and type of lesions, anatomical sites, and presence of scarring
- Skin of colour is more prone to post-inflammatory hyperpigmentation and keloid formation, so consider initiating systemic treatment at an early stage

Perioral dermatitis

(D) Perioral dermatitis is an eruption of small, monomorphic papules that begins around the mouth and may spread towards the cheeks (see Figure 40). Periorbital dermatitis is a variation of perioral dermatitis, characterised by monomorphic papules around the eyes.

(E) Perioral dermatitis occurs worldwide, most prevalent in females aged 20-45. Exact prevalence unknown.

(Ae) Local corticosteroid use, contact dermatitis ⊖, cosmetic use ⊖, idiopathic

(R) ♀, contact dermatitis, local corticosteroid use, use of oily cosmetics

(Hx) Red bumps and pimples around the mouth, itching, burning sensation

(PE) (P) Chin and vermillion border are unaffected
- (A) Grouped, circumscribed
- (S) Dozens of miliar lesions
- (S) Round, raised
- (O) Moderately well-demarcated
- (N) Skin-coloured to red
- (E) Erythematous papules, vesicles, and papulopustules, sometimes with scaling

(Dx) No added value

(Tx) Educate on cosmetics use; discontinue topical corticosteroids and skin irritants (e.g. certain types of skin care and dental hygiene products)
- Mild: topical ABx (erythromycin or metronidazole) or calcineurin inhibitors (pimecrolimus)
- Moderate-to-severe: oral ABx for 6 wk, preferably tetracycline (clarithromycin or erythromycin when tetracycline is contraindicated)

(P) Small risk of recurrence after successful treatment and elimination of causal factors

(!) • Consider gradual tapering regimen for topical corticosteroids as sudden

discontinuation may cause perioral dermatitis to flare up
- Warn patients that after withdrawal of the steroid, symptoms are likely to get worse before improving

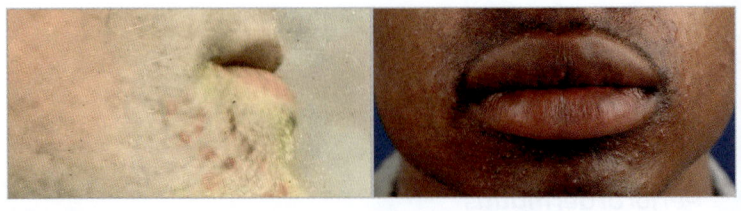

Figure 40A and 40B // Perioral dermatitis

Hidradenitis suppurativa (HS)

(D) HS, also known as acne ectopica or acne inversa, is a chronic inflammation emanating from the hair follicles. It is found primarily in the flexures (see Figure 41).

(E) Prevalence 0.4-4%

(Ae) Multifactorial disorder → blockage of sebaceous glands by keratin or a sebum plug → dilatation and secondary inflammation of glands and surrounding area

(R) Smoking (>95% of patients with severe hidradenitis suppurativa are smokers), obesity, heavy sweating, ♂:♀ = 1:2-5, genetic predisposition (approx. 40% of patients with a 1st degree relative)

(Hx) Painful swelling and extensive inflammation

(PE) (P) In flexures, e.g. armpits and groin
- (A) Grouped
- (S) Highly variable: from several lesions to large areas covered with inflammatory infiltrates and fistulas
- (S) Depends on severity, severe forms present with a gyrate network of lesions
- (O) Moderately well-demarcated
- (N) Red, dark brown in darker skin types
- (E) Pustules, small and large nodules, abscesses, fistulas, scarring

(Dx) Clinical diagnosis, consider culture to rule out staphylococcal infection or biopsy to rule out other conditions

(Tx) Lifestyle changes: smoking cessation, weight loss
- Treatment is based on Hurley-stage disease severity (see Table 25):
  - Mild HS: topical antiseptic washes, e.g. chlorhexidine 4%, benzoyl peroxide, zinc pyrithione, topical exfoliants (e.g. resorcinol), topical clindamycin

- Moderate-to-severe HS: systemic ABx (tetracycline or dual-therapy clindamycin-rifampicin), TNF-alpha inhibitors (adalimumab or infliximab), or biologicals
- Adequate adjuvant pain management in all stages
- 🔬 Acute lesions: intralesional corticosteroid injections or punch debridement
- Severe or refractory HS: wide surgical excision

(P) Prolonged course with severe inflammatory reactions

(!) Associated with high morbidity (pain symptoms)

HURLEY STAGE	FEATURES	EXAMPLE	TREATMENT
I	Abscess formation, single or multiple, without sinus fistulas or cicatrisation		Topical antiseptic washes, topical clindamycin, or oral tetracycline (for widely spread Hurley I)
II	Recurrent abscesses with fistula formation and cicatrisation, single or multiple, widely separated lesions		Oral tetracycline or oral clindamycin and rifampin, TNF inhibitors (adalimumab), or surgical excision (refractory disease)
III	Diffuse or near-diffuse involvement, or multiple interconnected fistulas and abscesses across the entire area		Surgical excision or partial deroofing in case of large lesions

Table 25 // Hurley-stage disease severity

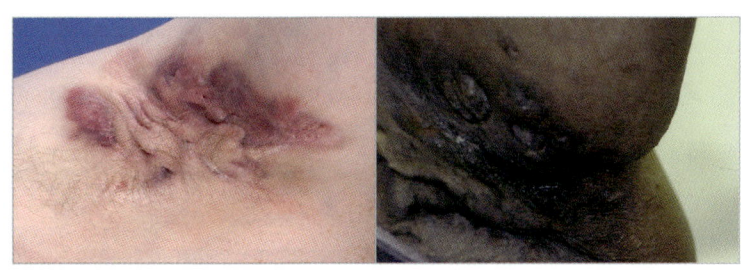

Figure 41A and 41B // Hidradenitis suppurativa with fistulas

Rosacea

D Rosacea is a chronic skin disorder of the face associated with erythema and inflammation. There are several subtypes of rosacea, the most common being the telangiectatic (see Figure 42 and 45) and papulopustular forms (see Table 26).

E Estimated prevalence 5%, ♀>♂

Ae • Genetic predisposition: dysregulated immune response and neurovascular dysfunction
- Triggers: exposure to sunlight, heat, cold, alcohol, spicy food

R Light skin types, peak age 30-50

Hx Facial redness and pimples with burning sensation, eye symptoms

PE (P) Face, often central, symmetrical
- (A) Grouped, circumscribed
- (S) Nummular to adult/child palm-sized area
- (S) Round, oval, may run along skin lines
- (O) Moderately well-demarcated
- (N) Red, dark brown in darker skin types
- (E) Depends on subtype: either predominantly telangiectatic or papulopustular

Dx No added value

Tx 🗨 Avoid triggers, use neutral skin care products, sun protection

💊 Treatment according to predominant clinical features:
- Erythematotelangiectatic rosacea (vascular rosacea): topical vasoconstrictive agents (brimonidine), oral propranolol
- Mild papulopustular rosacea (inflammatory rosacea): topical metronidazole, ivermectin cream (helps against *Demodex* and has anti-inflammatory properties), or azelaic acid
- Moderate-to-severe papulopustular rosacea: systemic ABx (tetracycline or doxycycline)
- Severe or therapy-resistant papulopustular rosacea: low-dose isotretinoin

🔪 Pulsed dye laser, Nd:YAG laser, or intense pulsed light laser for persistent facial erythema

P Chronic with remissions and exacerbations
- The presence of telangiectasias and the absence of comedones are important features that distinguish rosacea from acne
- Other variants: fibromatous variant (rhinophyma, esp. in men; see Figure 43), ocular variant (always ask, $^2/_3$ of patients with rosacea have ocular

- symptoms without making the link themselves)
- Although rosacea is more common in people with pale to fair skin type, it also affects those with darker skin types. Beware of underdiagnosis.

> 🔔 Note that red discolouration can present as dark brown in darker skin types (i.e. type 1 very light beige to 5 very dark brown)

	ERYTHEMATOTELANGIECTATIC ROSACEA	**PAPULOPUSTULAR ROSACEA**
D	Rosacea subtype presenting with persistent erythema with intermittent flushing of nose and cheeks.	Rosacea subtype presenting with eruptions of papules and pustules on the affected facial area (see Figure 44).
E	Prevalence ± 57% of all rosacea cases	Prevalence ± 43% of all rosacea cases
Ae	See Rosacea	
R		
Hx	Facial redness with burning sensation, eye symptoms	Facial redness and pimples with burning sensation, eye symptoms
PE	(P) Central face, esp. on cheeks, symmetrical (A) Circumscribed (S) Nummular to adult/child palm-sized area (S) Round, oval, may run along skin lines (O) Moderately well-demarcated (N) Erythema (E) Telangiectasias	(P) Face, often central, symmetrical (A) Grouped (S) Miliar to lenticular-sized (S) Round, oval, may run along skin lines (O) Moderately well-demarcated (N) Red (E) Papules, sometimes extending outward beyond the follicular unit to form plaques, and pustules
Dx	Histology: solar elastosis, telangiectasia, oedema, and perivascular lymphohistiocytic infiltration	Histology: neutrophilic infiltration in hair follicles
Tx	• Brimonidine tartrate (alpha-2 agonist) 0.33% gel • Oxymetazoline hydrochloride (alpha-1 agonist) 1% cream • Propranolol, carvedilol for flushing	Topical therapies, e.g.: • Ivermectin 1% cream • Azelaic acid 15% gel, foam, or 20% cream • Metronidazole 0.75% and 1% gel or cream • Systemic oral AB (preferably doxycycline)
P	See Rosacea	
!	Subtypes are not exclusive. Patients can present with features of multiple subtypes, and the predominant features and areas of involvement can change over time.	

Table 26 // Rosacea subtypes

> The typical patient with rosacea is a middle-aged female with a light skin type presenting with bright red cheeks and nose.

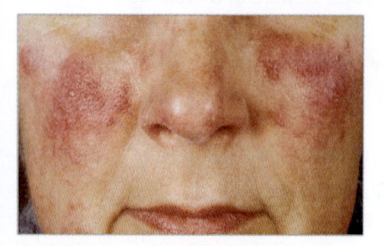

Figure 42 // Rosacea telangiectasia

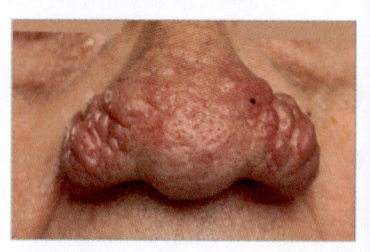

Figure 43 // Rhinophyma

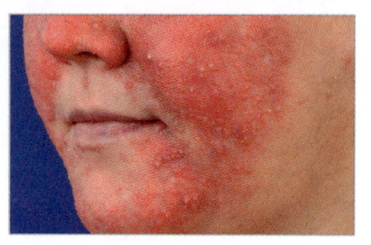

Figure 44 // Rosacea papulopustulosa

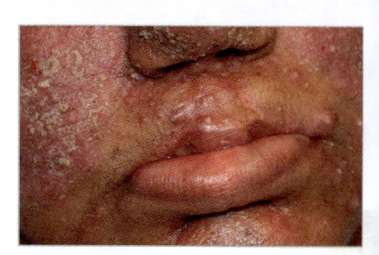

Figure 45 // Rosacea

Pyodermas

Folliculitis

- (D) Folliculitis is a collective term for inflammation of the hair follicles secondary to infection, chemical irritation, or damage (see Figure 46). The most common cause of folliculitis is *Staphylococcus aureus*.
- (E) Very common, specific incidence and prevalence unknown
- (Ae) *Staphylococcus aureus* ☉, *Pseudomonas aeruginosa* ☉, *Malassezia* (♂>♀), and HSV, provoked by occlusive factors (e.g. bandages or high-fat ointment)
- (R) Shaving/waxing/depilation, prolonged use of oral AB or topical corticosteroids, warm and humid weather, atopic dermatitis, DM, obesity, immunosuppressed or immunocompromised patients
- (Hx) Papules and pustules in areas where hair grows
- (PE) (P) Parts of the skin with terminal hair
  - (A) Solitary or grouped, follicular
  - (S) Multiple, often miliar, circumscribed

- (S) Round
- (O) Ill-demarcated
- (N) White to yellow surrounded by redness, hyperpigmentation
- (E) Erythematous papules or papulopustules surrounded by a red ring, hair may protrude from the lesion

(Dx) Pus culture to detect pathogens (often negative). The pus culture can include: HSV 1 and 2, general culture, fungus and yeast.

(Tx) 💬 Generally no treatment; recommend to avoid occlusive factors or take hygienic measures (wash daily with betadine scrub)
- 💊 For persisting *Staphylococcus aureus* folliculitis, topical ABx (mupirocin or clindamycin) may be given
  - For extensive *Staphylococcus aureus* folliculitis, systemic ABx (cephalexin or flucloxacillin)

(P) Heals spontaneously in <2 wk, often followed by a period with post-inflammatory hyperpigmentation

(!) Bacterial overgrowth in patients with known immunodeficiency may mimick folliculitis

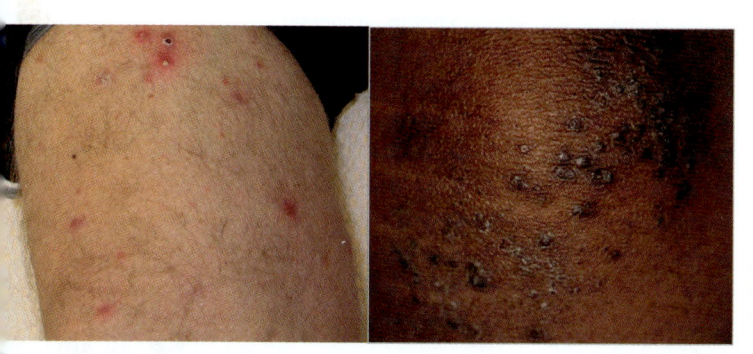

Figure 46 // Folliculitis

Pseudofolliculitis barbae

(D) Pseudofolliculitis barbae, also called 'razor bumps' or 'ingrown hairs', is a common skin condition resulting from the removal of facial hair, esp. shaving. It is a form of irritant folliculitis (see Figure 47).

(E) Predominantly affects men of African descent, approx. 45-80%

(Ae) Inflammatory reaction against hair penetrating the interfollicular skin prior to (transfollicular) or after exiting the follicular orifice (extrafollicular)

- (R) Hair removal (shaving, plucking, waxing), postpubertal males, populations with naturally curly hair
- (Hx) May itch, review patient's hair removal practices and observed associations between lesion development
- (PE) (P) Anterior neck, mandible, cheeks, and chin
  - (A) Grouped, follicular
  - (S) Miliar
  - (S) Round
  - (O) Ill-demarcated
  - (N) Skin-coloured, erythematous, or hyperpigmented
  - (E) Papules, loops of hair emerging from the follicular orifice and re-entering the skin
- (Dx) Skin biopsy if clinical diagnosis unclear: intraepidermal neutrophils, abscess formation in the dermis, and granulomatous inflammation with foreign-body giant cells surrounding the tip of penetrating hairs
- (Tx) 💬 Discontinue shaving or other hair removal practice, if not possible (e.g. due to occupational requirements, cultural values) adjust hair removal methods (e.g. laser, do not use a shaving device using the 'lift and cut' technique)
  - 💊 Low-potency topical corticosteroids for acute lesions
  - Intralesional corticosteroid injections for highly inflamed lesions
- (P) Hyperpigmentation, keloids, and secondary infection are potential complications of pseudofolliculitis barbae

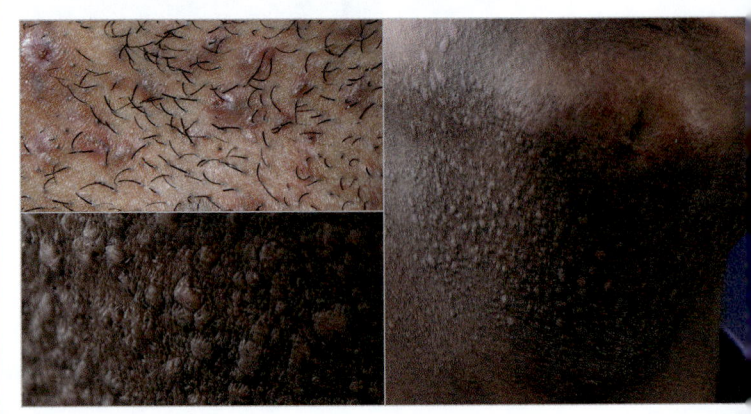

Figure 47 // Pseudofolliculitis barbae

Furuncle and carbuncle

- (D) A furuncle, or boil, is an infected hair follicle (see Figure 48). It is accompanied by a deep infiltrate that leads to necrosis and pus formation. The skin is tender at first, but pain decreases after a rupture, pus discharge, or resorption. A carbuncle is a cluster of furuncles (see Figure 49).
- (E) Incidences and prevalences unknown
- (Ae) *Staphylococcus aureus*
- (R) • ♂, obesity, poor hygiene, hyperhidrosis, immunodeficiency, anaemia, DM
  - Local risk factors: staphylococcus carrier, friction, trauma, occlusive factors
- (Hx) • Furuncle: acute onset, single lesion
  - Carbuncle: sometimes general malaise and fever ⊖
- (PE) (P) Face, neck, armpits, buttocks, thighs and perineum, neck and back
  - (A) Solitary or disseminated (furunculosis), coalescent (carbuncle)
  - (S) Single or several, lenticular to nummular
  - (S) Round
  - (O) Ill-demarcated
  - (N) Red, occasionally with white pus or black necrosis
  - (E) Raised erythematous erosion, possibly with central necrosis and purulent drainage
- (Dx) Nose/throat/perineal culture in recurrent infections to detect *Staphylococcus aureus*
- (Tx) • Treatment may not be needed
  - Prevention of recurrent furuncles with topical antiseptic agents (benzoyl peroxide, chlorhexidine, mupirocin cream)
  - Systemic ABx (oral dicloxacillin, flucloxacillin, cefalexin, clindamycin, or erythromycin) for fever, lymphadenitis, or cellulitis
  - Incision and drainage
- (P) • Furuncle: heals spontaneously, slight scarring
  - Carbuncle: heals slowly, always scarring
- (!) Watch out for cavernous sinus thrombosis in patients with a furuncle of the nose or upper lip, as direct drainage into the cavernous sinus poses a risk of bacteraemia and sepsis in patients with a poor general condition

Figure 48 // Furuncle

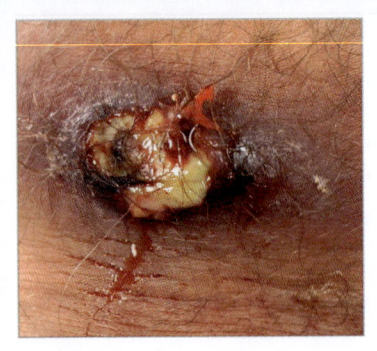

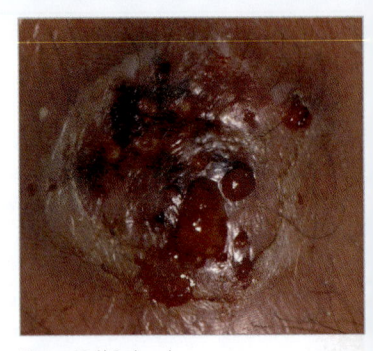

Figure 49 // Carbuncle

Impetigo vulgaris

- D Impetigo vulgaris, also known as impetigo contagiosa or simply (nonbullous) impetigo, is an infection of the superficial layers of the skin without the production of toxins. It is extremely contagious and is the most common skin infection in children.
- E Prevalence 8.4-19.4% of children, 70% of all impetigo cases are nonbullous
- Ae *Staphylococcus aureus* (90%) and/or *Streptococcus pyogenes* (10%) de novo or transmitted after direct contact with an infected person
- R Heat, high humidity, poor hygiene, atopy, trauma, *Staphylococcus aureus* colonisation
- Hx Severe infection: general malaise, fever, regional lymph node swelling
- PE
  - P Face (around nose and mouth), limbs ⊖
  - A Solitary or coalescent
  - S Multiple, 2-4 mm, regional
  - S Round, polycyclic after coalescence
  - O Ill-demarcated or jagged borders
  - N Red with mainly honey yellow, but also brown or black crusts (see Figure 50)
  - E Erythematous papules and plaques → vesicles or pustules → erosions and honey yellow crusts
- Dx Culture if patient does not respond to standard treatment
- Tx 💬 Explanation of onset and course, hygiene recommendations, explain that it is highly contagious
  - 💊 • Topical ABx mupirocin 2%, retapamulin, or fusidic acid
    - Systemic ABx cephalexin, dicloxacillin, or flucloxacillin (during hospital admission erythromycin, clindamycin) for extensive lesions

- (P) Spontaneous healing without scarring within 2-3 wk, complications such as post-streptococcal acute glomerulonephritis are rare
- (!) Increasing resistance of *Staphylococcus aureus* to fusidic acid in locations where topical fusidic acid use is common

> 💡 Secondary impetigo accompanying pre-existing skin conditions (e.g. dermatitis) is called impetiginisation.

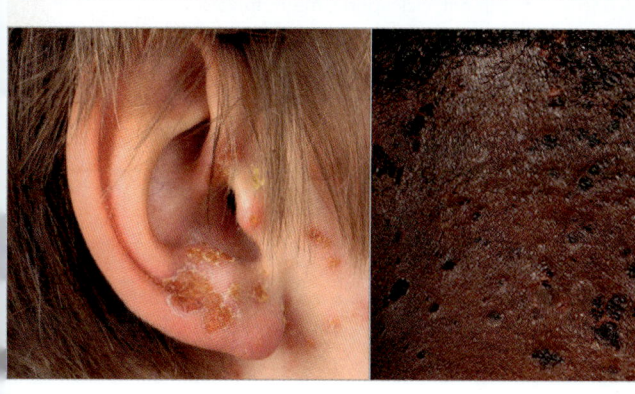

Figure 50 // Impetigo vulgaris

Palmoplantar pustulosis (PPP)

- (D) PPP, or Andrews-Barber's disease, is an inflammatory skin condition characterised by erythema, pustules, and scaly skin on the hands and soles of the feet.
- (E) Prevalence 0.05-0.12%, peak incidence in middle age
- (Ae) Unknown
- (R) ♀:♂ = 4:1, smoking
- (Hx) Asymptomatic 😊, can be itchy/painful (esp. in cases with deep cracks in the skin)
- (PE) (P) Palms of hands, soles of feet
  - (A) Disseminated across palms and soles of feet
  - (S) 2-5 mm pustules
  - (S) Round
  - (O) Well-demarcated
  - (N) Red with white, green, or yellow pustules that fade into brown spots
  - (E) Erythematosquamous skin with pustules, hyperkeratosis and skin cracks

- Dx Biopsy: epidermal changes (loss of granular layer, suprapapillary plates thinning, tortuous capillaries), spongiosis, pustule, dermal infiltrate
- Tx Smoking cessation, number of pustules is correlated with number of cigarettes smoked daily, avoidance of skin irritants
  - First-line treatment: topical high-potency corticosteroids (under occlusion), salicylic acid cream 10%, oral retinoids (e.g. acitretin), and photochemotherapy (psoralen plus PUVA therapy)
  - Second-line treatment: ciclosporin, methotrexate
  - TNF-alpha inhibitors for severe recalcitrant disease
  - Adjuvant therapy with skin moisturisers
- P Highly therapy-resistant disease, spontaneous remission is possible but rare
- ! Tonsillectomy may provide relief when combined with recurrent tonsillitis

Bullous dermatoses

> Biopsy site in blistering skin disease:
> - Histopathological staining (H&E staining): at edge of blister
> - Immunofluorescence testing: normal perilesional skin

Bullous pemphigoid

- D Bullous pemphigoid is a skin condition that causes large blisters and is characterised by severe itching (see Figure 51). It is the most common autoimmune blistering disease in Western Europe and North America.
- E Incidence 0.6-4.3:100,000 per year
- Ae Autoimmune disease: antibodies to hemidesmosome components (BP180, BP230)
- R Age >60, certain HLA alleles (DQB1*0301), medication (e.g. diuretics, analgesics, AB)
- Hx Firm blisters on body or mucous membranes
- PE P Flexural surfaces of arms and legs, less commonly on torso, knees (see Figure 52), extensor surface of thighs, and oral mucosa
  - A Symmetrical, disseminated or grouped
  - S Dozens, 1-4 cm
  - S Round
  - O Well-demarcated
  - N Blister fluid is usually clear and yellowish, sometimes haemorrhagic

(E) Firm bullae on erythematous surface, urticarial plaques, erosions, crusts

Dx
- Biopsy and H&E stain of recent intact bulla: subepidermal cleavage, dermal infiltrate of eosinophils and/or neutrophils
- IF test of perilesional erythematous or normal-appearing skin: linear depositions of IgG and/or C3 in basal membrane (direct IF), Salt-split positive for IgG anti-basement membrane antibodies (indirect IF)
- Serology: 70-80% of patients have circulating antibodies to BP180 or BP230 (ELISA)

Tx
- First-line treatment: superpotent topical or oral corticosteroids at an initial dose of 0.5 mg/kg/d prednisone (think of osteoporosis prevention when using high dosages of prednisone for longer than 3 mo)
- Relapsing or treatment-recalcitrant BP: methotrexate, azathioprine, mycophenolate mofetil (MMF), or in case of contraindications to immunosuppressive drugs: doxycycline, dapsone, or omalizumab

P Chronic disease, spontaneous exacerbations and remissions

- Bullous pemphigoid has multiple clinical variants: e.g. pemphigoid gestationis (during pregnancy), pemphigoid vegetans, nodularis, Brunsting-Perry pemphigoid, and anti-p200 pemphigoid
- Solitary recurrent bulla mistaken for a mechanical bulla

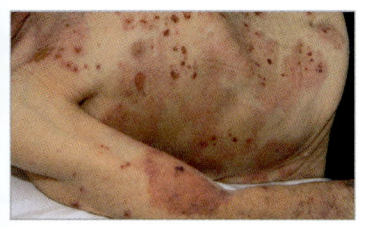

Figure 51 // Bullous pemphigoid

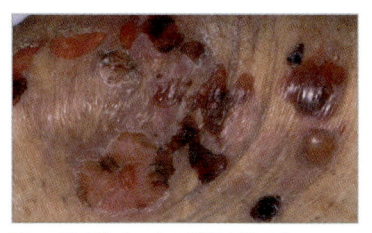

Figure 52 // Bullous pemphigoid (knee)

> Non-bullous pemphigoid is characterised by the absence of blisters and is particularly difficult to identify.

Dermatitis herpetiformis

D Dermatitis herpetiformis, or Duhring's disease, is a severely itchy skin condition secondary to gluten hypersensitivity. About 20% of people with dermatitis herpetiformis have GI symptoms.

E Prevalence 10-75:100,000 and incidence 1.0-3.5:100,000 per year

Ae Coeliac disease → formation of IgA antibodies in intestinal mucosa against transglutaminase → immune complexes precipitate in dermal papillae → neutrophilic inflammatory response

- (R) ♂, age 20-55, North European descent, positive PMHx, coeliac disease, associated with human leukocyte antigen (HLA)-DQ2 (85%) or HLA-DQ8 (15%)
- (Hx) Severe itching, GI complaints
- (PE)
  - (P) Extensor surface of elbows (see Figure 53), forearms, knees, buttocks, sacral region, and shoulder girdle
  - (A) Herpetiform
  - (S) Multiple simultaneous lesions, symmetrical
  - (S) Variable, often lenticular to nummular
  - (O) Moderately well-demarcated
  - (N) Skin-coloured to red
  - (E) Papules and vesicles, however often masked by less specific manifestations such as excoriations, erosions, and crusts due to pruritic nature
- (Dx)
  - Lesional biopsy: neutrophilic microabscesses and oedema in dermal papillae
  - Perilesional direct IF (gold standard): microgranular fibrillar IgA deposits in dermal papillae and dermo-epidermal junction
  - Serology: detection of IgA EMA (IF microscopy) or IgA antibodies against TG2 and TG3 (ELISA)
  - Consider referral for duodenal biopsy or HLA testing
- (Tx)
  - 🗨 Gluten-free diet → effect after months to years
  - 💊 Dapsone
- (P) Depends on gluten intake, chronic disease with fluctuating activity. IgA deposits may remain in dermis several years after starting a gluten-free diet.
- (!) There is an association between dermatitis herpetiformis and autoimmune disorders (thyroiditis, gastritis, SLE, RA, DM, etc.), and T-cell lymphoma

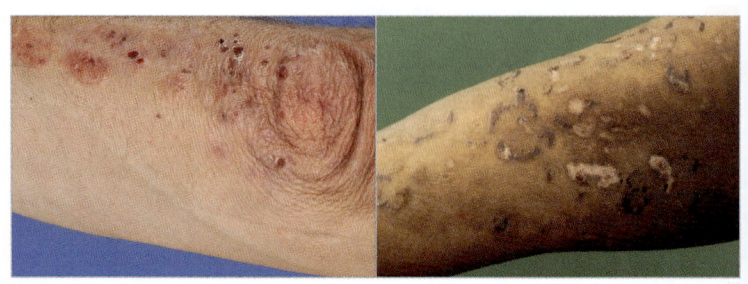

Figure 53 // Herpetiform dermatitis

Bullous impetigo

- (D) Bullous impetigo is a superficial skin infection caused by strains of *Staphylococcus aureus* ⊕ or *Streptococcus pygenes* ⊖ that produce epidermolytic toxins (see Figure 54).
- (E) Rare; exact incidence unknown, 30% of impetigo cases are bullous
- (Ae) Cleavage of the stratum granulosum by epidermolytic toxins → blister formation
- (R) Heat, high humidity, poor hygiene, atopy, trauma, *Staphylococcus aureus* colonisation, young age
- (Hx) Sick appearance ⊖, fever ⊖, swollen lymph nodes ⊖
- (PE) (P) Trunk, limbs, face ⊖
  - (A) Coalescence
  - (S) Several, ≥1-2 cm before coalescence, ≥8 cm after coalescence, regional
  - (S) Annular and polycyclic due to coalescence and central healing
  - (O) Well-demarcated due to deroofed blisters
  - (N) Red with brown crusts
  - (E) Vesicles or bullae with clear or cloudy contents, erosions, crusts
- (Dx) • Bacterial cultures for recurrent or recalcitrant impetigo
  - HIV testing can be considered in adults
- (Tx) 💬 Good hygiene
  - 💊 • Mupirocin cream, antibacterial soap
    - Systemic treatment with AB (cephalexin, dicloxacillin)
    - Treat recurrent infections with mupirocin intranasal (common reservoir)
- (P) Spontaneous recovery within 2-3 wk on average, chronic courses with recurrences are common if untreated

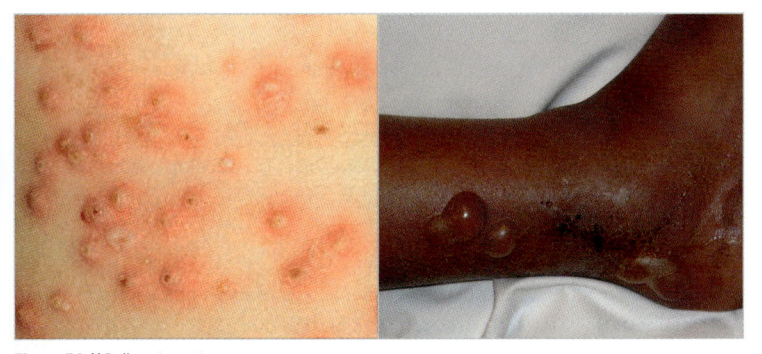

Figure 54 // Bullous impetigo

Pemphigus vulgaris (PV)

- PV is an autoimmune blistering disease that can be categorised into two subgroups: the mucosal dominant type with mucosal erosions and minimal manifestations on the skin and the mucocutaneous type with extensive blisters and erosions in addition to mucosal erosions (see Figure 55).
- Incidence 0.1-0.5:100,000 per year
- Autoantibodies to desmoglein 3 (and sometimes later to desmoglein 1) → deterioration of intraepidermal adhesion → blister formation
- Age 50-60
- Painful lesions on the oral mucosa, pain on eating and swallowing, affects conjunctiva, nose, genitalia, and anus
- Mucosal dominant type:
  - Palate, inner cheeks
  - Regional
  - Multiple lesions, varying in size
  - Irregular
  - Ill-demarcated
  - Red
  - Painful, erosions, intact bullae are rare due to fragility
- Lesional biopsy for histopathology: intraepidermal suprabasal acantholysis
- Perilesional skin or mucosal biopsy for DIF: IgG and/or C3 deposits at the surface of epidermal/epithelial keratinocytes
- Serology: desmoglein 1 and 3 autoantibodies (anti-Dsg1 or anti-Dsg3) autoantibodies (ELISA)
- Systemic corticosteroid therapy 0.5–1.0 mg/kg/d prednisone (in combination with azathioprine, MMF, or mycophenolate sodium) or rituximab
- Refractory PV: intravenous immunoglobulins, intravenous corticosteroid pulses, or immunoadsorption
- Chronic
- Over 50% of patients with mucosal erosions also develop cutaneous manifestations: flaccid bullae that rupture and develop into painful erosions with crusts
- Risk of secondary infections, fluid loss
- Pemphigus also has other rare variants, e.g. pemphigus vegetans, pemphigus foliaceus, and paraneoplastic pemphigus
- It is recommended to quantify the extent of skin and mucosal lesions using

one of the two validated scoring systems: the Pemphigus Disease Area Index (PDAI) or the Autoimmune Bullous Skin Intensity and Severity Score (ABSIS)

- **Nikolsky sign**: rubbing healthy-looking skin causes the superficial layers of the epidermis to separate from the deeper layers resulting in detachment or forming of blisters (often positive in conditions characterised by more superficial cleavage e.g. PV).
- **Nikolsky-II sign** (or Asboe-Hansen sign): pressing an intact blister causes it to extend laterally (often positive in conditions characterised by deep cleavage and firm blisters e.g. bullous pemphigoid).

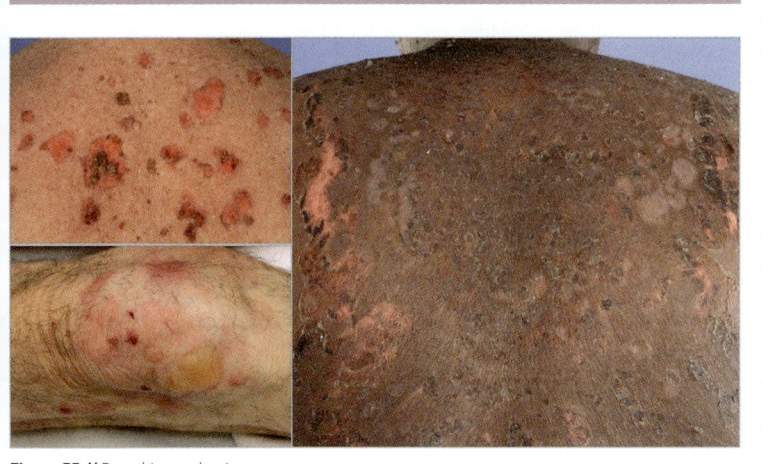

Figure 55 // Pemphigus vulgaris

Toxic epidermal necrolysis (TEN)

- D TEN is a rare, unpredictable, and life-threatening disease that is almost always caused by medication (80% of cases) (see Figure 56). Other rare causes are infections and vaccinations.
- E Incidence 0.1-0.6:100,000 per year
- Ae The aetiology of TEN is not fully understood but is associated with an impaired medication detoxification mechanism
- R Medication use (esp. allopurinol, antiepileptics, sulfonamides, oxicam, nevirapine), HIV-positive, malignancy
- Hx Prodromal phase with malaise, fever, and myalgia, followed by a painful rash and blisters in later stage

- (PE) General malaise ☺, T ↑, inflammation of the internal mucosa
  - (P) Widespread and diffuse
  - (A) Isolated lesions, coalescent ☺
  - (S) >30% of body surface and mucous membranes affected
  - (S) Variable
  - (O) Ill-demarcated
  - (N) Red, hyperpigmentation
  - (E) Ill-demarcated erythematous plaques, extensive necrosis, epidermal detachment (spontaneous or due to friction)
- (Dx)
  - Lab: complete blood count (increased risk of infections), electrolytes (risk of electrolyte imbalance due to fluid loss), glucose, liver function tests (multi-organ failure)
  - Skin biopsy for histopathology: keratinocyte apoptosis, epidermal necrolysis, and separation of the epidermis at the dermo-epidermal junction
  - Swabs for bacteriology and virology (due to high risk of superinfection or sepsis): *Mycoplasma pneumoniae* serology
  - Chest X-ray to check for pulmonary involvement of TEN: pneumonia and interstitial pneumonitis
- (Tx) 💬 Discontinue all potentially triggering medication, transfer to intensive care unit (ICU) or specialised burn unit
  - 💊 High dose corticosteroids or ciclosporin, fluid, electrolyte, temperature and pain management, infection prevention, and nutritional support
- (P) Depends on how quickly the offending medication is stopped, mortality ±25-35%
- (!) TEN exists as a continuum with Stevens-Johnson syndrome (SJS) and can be classified based on body surface area involvement, with <10% affected indicating SJS and >30% indicating TEN

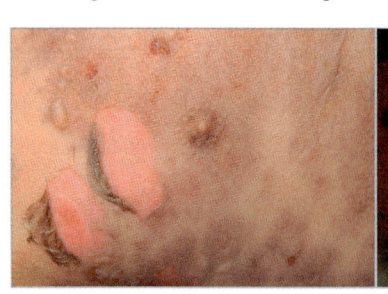

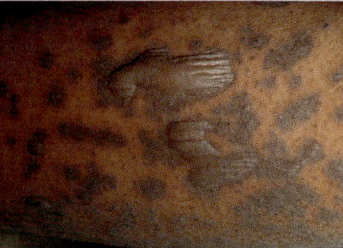

Figure 56 // Toxic epidermal necrolysis

Nodular dermatoses

Erythema nodosum (EN)

- EN is an inflammation affecting subcutaneous fat (panniculitis) (see Figure 57).
- Incidence 1-5:100,000 per year
- Idiopathic in 33% of cases
  - Hypersensitivity reaction to microbial antigens (primarily streptococci, TB) → perivascular inflammation → lobular inflammation of subcutaneous adipose tissue
  - In adults commonly caused by sarcoidosis, rheumatoid arthritis (RA), or Crohn's disease, in children by an underlying streptococcal infection. Other triggers are fungal and viral infections, chlamydia infections, medication, pregnancy, and malignancies.
- ♀, young adulthood
- Sometimes preceded by general malaise, fever, headache, joint pains, or GI symptoms
- Extensor surface of lower legs, usually bilateral, sometimes upper legs or arms
  - Several solitary
  - 2-6 cm
  - Oval or round
  - Moderately well to ill-demarcated
  - Red or purple
  - Small or large nodules, often painful or warm to the touch
- Labs: erythrocyte sedimentation rate (ESR) =/↑, CRP =/↑, leukocytes =/↑
  - Biopsy is often unnecessary. If performed, it must reach the subcutaneous adipose tissue for reliable sampling: septal oedema with mild lymphocytic infiltrates.
  - Duplex ultrasound: rule out DVT
- Limit physical exercise, relieve pressure on the legs (through mild compression), and cold compresses
- Pain management (NSAIDs)
  - If more severe or recurrent: corticosteroids intralesionally or systemically (short-term), oral AB (preferred option: doxycycline), colchicine, hydroxychloroquine, or dapsone
- Heals spontaneously after 2-6 wk, however common relapse
  - Joint symptoms affect 50% of patients, may precede EN and go away

spontaneously

!) Persistent EN: further testing for cause, DDx includes sarcoidosis, inflammatory disease, and malignancy

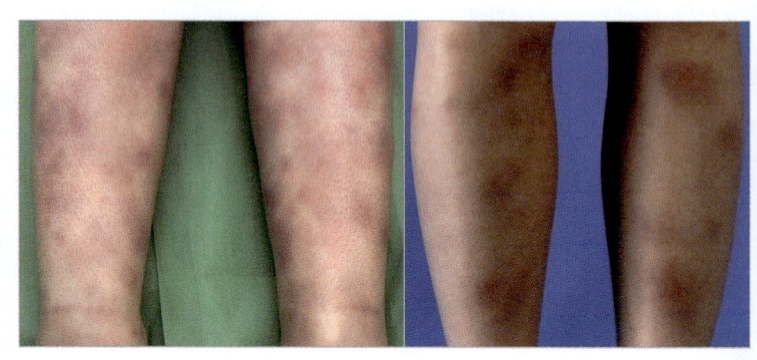

Figure 57 // Erythema nodosum

Prurigo nodularis (PN)

D) PN is a condition characterised by the presence of numerous firm, itchy nodules that are symmetrically distributed. It typically appears in individuals with chronic itching (see Figure 58).

E) Prevalence 72:100,000 per year

Ae) The exact mechanism of origin is unknown, and it remains unclear whether the itching/scratching or the nodules appeared first. However, it is evident that scratching contributes to skin thickening and inflammation, thereby sustaining the disease.

R) Atopic dermatitis and other diseases associated with chronic pruritus

Hx) Chronic, severe itching, with hard bumps and rash on the skin

PE) P) Extensor surfaces of the extremities
- A) Symmetrically distributed
- S) Few to hundreds of lesions, miliar to nummular
- S) Round
- O) Well-demarcated
- N) Skin-coloured, erythematous, or brown/black
- E) Pruritic nodules

Dx) • Labs: complete blood cell count, urea, creatinine, liver enzymes, glucose
- Biopsy is rarely needed
- Rule out systemic cause of chronic itching in patients without atopic der-

matitis or other pruritic skin conditions

- Tx • Avoid scratching, apply emollients to reduce dryness
  - Psychological counselling from medical psychologist (scratch therapy)
  - Local or intralesional corticosteroids, other topical therapies (tacrolimus, capsaicin, vitamin D analogue), occasionally under occlusion
  - Refractory disease: phototherapy, systemic immunosuppressive therapy (e.g. ciclosporin, methotrexate, dupilumab)
- P Full resolution of lesions ⊖, recurrence ⊕
- ! Potential initial symptom of an underlying systemic condition, e.g. HIV or a mycobacterial infection, parasitic infestation, or lymphoma

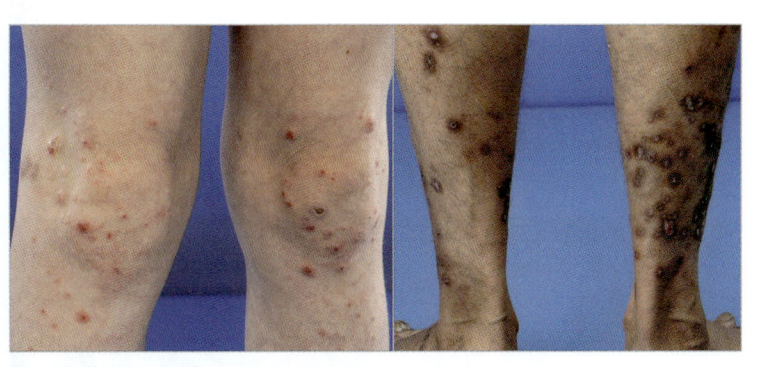

Figure 58 // Prurigo nodularis

Papulomatous dermatoses

Granuloma annulare

- D Granuloma annulare is a skin condition characterised by early-stage papules that may gradually coalesce into an annular papular lesion (see Figure 59).
- E Prevalence among new patients seen by a dermatologist 0.1-0.4%
- Ae Idiopathic, possible response to triggers such as trauma, vaccinations, or sunlight exposure; generalised form may be associated with DM
- R DM, ♀:♂ = 2:1, age <30
- Hx Asymptomatic ⊕, itchy ⊖, annular elevation of the skin
- PE P Fingers, backs of hands, arms, backs of feet, around joints
     A Solitary, disseminated
     S Single lesion, sometimes multiple, several to dozens of cm across

- (S) Circular, annular, or arciform with central healing
- (O) Moderately well to well-demarcated, raised margin
- (N) Skin-coloured to red
- (E) Annular plaques, absent scaling

(Dx) Consider biopsy of the active margin: dermal lymphocytic infiltrate, focal degeneration of collagen and mucin depositions in an interstitial or palisading pattern

(Tx) 💬 Generally no treatment needed as it is self-limiting and symptom-free
- 💊 Local or intralesional corticosteroids, topical tacrolimus, phototherapy
- Systemic treatment: e.g. hydroxychloroquine, methotrexate, ciclosporin
- 🔪 Cryotherapy

(P) Lesions may regress due to certain stimuli (e.g. biopsy), or spontaneously within 1-2y, high recurrence rate (40%)

(I) Some treatments can provide improvement in disseminated granuloma annulare, but none are guaranteed to provide resolution and there may be side effects

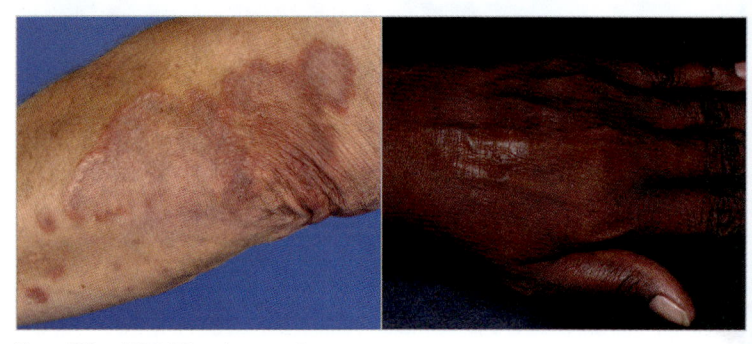

Figure 59A and 59B // Granuloma annulare

Lichen planus (LP)

(D) LP, or lichen ruber planus, is an inflammatory condition of the mucosa and skin (see Figure 60).

(E) Prevalence of local, cutaneous LP 0.14-1.27%, oral lesions 1.5%

(Ae) Idiopathic, possibly autoimmune cause given association with autoimmune disorders, hepatitis B and C infection, and medication

(R) Autoimmune disorders (e.g. thyroid disease, vitiligo, inflammatory bowel disease (IBD), SLE), age 25-70, positive PMHx

- **Hx** Itching ⊕, severe eruptions may present with nail defects, occasionally accompanied by cicatricial alopecia, medication use inventory
- **PE**
  - **P** Mucosa, flexor surface of wrists, forearms, backs of hands, lower legs, sacral region, tip of the penis
    - **A** Often grouped, sometimes solitary or linear (in Köbner phenomenon)
    - **S** Single to several lesions, miliar to lenticular
    - **S** Polygonal
    - **O** Well-demarcated
    - **N** Violaceous with whitish streaks on the surface (Wickham striae)
    - **E** Papules and plaques
- **Dx**
  - Biopsy: band-like lymphocytic infiltrate with cytotoxic T lymphocytes acting on the epidermis
  - Direct immunofluorescence (DIF): globular deposits of IgM and complement or fibrogen mixed with apoptotic keratinocytes
  - If indicated, consider testing for associated hepatitis B and C infections (hepatitis B and C serology: anti-HBS, anti-HBc, anti-HCV) and liver enzymes
- **Tx** Local corticosteroids. If ineffective, consider systemic (oral or IM) or intralesional corticosteroids, UVB, ciclosporin, systemic retinoids, methotrexate, azathioprine, and hydroxychloroquine.
- **P** Usually heals spontaneously within 1-2y
- **!** There are many other variants of LP besides mucosal and cutaneous LP, e.g. medication-induced LP (by e.g. NSAIDs, angiotensin-converting enzyme (ACE) inhibitors, beta blockers, hydroxychloroquine), nail LP, hair LP (lichen planopilaris), linear/annular/bulbous/verrucous variants of LP, LP pigmentosus

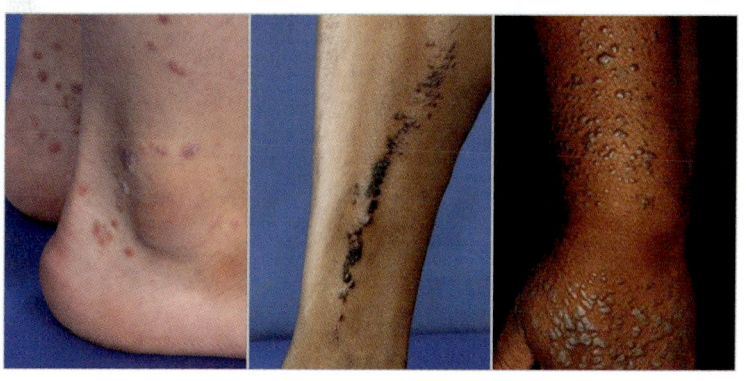

Figure 60A, 60B, and 60C // Lichen planus

> The **6 Ps** are a mnemonic for the lesions associated with LP: **p**apula, **p**laque, **p**lanar, **p**olygonal, **p**urple, and **p**ruritus.

Keratosis pilaris (KP)

(D) KP is a skin condition characterised by follicular papules, sometimes erythematous, primarily on the extensor surface of proximal arms and legs, and occasionally on the face, buttocks, or trunk. It results from keratotic plugs in hair follicles. Due to its high prevalence, it is considered a physiological phenomenon (see Figure 61).

(E) Typically in atopic children and adolescents, prevalence 2-12%

(Ae) An error in the keratinisation process (e.g. genetic) → keratin plug formation within the hair follicle duct → development of the papule with hyperkeratosis and hypergranulosis of the surrounding epidermis

(R) Atopic patients ☺

(Hx) Asymptomatic ☺, some patients may report a rough texture and a cosmetically disruptive appearance of their skin

(PE) (P) Extensor surface of the proximal arms and thighs, cheeks
- (A) Follicular
- (S) Miliar
- (S) Spiny
- (O) Well-demarcated
- (N) Skin-coloured, erythematous
- (E) Papules or pustules

(Dx)
- Dermoscopy: keratinous plugging of the hair follicles
- Biopsy generally not required: if conducted, it typically shows a dilated follicular infundibulum and an orthokeratotic keratin plug

(Tx) 👁 Mostly does not require any treatment

💊 If the patient has cosmetic concerns, the following treatments can be considered:
- Moisturising cream containing urea, salicylic acid, or lactic acid (first-line therapy)
- Topical corticosteroids (short-term)
- Topical/systemic retinoids

(P) Mostly resolves spontaneously with age. In some cases, it persists in adults.

(!) Often exacerbations in winter, most likely due to outdoor cold temperatures and dry, heated interiors

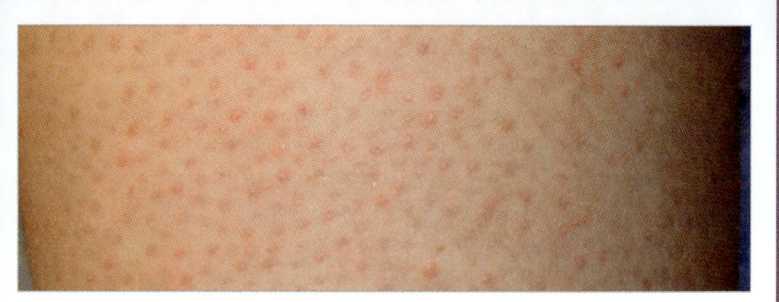

Figure 61 // Keratosis pilaris

Eczematous dermatoses

> Eczema is an efflorescence and an umbrella term for polymorphic, itchy skin conditions with erythema, oedema, papules, vesicles, crusts, scaling, and/or lichenification due to a non-infectious inflammatory skin reaction.

Constitutional dermatitis

- D Constitutional dermatitis, or atopic eczema, is an itchy variant of eczema and part of the atopic triad of asthma, rhinitis, and eczema (see Figure 62). Constitutional dermatitis is caused by a type I hypersensitivity reaction.
- E Most frequent form of eczema, prevalence 5-25% in children and 2-7% in adults
- Ae Congenital impaired skin barrier function (e.g. due to a genetic filaggrin defect) → dry skin → constitutional dermatitis
- R Atopic constitution, PMHx for atopy, dry skin, frequent washing
- Hx Itching, allergies, atopy in family
- PE P • Infants: face and scalp, possibly extending to torso
  - Childhood age: elbow folds and backs of the knees
  - Adult form: recurrences, exacerbations, and remissions, esp. on flexor side of elbows and knees, face, neck, hands, and genital region
- A Symmetrical
- S Present in multiple folds simultaneously ⊕
- S Oval, round, jagged
- O Moderately well-demarcated
- N Red, hyperpigmentation, and lichenification in darker skin types
- E Erythema, oedematous papules, scaling, vesicles, occasional weeping

- **Dx** Differentiate between contact dermatitis and constitutional dermatitis: contact allergological testing
- **Tx** 💬 Washing recommendations include lukewarm water, no soap, applying emollient daily, eliminate potential exac-erbating factors
  - 💊 Pulse therapy with local corticosteroids (potency depending on location and severity), possibly with local immunotherapy (pimecrolimus, tacrolimus), coal tar solution
  - Narrowband UVB therapy as second-line therapy
  - Patients with very severe forms can be started on systemic immunosuppressants (e.g. ciclosporin or methotrexate) or a biological (dupilumab, tralokinumab)
- **P** Usually begins 3-4 mo after birth, disappears by age 15 in 80%
- **!** Secondary bacterial or HSV infections

> 💡 30-35% of children with constitutional dermatitis will develop asthma later in life, 50% will develop rhinitis.

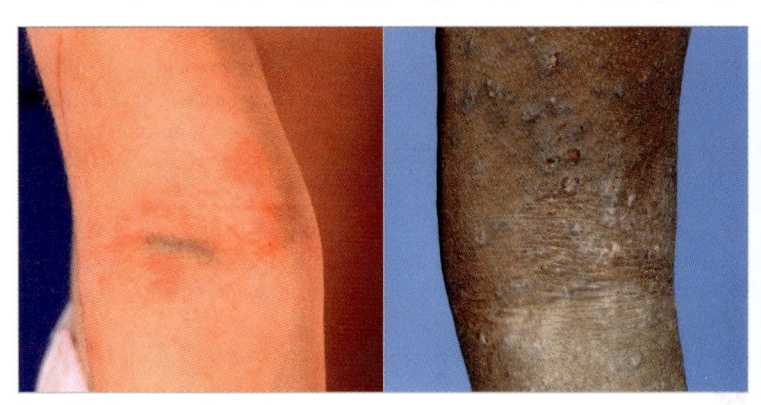

Figure 62 // Constitutional/atopic dermatitis

Acrovesicular eczema

- **D** Acrovesicular eczema, or dyshidrotic eczema, is a highly itchy variant of eczema with firm vesicles (see Figure 63). It is often a manifestation of other types of eczema.
- **E** Overall prevalence unknown, accounts for 5-20% of all hand eczema cases
- **Ae** Manifestation of atopic, irritative, or allergic contact dermatitis or in response

to a mycosis (mycid reaction)

- **R** Atopy, sweaty hands, smoking, stress, ♀:♂ = 2:1, age 20-40
- **Hx** Itching, redness on hands and feet
- **PE** **P** Sides of fingers and toes, palms, soles of feet
  - **A** Often symmetrical
  - **S** Several to dozens, size of a pinhead to several cm
  - **S** Convex
  - **O** Well-demarcated
  - **N** Skin-coloured
  - **E** Vesicles or papules
- **Dx** Biopsy rarely needed: intraepidermal spongiotic vesicles or bullae along superficial perivascular infiltrate of lymphocytes
- **Tx** 💬 Antipruritic emollients against itching, avoid contact with exacerbating agents, and wear gloves as needed
  - 💊 • High-potency topical corticosteroids (preferably in ointment vehicle) as first-line treatment, sometimes in combination with topical tacrolimus
    - Refractory disease: psoralen plus UVA or narrowband UVB therapy, systemic medication (e.g. ciclosporine or methotrexate)
    - Treat underlying mycosis (often tinea pedis) in case of mycid reaction
  - **P** • Depends on underlying cause: may recur or evolve into chronic dermatitis
    - Vesicles disappear spontaneously, sometimes accompanied by desquamation and fissures
- ❗ Coalescence of vesicles into bullae (pompholyx)

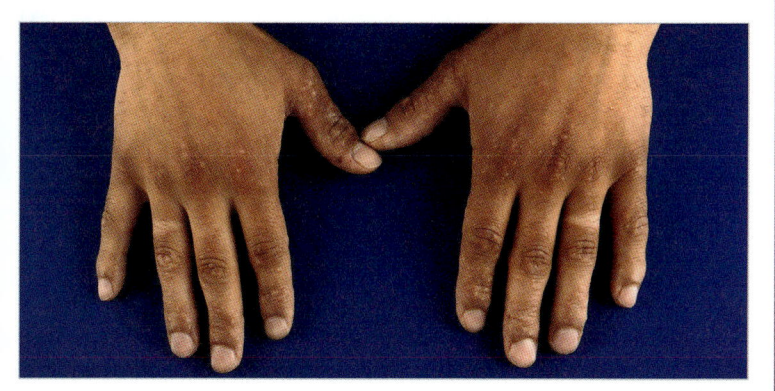

Figure 63 // Acrovesicular eczema

Allergic contact dermatitis

(D) Allergic contact dermatitis is caused by a type IV hypersensitivity reaction to an allergen penetrating the skin (see Figure 64). Initial exposure will be followed by a period of sensitisation lasting 10-14 days. Contact dermatitis may subsequently develop within a few hours to days after contact with the allergen. Common allergens are rubber, nickel, perfume, leather, acrylates, and hair dye.

(E) Estimated prevalence 7-27%, nickel allergy ☺ (prevalence 8.6-17.0%), mostly in children and ♀

(Ae) Contact allergen binds to epidermal Langerhans cells → antigen presented to T helper cells → T lymphocytes migrate to epidermis → local inflammatory reaction

(R) Constitutional dermatitis (due to impaired skin barrier function)

(Hx) Occupation, hobbies, positive PMHx, atopic constitution, explore possible contact allergies with patient, enquiring about everything the patient uses on the hands or uses to apply products, check out ingredients

(PE) (P) Site exposed to allergen, often the hands. The back of the hand is a common site (acral, interdigital).

- (A) Depends on allergen
- (S) Depends on allergen
- (S) Depends on allergen
- (O) Mostly well-demarcated
- (N) Red
- (E) Erythematosquamous lesion with oedema and vesicles in acute phase, lichenised erythematosquamous lesion in chronic phase. In darker skin hyperpigmentation and lichenification.

(Dx) Epicutaneous allergy testing (patch tests) to detect allergies

(Tx) ● Strict allergen avoidance

    💊
- High-potency topical corticosteroids on hands, feet, and non-flexural areas, medium-low potency topical corticosteroids or topical tacrolimus on face and flexural areas
- Short-term systemic prednisone when >20% of body surface area affected

(P) Depends on degree of allergen contact: new contact → recurrence

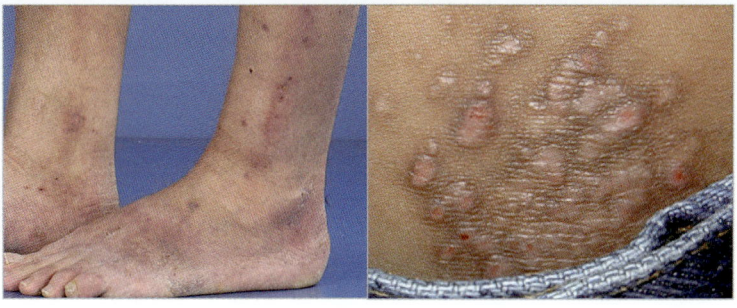

Figure 64A // Allergic contact dermatitis

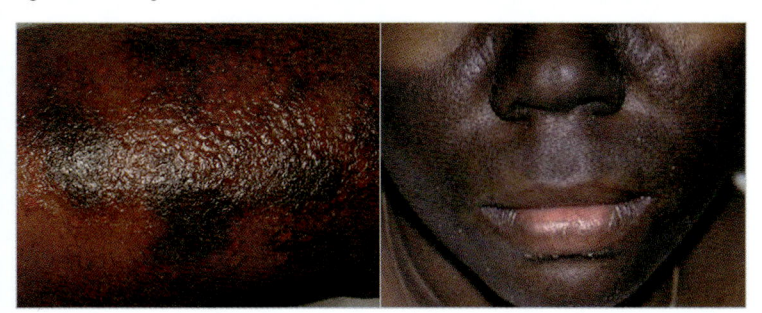

Figure 64B // Allergic contact dermatitis

> 🔔 The severity of dermatitis may be underestimated in people of colour, on whose skin erythema is less visible. Lichenification and hyperpigmentation, by contrast, are often more prominent.

> 💡 In addition to visible features, it is also important to consider itching and sleep problems when assessing the severity of dermatitis.

Irritant contact dermatitis

- D Irritant contact dermatitis is a variant of contact dermatitis resulting from direct skin irritation after exposure to chemical, physical, or mechanical factors (see Figure 65). Irritant contact dermatitis is not an allergy!
- E Incidence 45:100,000 per year, esp. in hairdressers, bakers, health care workers and cooks
- Ac Excessive washing with water/soap → dehydration → risk of irritant contact dermatitis

- (R) Atopic constitution, 'wet work' (e.g. cleaner or hairdresser)
- (Hx) Exacerbations linked to exposure to certain substances, remission in off-work periods (occupational contact dermatitis), itching, pain, burning sensation
- (PE)
  - (P) Dorsal side of the fingers, interdigital, and on the tips
  - (A) Depends on exposure to irritant
  - (S) Hands only
  - (S) Jagged
  - (O) Moderately to well-demarcated
  - (N) Red
  - (E) Erythematosquamous lesions, rhagades
- (Dx) Epicutaneous allergological testing (patch tests) to rule out contact allergies
- (Tx) Avoid irritants if possible, wash less frequent with soap (alternative: wash oil), apply emollient after washing hands
  - Super-high potency topical corticosteroids for non-facial/non-flexural areas
  - Medium-to-low potency topical corticosteroids for mild irritant contact dermatitis or facial/flexural areas
- (P) Complete remission if irritant is avoided
- (!) Symptoms disappear or improve in off-work periods, chronic irritant contact dermatitis is characterised by fissures and lichenification

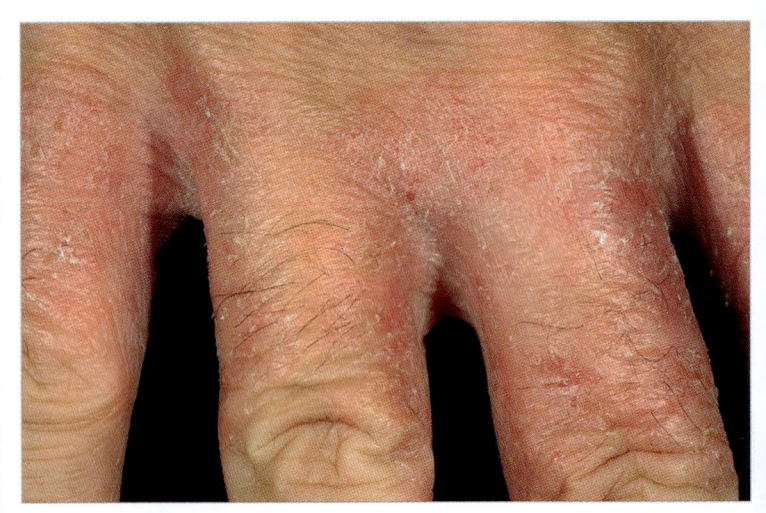

Figure 65 // Irritant contact dermatitis

Intertriginous dermatitis

(D) Intertriginous dermatitis, or intertrigo, is an inflammatory reaction caused by sweating and friction.

(E) Prevalence 2.0-2.5% in hospitals and 3.4-9.6% in geriatric institutions or nursing homes

(Ae) Combination of heat, moisture, and friction → maceration due to moisture and possible fungal (*Candida albicans*) and bacterial (*Staphylococcus aureus*) overgrowth

(R) Obesity, excessive perspiration, poor hygiene, tight-fitting clothing, incontinence (anogenital intertrigo), DM, infant age, immune deficiency

(Hx) Itching, burning pain, unpleasant odour

(PE) (P) Common sites (see Figure 66): skin folds (under the breasts, intergluteal cleft, groin, abdominal folds, armpits, between toes)
- (A) Depends on maceration surface, symmetrical
- (S) Proportionate to site
- (S) Oval, linear, follows fold
- (O) Moderately well-demarcated
- (N) Bright red to pink
- (E) Weeping, partially scaly, erythematous plaques

(Dx)
- Wood's lamp: distinguish from erythrasma
- KOH test: confirm/rule out candida infection

(Tx) 💬 Prevent maceration (clean and dry skin properly, weight loss)
- 💊 Use of mild cleansers and dry skin afterwards: ↓ risk of secondary infection
- Topical zinc oxide or dimethicone: ↓ moisture
- Topical antifungal agents (e.g. ketoconazole or miconazole) 1-2x/d for 2-6 wk
- Low-potency topical corticosteroids for pruritic lesions
- Consider a combination of the pharmacological treatment above

(P) Depends on ability to eliminate triggers, recurs easily

(I) Consider psoriasis inversa in DDx, characterised by sharper demarcation than intertriginous dermatitis

> 💡 Secondary *Candida albicans* infections present with satellite lesions immediately outside the intertriginous area.

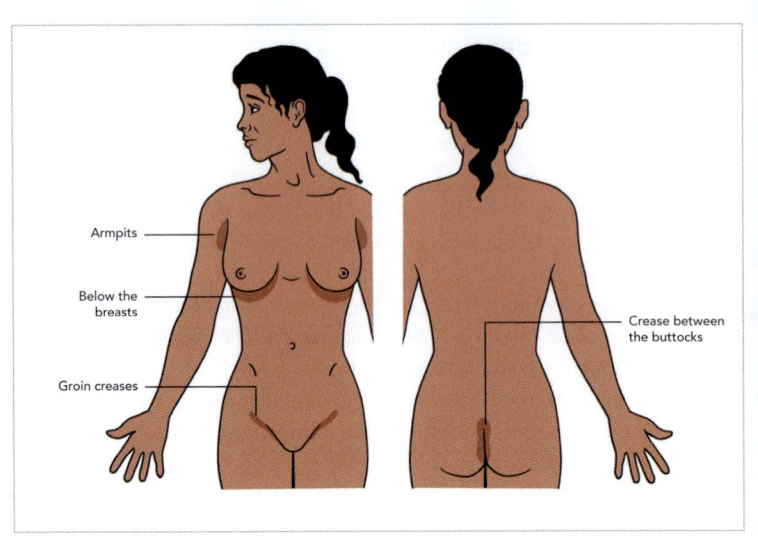

Figure 66 // Intertriginous dermatitis: common sites

Nummular dermatitis

- (D) Nummular dermatitis is a variant of dermatitis characterised by itchy, coin-shaped patches (see Figure 67). In small children, it is usually a nummular variant of constitutional dermatitis.
- (E) Prevalence 0.1-9.0%, peak incidences around age 50-60
- (Ae) Manifestation of atopic dermatitis, triggered by stress or fungal reaction (mycid reaction)
- (R) Atopic constitution
- (Hx) Itching, widespread rash, atopic constitution in childhood (asthma, dermatitis, rhinoconjunctivitis)
- (PE) (P) Extensor surfaces of extremities, torso
  - (A) Solitary
  - (S) Nummular (1-4 cm), several to multiple lesions
  - (S) Round or oval
  - (O) Moderately well-demarcated
  - (N) Red
  - (E) Erythematosquamous plaques. In dark skin there is hyperpigmentation.
- (Dx) KOH test: rule out mycosis
- (Tx) 💬 Emollient, washing and showering recommendations

- High or super-high potency topical corticosteroids as first-line treatment
- Narrowband UVB therapy or systemic immunosuppressants for refractory disease

Chronic with remissions and exacerbations (at higher age of onset)

With sudden expansion, consider secondary infection with *Staphylococcus aureus* (impetiginisation)

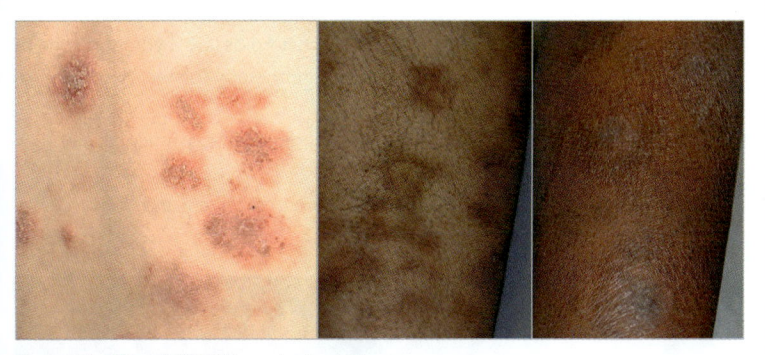

Figure 67A, 67B, and 67C // Nummular dermatitis

Seborrhoeic dermatitis

Seborrhoeic dermatitis is a common, chronic, and relapsing form of mild dermatitis that can range in severity from asymptomatic to more severe. It is thought to be caused by, or associated with, the yeast *Pityrosporon* (*Malassezia furfur*). This commensal yeast, which is part of the normal skin flora, can trigger an inflammatory reaction, leading to seborrhoeic dermatitis. A distinction is made between the adult and childhood variant (see Figure 68).

Prevalence 3-7% with a biphasic incidence (<1y and 30-60y)

Inflammatory reaction caused by the commensal yeast *Malassezia furfur*, not by increased sebum production

♂>♀

Oily skin, scaling, aggravated by scratching

Sites with sebum production (scalp, eyebrows, nasolabial fold, eyelid margins, retroauricular region, ear canal, presternal region) (see Figure 69)

Symmetrical ⊙ (esp. in the face)

Highly variable, from lenticular lesions in the eyebrows to widespread erythroderma ⊖

Round, oval, jagged

- (O) Ill-demarcated to moderately well-demarcated
- (N) Yellow-red
- (E) Erythematosquamous papules and plaques, hypopigmentation in darker skin types

(Dx) No added value

(Tx)
- Scalp: antifungal shampoos 2-3x/wk (e.g. ketoconazole 2%, ciclopirox 1%)
- Face/trunk: low-potency topical corticosteroids (e.g. hydrocortisone or triamcinolone acetonide), local immunotherapy (pimecrolimus, tacrolimus), or topical antifungal agents
- Severe or recurrent: oral antifungal medication (e.g. itraconazole)

(P) Chronic, recurrent course

(!) For extensive and therapy-resistant forms, consider an underlying cause, such as HIV or Parkinson's disease

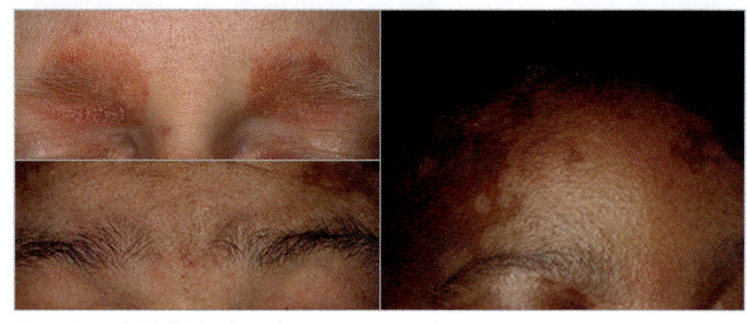

Figure 68A and 68B // Seborrhoeic dermatitis

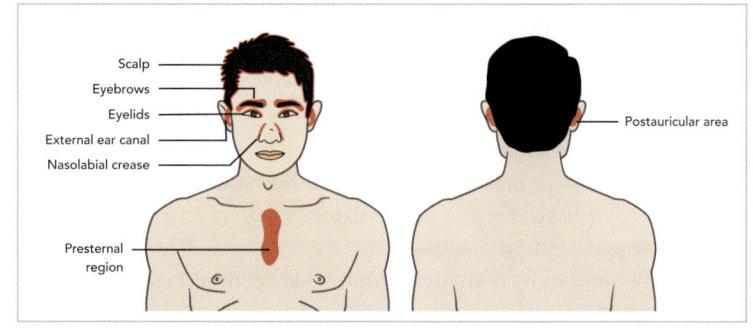

Figure 69 // Seborrhoeic dermatitis: common sites

Labels:
- Scalp
- Eyebrows
- Eyelids
- External ear canal
- Nasolabial crease
- Presternal region
- Postauricular area

Lichen simplex chronicus

(D) Lichen simplex chronicus is a chronic skin condition characterised by itchy, dry, scaly, and thickened skin patches, typically resulting from recurrent rubbing or scratching (see Figure 70). The disorder's primary cause may be a psychological factor or be associated with other dermatological issues like dermatitis or psoriasis.

(E) ♂:♀ = 1:2, prevalence 12%

(Ae) Reaction to chronic scratching

(R) Atopic dermatitis, psoriasis, emotional stressors

(Hx) Chronic itching and scratching

(PE) (P) Head, neck, arms, scalp, and genitals (easy-to-reach areas)
- (A) Regional
- (S) Variable
- (S) Variable
- (O) Moderately well-demarcated
- (N) Yellow, brown, varying degrees of erythema
- (E) Plaques

(Dx) No added value

(Tx) 💬 Psychological counselling from medical psychologist (scratch therapy)
- 💊 Emollients
- High potency topical corticosteroids (under occlusion), can be combined with salicylic acid 10-30% and coal tar solution
- Intralesional corticosteroids
- Phototherapy

(P) Often improves with treatment

(!) The constant scratching can cause infections and structural changes in the affected skin tissues. In rare cases it could even lead to the development of malignant cells.

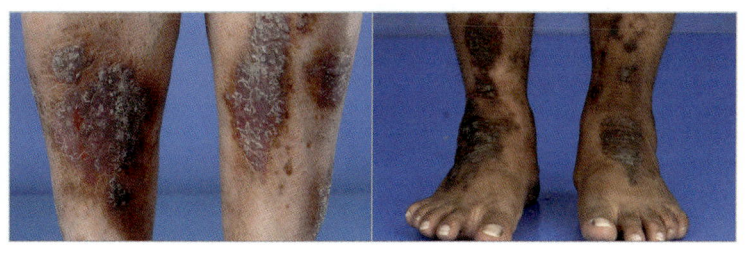

Figure 70 // Lichen simplex chronicus

Prurigo

Xerosis cutis

- (D) Xerosis cutis means dry skin. It is caused by an insufficient amount of hydrolipids in the skin. This can result in rough, tight, flaky, and scaly skin, and may be influenced by factors such as ageing, underlying health conditions, medications, and environmental shifts (see Figure 71).
- (E) Prevalence ↑ ≥60y
- (Ae) Natural moisturising factors constitute approx. 10% of the dry weight of the stratum corneum and are derived from the breakdown of filaggrin. Any alterations in these components can lead to reduced stratum corneum hydration.
- (R) Old age, exposure to cold weather and low humidity, skin disorders (e.g. atopic dermatitis, psoriasis, scabies), systemic diseases (e.g. DM, thyroid disorder, renal failure), pregnancy, menopause, malnutrition, certain medications (e.g. diuretics, beta blockers, retinoids)
- (Hx) Skin roughness, burning sensation, tightness, fissuring, flaking, scaling, itching
- (PE) (P) Lower legs, forearms, hands, and feet
  - (A) Generalised
  - (S) Variable
  - (S) Variable
  - (O) Ill-demarcated
  - (N) Skin-coloured, greyish tone
  - (E) Squama
- (Dx) No added value
- (Tx) 🗨 Adjust bathing habits (limit baths and showers, use lukewarm water, avoid too much soap), adequate hydration
  - 💊 Emollients and moisturisers
- (P) Favourable when avoiding triggers and following a skincare routine
- (!) On occasion, dry skin may be linked to a genetic condition (e.g. xeroderma pigmentosum) associated with e.g. a higher likelihood of developing skin cancer

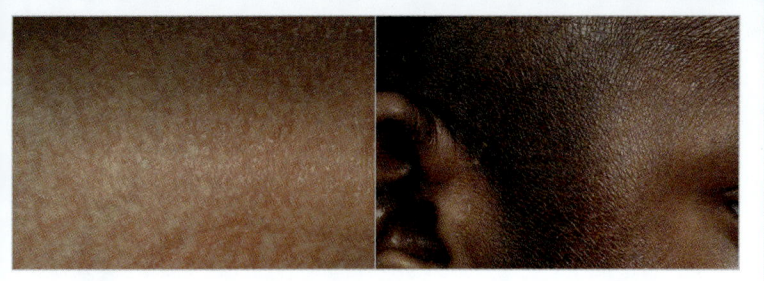

Figure 71 // Xerosis cutis

Notalgia paresthetica

(D) Notalgia paresthetica is a chronic neuropathic pruritus over the medial part of the lower scapula. It is typically unilateral and persists for months to years. There are no primary skin abnormalities, only secondary alterations caused by prolonged scratching (see Figure 72).

(E) Lifetime incidence 20%, highest prevalence in middle-aged ♀

(Ae) Unknown, possibly related to entrapment of the posterior rami of spinal nerves from Th2 to Th6

(R) Degenerative cervical/thoracic spine

(Hx) Chronic, intermittent itching, typically over the medial to the lower two-thirds of the scapula contralateral to the dominant hand, rarely bilateral; sensations of pain, heat, cold, a foreign body, tingling, and numbness

(PE) No primary lesions; in long-standing cases, secondary changes such as hyperpigmentation and lichenification due to chronic scratching can be seen

(Dx) No added value

(Tx)
- Topical antipruritic agents (pramoxine, capsaicin, compounded topical ketamine, lidocaine, amitriptyline)
- Refractory disease: oral anti-seizure medication (gabapentin, pregabalin), botulinum toxin type A injection

(P) Notalgia paresthetica typically does not go away completely, but it can be managed

(!) Potential complications of chronic scratching are secondary skin infection, lichen amyloid, lichen simplex chronicus, and prurigo nodules

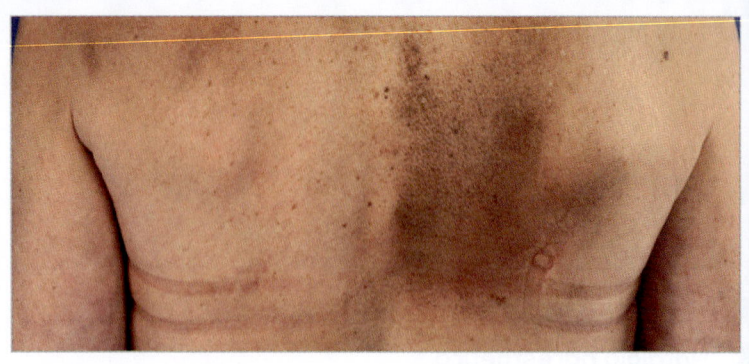

Figure 72 // Notalgia paresthetica

Erythematous dermatoses

Acute urticaria and angioedema

- D Urticaria, or hives, is a type I hypersensitivity reaction that manifests as itchy wheals (see Figure 73). Urticaria is a vascular reaction characterised by rapid onset (within 30 minutes) of erythema (vasodilation), oedema and angioedema (increased vascular permeability; see Figure 74) that disappears spontaneously within 24 hours. Urticaria can become chronic when it lasts for more than six weeks.
- E Lifetime prevalence of ±20%
- Ae Release of vasoactive substances (i.e. histamine, bradykinin, kallikrein) from mast cells (and basophils) in superficial (urticaria) or deeper (angioedema) dermis → capillary and venous vasodilation → intradermal oedema
- R Idiopathic ⊕, combined with physical triggers, medications, foods, plant contact, insect bites, hereditary factors, internal pathology, psychological factors
- Hx Itching, facial, oral, or pharyngeal swelling, dyspnoea, redness, medication (ACE inhibitors and NSAIDs), or other triggering factors
- PE P Urticaria: may appear anywhere on the skin; angioedema: esp. in the face or extremities
  - A Coalescence
  - S Multiple, several mm to cm, regional
  - S Jagged
  - O Well-demarcated
  - N Red with a pale-red edge and pale centre, pale or skin-coloured in darker skin types

- (E) Wheal
- (Dx) No added value
- (Tx) 💬 Trigger avoidance
  - 💊 Second-generation antihistamines (against itching, in combination with H2 antihistamines like cimetidine, famotidine, ranitidine), oral corticosteroids (0.5-1.0 mg/kg/d for 3-10d) if ineffective
    - Intramuscular epinephrine and airway management for symptoms of airway obstruction
    - In cases of chronic severe persistent urticaria: systemic therapy omalizumab
- (P) Life-threatening with severe symptoms, e.g. respiratory (anaphylactic reaction)
- (!) • Acute urticaria and angioedema may be part of an anaphylactic reaction
  - Use ABCDE approach to assess patient
  - IM adrenaline (epinephrine auto injector) for anaphylactic reaction

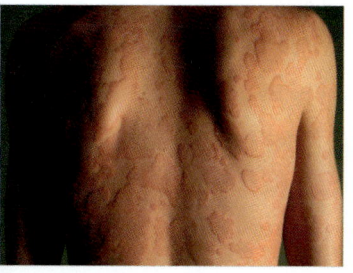

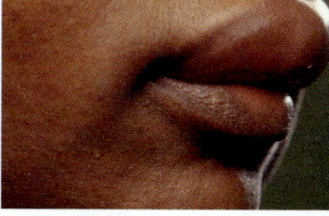

Figure 73 // Urticaria

Figure 74 // Angioedema

Erythema chronicum migrans (ECM)

- (D) ECM is a skin condition caused by the bacterium *Borrelia burgdorferi*, which is transmitted by a tick bite (see Figure 75). It is an early manifestation of Lyme disease (on average 7-14 days after the bite).
- (E) Approx. 80% of patients with Lyme disease have ECM, on average 128,888 cases annually in Europe
- (Ae) Borrelia burgdorferi, a spirochete found in 5-40% of ticks in Europe
- (R) Gardeners, walkers
- (Hx) Red ring, forest walk, tick bite
- (PE) (P) At site of bite, often on the flexor surfaces of joints, legs, or groin
  - (A) Solitary

- (S) Ankle, tens of cm (>5 cm for diagnosis)
- (S) Round or annular
- (O) Well-demarcated, jagged borders
- (N) Bluish red, occasionally with a pale centre, hyperpigmentation in darker skin types
- (E) Blanching erythema with centrifugal enlargement, may begin with a papule or plaque

Dx
- Labs: IgM+ up to 6 wk after infection, >6 wk IgG+, C6-peptide K
- Polymerase chain reaction (PCR) or skin biopsy for pathogen: *Borellia burgdorferi*

Tx
- Oral doxycycline 10d (first choice), or amoxicillin or cefuroxime axetil for 14d
- Azithromycin 5-10d (7d course preferred in the US) in case of contraindications

Tick removal

P ECM heals spontaneously within a few months

- Ineffective treatment poses a risk of late Lyme disease complications in nervous system, joints, heart, or skin
- Beware of underdiagnosis: redness may be less noticeable on skin of colour

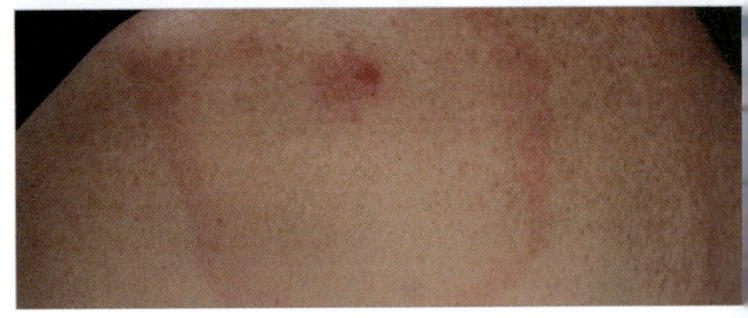

Figure 75 // Erythema chronicum migrans

Erythema multiforme minor (EMm)

D EMm is an acute-onset (within 72 hours) eruption of the skin and mucous membranes (see Figure 76) resulting from a toxic-allergic reaction. EMm is characterised by minimal or absent mucosal defects, which are very severe in EM major (EMM).

E Annual incidence of erythema multiforme is <1%, exact incidence of EMm

is unknown
- (Ae) Immunological response to infections (HSV ⊕, *Mycoplasma pneumoniae*) or medication (e.g. NSAIDs, AB) ⊖
- (R) Young adults (>50% <20y)
- (Hx) Cold sore, sore throat, malaise ⊖, fever ⊖, GI symptoms ⊖
- (PE) (P) Face and extremities (esp. distal parts)
  - (A) Grouped, coalescent
  - (S) <3 cm, multiple lesions
  - (S) Concentric target lesions (red centre, pale inner ring due to oedema and red outer ring)
  - (O) Well-demarcated
  - (N) Red
  - (E) Erythema, papules, plaques, may be accompanied by oedema and vesicles
- (Dx) • Labs: exploratory, further testing for underlying infection if indicated
  - Skin biopsy if unsure about diagnosis: spongiosis or intraepidermal vesicles, basal layer liquefaction and/or subepidermal blister, mixed perivascular inflammatory infiltrate, red blood cell extravasation
- (Tx) 🗨 Wait-and-see, sometimes symptomatic treatment such as incision and drainage of large bullae, topical corticosteroids, and oral antihistamines
  - 🔗 Recurrent EMm may be minimised or prevented with prophylactic oral aciclovir
- (P) Heals spontaneously <3 wk, recurrences possible
- (!) Possible complications affecting mucous membranes (erosions, ulcers, membranous patches, foetor ex ore), eyes (keratitis, severe corneal damage), skin (generalised eruption)

Erythema multiforme major (EMM)

- (D) EMM is predominantly a mucosal eruption of erosions and blisters in the oropharynx, on the lips, conjunctivae, and genitalia. EMM can be very severe, with mortality around 15%.
- (E) Annual incidence of erythema multiforme <1%, incidence of EMM is unknown (EMM<EMm)
- (Ae) Reaction to medication or underlying infection
- (R) Young adult age, HSV infection
- (Hx) Sore throat, malaise ⊖, fever ⊖, GI symptoms ⊖
- (PE) (P) Acral target lesions (on palms and soles)

- (A) Regional
- (S) Multiple lesions, max. 3 cm in size, up to 10% of body surface area
- (S) Raised, round, consisting of two concentric targets
- (O) Well-demarcated
- (N) Red
- (E) Oedematous macule with erythematous centre

(Dx)
- Labs: exploratory, further testing for underlying infection if indicated
- Consider skin biopsy: necrotic keratinocytes ⊕ (see EMm)

(Tx)
- Wait and see
  - Consider treating infection
  - Consult an ophthalmologist or ENT specialist if eyes or oral cavity/throat are affected
- IV fluid therapy
  - Systemic corticosteroids for severe cases
  - Valaciclovir or aciclovir for suspected underlying herpes infection

(P) Self-limiting, may cause permanent damage to mucous membranes

(!) EMm/EMM, SJS, and TEN can be distinguished by their clinical presentation, the body surface area involved, and pathogenesis (infectious or medicinal); see section on *TEN*

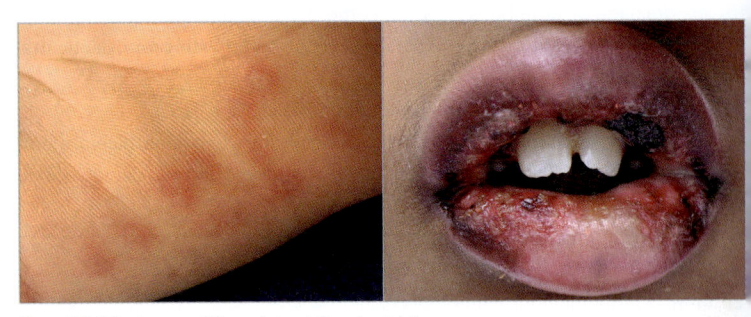

Figure 76 // Erythema multiforme (minor left, major right)

Polymorphous light eruption (PMLE)

(D) PMLE is a common and benign photodermatosis characterised by the development of erythematous papules, plaques, or vesicles on sun-exposed skin, typically occurring in the spring or early summer following unaccustomed sun exposure (see Figure 77). The pathogenesis of PMLE is not fully understood but is thought to involve an abnormal immune response to UV radiation.

- (E) Prevalence 1-20%
- (Ae) In healthy individuals, UV radiation suppresses T cell immune reactions in the skin. Hypothesis for PMLE: no suppression of T cell immune reaction in the skin → inflammatory reaction to a photo-induced antigen.
- (R) Positive PMHx
- (Hx) Skin eruption following the initial exposure to strong sunlight in the spring or early summer, itching ⊙, remains several days until it disappears without scarring
- (PE) (P) Low neckline, forearms, backs of hands, lower legs (areas newly exposed to the sun)
  - (A) Regional
  - (S) Variable
  - (S) Polymorphous
  - (O) Variable
  - (N) Erythematous
  - (E) Papulovesicles, vesicles, bullae, or confluent oedematous plaques
- (Dx) No added value. Skin biopsy (lymphohistiocytic infiltrate, dermal oedema, epidermal spongiosis) and photo-testing can be considered.
- (Tx) 🕮 Sun protection (avoidance, protective clothing, sunscreen)
  - 💊 • Prophylactic phototherapy (low dose UVB) in late winter or early spring
  - Topical corticosteroids, oral antihistamines
- (P) May persist for several years, though the severity diminishes with time
- (!) Primary DDx: photosensitivity associated with lupus erythematosus → similar symptoms but more persistent, solar urticaria that develops during or shortly after exposure and dissipates <1h after covering up

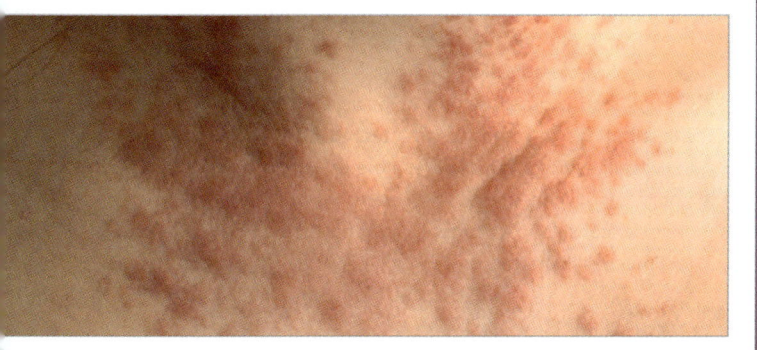

Figure 77 // Polymorphous light eruption

Lichen sclerosus

(D) Lichen sclerosus is a chronic inflammatory skin condition associated with white sclerotic lesions. Long-standing complaints may present with atrophy and scarring.

(E)
- Prevalence 0,1% in children and 3% in elderly women (age >80)
- Incidence ♀ 15-20:100,000 per year

(Ae)
- Idiopathic, suspected correlation with autoimmune disorders
- Associated with infectious, hormonal, and genetic factors
- May arise due to Köbner phenomenon following episiotomy or local friction

(R) Peaks around prepubertal and postmenopausal ages

(Hx) Itching, painful or burning sensation in the anogenital region, micturition problems, constipation, painful defecation, risk of phimosis when located on the penis, dyspareunia

(PE) (P) 90% in genital or perianal area (see Figure 78), vaginal mucosa are never affected
- (A) Predominantly solitary
- (S) Variable
- (S) Symmetrical
- (O) Well-demarcated
- (N) Pearlescent
- (E) Pearly macules, papules, and plaques, white atrophic lesions, hyperkeratosis, fibrotic changes in longstanding disease

(Dx) Skin biopsy: if needed for diagnosis and to rule out malignancy (SCC)

(Tx)
- Topical emollients (always in combination with an active treatment such as corticosteroids)
- Topical corticosteroids (class III-IV)
- Topical calcineurin inhibitors

Surgical: de-adhesion, perineoplasty (♀), circumcision (♂)

(P) Chronic and progressive, no cure, asymptomatic periods alternating with exacerbations, maintenance treatment with topical corticosteroids indicated to prevent symptoms and reduce the risk of developing SCC

(I) Anogenital lichen sclerosus increases risk of vulvar and penile carcinoma consider consulting urologist or gynaecologist. Lichen sclerosus does not affect mucous membranes.

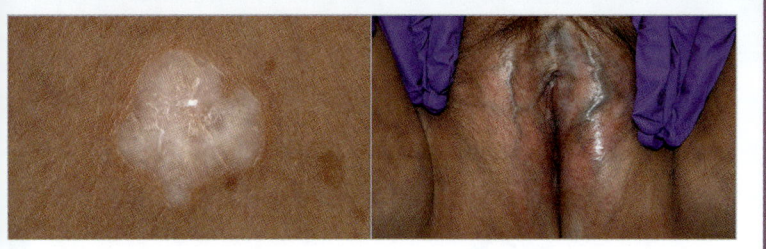

Figure 78A and 78B // Lichen sclerosus, extragenital (left) and genital (right) localisation

Infectious exanthem

- D Infectious exanthems are skin rashes that result from viral, bacterial, parasitic, and helminth infections (see Figure 79). They are often accompanied by other symptoms such as fever, malaise, and inflammation. The six classic infectious exanthems are measles, scarlet fever, rubella, varicella, erythema infectiosum (fifth disease), and exanthema subitum (sixth disease). These diseases are individually addressed in the Paediatrics section.
- E Peak incidence in childhood
- Ae Infectious exanthems can arise from the direct inoculation of the infectious agent into the cutaneous surface or through dissemination of the antigens from a distant site. Alternatively, they may result from an immune response against the infectious agents or cell-mediated reactions to the virus.
- R Unvaccinated
- Hx Systemic symptoms, e.g. fever, malaise, muscle aches, headache
- PE
  - P Face and trunk
  - A Diffuse, symmetrical
  - S Generalised
  - S Variable
  - O Well-demarcated
  - N Erythematous
  - E Maculopapular
- Dx Viral swab and/or blood tests (for viral culture, immunofluorescence, PCR, serology)
- Tx 💬 Wait-and-see
  - 💊 Topical corticosteroids or antihistamines in case of pruritus
- P Self-limiting
- ! To ensure early detection of serious complications (e.g. meningitis), it is important to look for petechial eruption and neurological signs

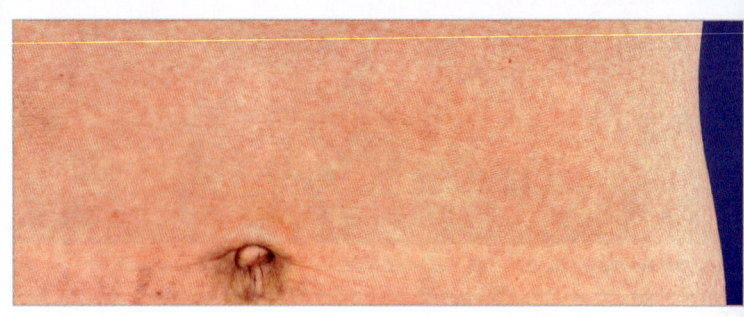

Figure 79 // Infectious exanthem

Cutaneous adverse drug reactions (CADR)

- D CADR encompasses various types of drug-induced skin responses, ranging from a relatively mild and unnoticeable rash to TEN, with potentially life-threatening consequences (see section on *TEN*).
- E Incidence 1-3% in patients who use multiple medications
- Ae Adverse drug reactions (ADR) can be divided into two main types: immunological and non-immunological. The majority of ADR (approx. 75%-80%) results from predictable, dose dependent, non-immunological effects; 20%-25% are due to unpredictable effects. 5%-10% of all ADR are immune-mediated and typically involve immediate or delayed immunological mechanisms, facilitated by cellular or humoral immune responses.
- R Systemic lupus erythematosus, HIV infection, non-Hodgkin's lymphoma
- Hx Rash or dermatitis in patients without a known skin disorder, 1-2h to weeks after exposure to a new drug. ADR resolve ≤2 wk following discontinuation of a medication.
- PE Variable depending on the type of reaction: maculopapular rash ☺ ("toxicodermia", generalised maculopapular lesions without mucosal involvement resembling an infectious/viral rash), urticaria, and fixed drug eruptions (round to oval-shaped, red to brown maculous lesions). See Figure 80.
- Dx • Biopsy can be considered: eosinophils, oedema, and inflammation
  • Skin prick testing and intradermal testing: test for IgE-mediated immediate hypersensitivity reactions
- Tx 💬 Withdrawal of the causative drug
  🩹 Topical corticosteroids, oral antihistamines
- P Variable
- I Most commonly seen in use of AB such as beta-lactams and sulfonamides,

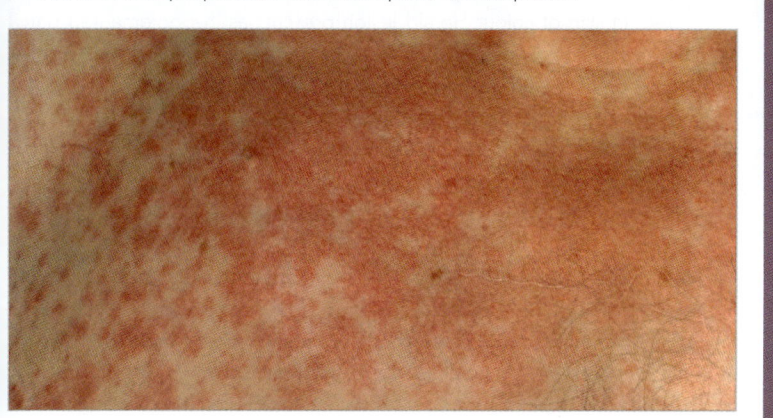

NSAIDs, antiepileptics like carbamazepine, and allopurinol

Figure 80 // Toxicodermia

Erythematosquamous dermatoses

Pityriasis rosea

- D Pityriasis rosea is a skin condition characterised by a highly recognisable clinical presentation and spontaneous recovery (self-limiting).
- E Incidence 170:100,000 per year (peaks in spring and autumn), predominantly between ages 15-30
- Ae Unclear, possible association with human herpes viruses (HHV-6 and HHV-7) and rotavirus
- R Children or young adults, age 10-35 (peak around 23), ♀>♂
- Hx Itching, scaly skin
- PE P Torso, neck, and proximal extremities (palms and soles unaffected)
  - A Symmetrical, disseminated, follows skin lines (Christmas-tree pattern; see Figure 81), atypical presentations (resembling erythema multiforme) may also occur
  - S Mother lesion (Herald patch): 2-5 cm, exanthema: dozens, lenticular to nummular, generalised
  - S Round, oval
  - O Well-demarcated, larger lesions show marginal flaking, flaking starts at the outer edge of the lesion and gradually moves toward the center (collerette, Herald lesion or plaque mère; see Figure 82)

- (N) Herald patch: pink margin and skin-coloured centre, exanthema: pinkish red. In skin of colour Herald lesion presents as: hypopigmented patch with sunken pale centre.
- (E) Erythematosquamous papules and plaques. In skin of colour plaques vary between hyperpigmented and gray plaques.
- (Dx)
  - Syphilis serology to rule out secondary syphilis ⊖
  - KOH test to rule out tinea corporis
  - Biopsy is often not necessary, but can be performed if the diagnosis is uncertain
- (Tx)
  - 💬 Often left untreated due to generally asymptomatic and self-limiting character
  - 🔗 If symptomatic: emollients, medium-potency topical corticosteroids for pruritic lesions, UVB therapy, or sedating antihistamines
- (P) Excellent, heals spontaneously <4-6 wk, 2% recurs after months or years
- (!) DDx: syphilis stage II (affecting palms and soles)

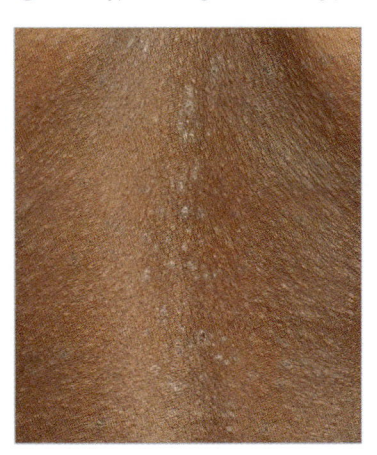

Figure 81 // Pityriasis rosea

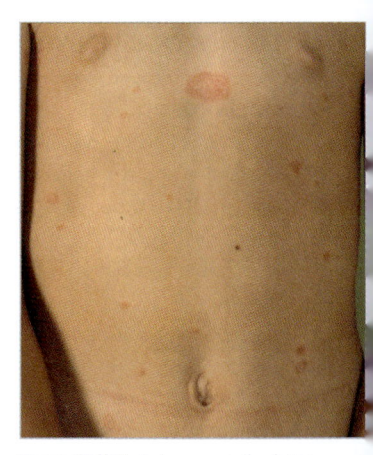

Figure 82 // Pityriasis rosea: mother lesion

Psoriasis vulgaris

Psoriasis vulgaris is a chronic inflammatory skin disease that tends to flare up and go into remission over time (see Figure 84). It may be accompanied by nail defects (see Figure 85) and arthritis in 10%. Psoriasis can be classified morphologically and topographically. Psoriasis vulgaris is the most common variant (see Table 27).

(E) Prevalence ±1.4% in paediatric patients, 0.5-11% in adults, distance from the equator ↑ → prevalence ↑

(Ae) Genetic predisposition, combined with cellular immune system (incl. IL-17 activation)

(R) European descent, genetic factors (both parents affected: 50% risk, one parent affected: 16% risk) combined with triggering factors, e.g. skin damage (Koebner phenomenon), infections, hormonal factors, psychological stress, medication, alcohol consumption, smoking, obesity

(Hx) Mild itching, medication use (beta blockers, lithium, chloroquine/nivaquine, renin-angiotensin system (RAS) inhibitors, terbinafine, or NSAIDs)

(PE) (P) Extensor surfaces of knees and elbows, tailbone, scalp (see Figure 83)
- (A) Grouped
- (S) Single or several, 1 mm to >20 cm, regional
- (S) Round or oval, often with polycyclic coalescence of plaques
- (O) Well-demarcated
- (N) Silvery white, red, dark grey on darker skin types
- (E) Erythematosquamous papules and plaques, scaling

(Dx) Biopsy: signs of inflammation with neutrophil accumulation in stratum corneum and dermal vasodilation (tortuous, dilated papillary capillaries), inflammation with accelerated keratinocyte proliferation and impaired maturation in the epidermis leading to hyperkeratosis and parakeratosis

(Tx)
- Mild disease: topical corticosteroids, tar, topical retinoids, vitamin D, tacrolimus, or pimecrolimus, emollients
- Moderate disease or insufficient response to topical therapy: phototherapy with adjuvant topical therapy
- Severe disease: systemic therapy with methotrexate, ciclosporin, oral retinoids, or biologicals (anti-TNF-alpha, anti-interleukin-23 or -17)

(P)
- Chronic skin disease with unpredictable course
- Risk ↑ for metabolic syndrome and cardiovascular disease

(!)
- Always enquire about joint symptoms to detect psoriatic arthritis → referral to rheumatologist
- DDx: cutaneous discoid lupus erythematosus and secondary syphilis

> The candle-grease sign, indicating psoriatic scales falling off revealing a shiny candle-like surface when scratched, and Auspitz's sign, showing pinpoint bleeding points upon removal of psoriatic scales, are typical findings of psoriasis vulgaris.

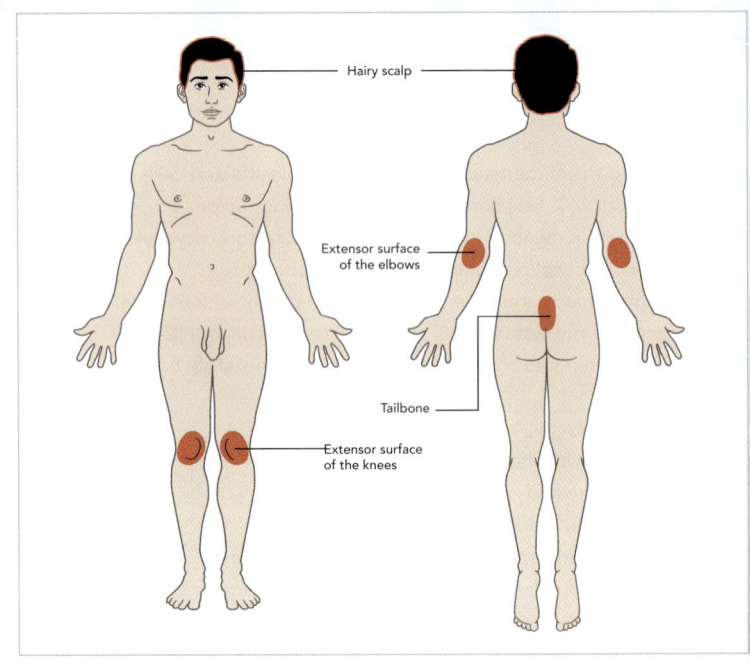

Figure 83 // Psoriasis vulgaris: common sites

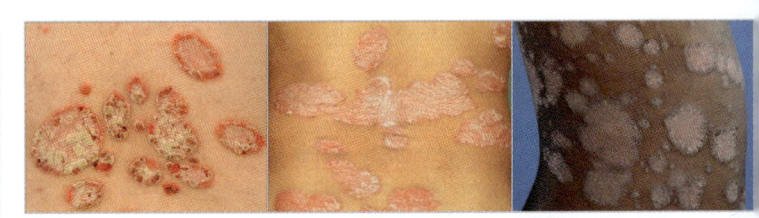

Figure 84 // Psoriasis vulgaris

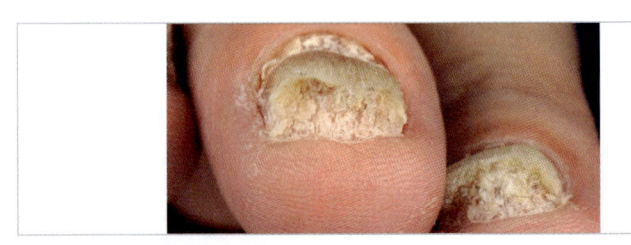

Figure 85 // Psoriasis vulgaris: nail defects

	GUTTATE PSORIASIS	**SCALP PSORIASIS**	**PSORIASIS INVERSA**
D	Form of psoriasis characterised by acute onset of numerous small, scaly plaques on the trunk and extremities (see Figure 86).	Form of psoriasis typically located on the scalp (see Figure 87).	Form of psoriasis involving the intertriginous areas. This presentation is called 'inverse', since it is the reverse of the typical presentation of plaque psoriasis on extensor surfaces (see Figure 88).
E	Prevalence 4%, most common among children and young adults	80% of psoriasis patients experience scalp involvement	20-30% of psoriasis patients develop inverse psoriasis
Ae	See Psoriasis vulgaris		
R	PMHx of streptococcal infection	See Psoriasis vulgaris	
Hx	Period of throat infection prior to skin complaints	Mild itching skin lesions on the scalp	Mild itching skin lesions around navel, buttocks, ear
PE	P Trunk, proximal extremities A Generalised S Multiple S Round or oval O Well-demarcated N Red E Erythematosquamous papules	P Scalp A Regional S Single or several S Oval, round, polygonal O Well-demarcated N Red, silvery-white E Patches or plaques, scaling	P Inguinal, perineal, genital, intergluteal, axillary, or inframammary regions A Grouped S Single or several, regional S Round, oval, polygonal O Well-demarcated N Red E Smooth, shiny plaques, with absent or minimal scaling
Dx	See Psoriasis vulgaris		
Tx	• Narrowband UVB therapy	• Topical keratolytic agents (i.e. salicylic acid or urea, or a dimethicone-based topical keratolytic) • Coal tar shampoos	• Calcineurin inhibitors
	Topical corticosteroids, topical vitamin D analogs (e.g. calcipotriol)		
P	See Psoriasis vulgaris		
!	• Often no nail involvement or joint complaints • May develop into chronic plaque psoriasis	• Scarring alopecia can develop due to chronic, relapsing scalp psoriasis • May be associated with psoriatic arthritis	Often misdiagnosed as intertriginous fungal or bacterial infections

Table 27 // Types of psoriasis

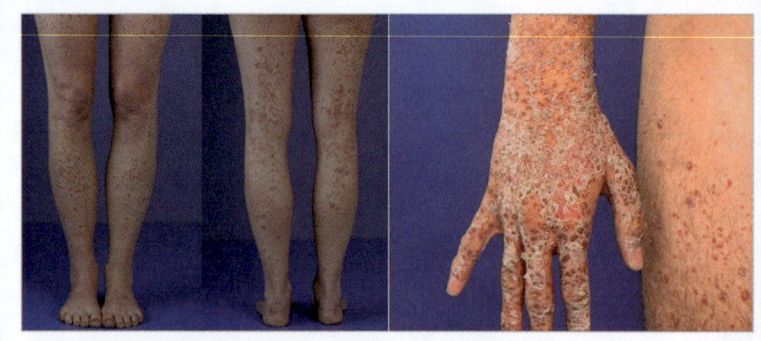

Figure 86 // Guttate psoriasis

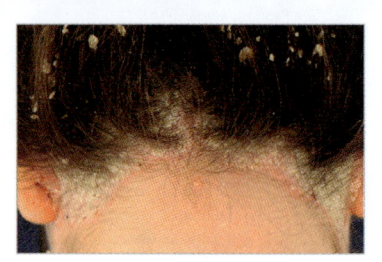

Figure 87 // Scalp psoriasis

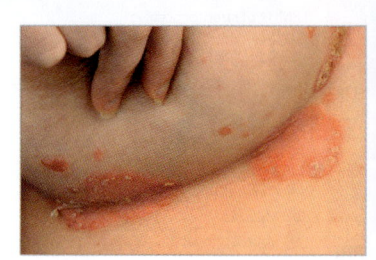

Figure 88 // Psoriasis inversa

Cutaneous lupus erythematosus

ACUTE CUTANEOUS LUPUS ERYTHEMATOSUS (ACLE)	SUBACUTE CUTANEOUS LUPUS ERYTHEMATOSUS (SCLE)	CHRONIC CUTANEOUS LUPUS ERYTHEMATOSUS (CCLE)
ACLE is a manifestation of SLE that can appear as a facial eruption (i.e. malar rash), occasionally as a generalised rash, and in rare cases as a TEN-like variant. ACLE may manifest before other symptoms of SLE by months or even years, or may coincide with other acute signs and symptoms of SLE.	SCLE occurs in 50% of patients with SLE. It can also occur as a result of drug exposure and commonly affects areas that are exposed to the sun, e.g. shoulders, forearms, neck, upper torso. Despite being aggravated by sunlight, the condition often spares the face.	CCLE is characterised by lesions that can last years without treatment. It is rarely associated with a systemic disease. The most prevalent subtype of CCLE is discoid lupus erythematosus (DLE), which accounts for 73-85% of all cases of CCLE. Less common subtypes, e.g. lupus erythematosus tumidus, lupus profundus, chilblain lupus erythematodes (LE), LE lichen planus.

Table 28A // Subtypes of lupus erythematosus

	ACUTE CUTANEOUS LUPUS ERYTHEMATOSUS (ACLE)	**SUBACUTE CUTANEOUS LUPUS ERYTHEMATOSUS (SCLE)**	**CHRONIC CUTANEOUS LUPUS ERYTHEMATOSUS (CCLE)**
E	Incidence 1-10:100,000 per year	Incidence 0.6:100,000 per year	• Incidence 3.6:100,000 per year • Prevalence of concurrent SLE in patients with localised or generalised DLE 5-28%
Ae	Chronic activation of inherent immune pathways → release of endogenous nucleic acids from perishing cells → various pattern-recognition receptors → IFN-driven inflammatory process → adaptive immune responses, esp. cytotoxic responses		
R	UV radiation, medications (e.g. antihypertensives, statins, antifungals, ACE inhibitors, NSAIDs, antiepileptics, biologicals, proton pump inhibitors), smoking, viral infections		
Hx	Localised or generalised rash lasting for hours to weeks, esp. after sun exposure	Extreme photosensitivity, exposure to certain drugs, rash lasting for months	Rash lasting for years, systemic symptoms ⊖
PE	(P) Localised (malar region with sparing of nasolabial folds) or generalised (mainly sun-exposed areas) (A) Malar distribution or generalised (S) Varies (S) Irregular (O) Well-demarcated (N) Erythematous (E) Macules and papules, sometimes progressing to vesicles or bullae	(P) Sun-exposed areas (e.g. upper back, shoulders, arms) (A) Generalised (S) Varies (S) Psoriasiform or annular (O) Well-demarcated (N) Erythematous (E) Macules and papules	(P) Sun-exposed areas (e.g. upper back, shoulders, arms) (A) Generalised (S) Varies (S) Round, oval (O) Well-demarcated (N) Erythematous, hyper-/hypopigmented (E) Plaques, scales, atrophy, scarring (see Figure 89)
Dx	• Biopsy: apoptotic keratinocytes, vacuolisation of the basement membrane, a lymphohistiocytic infiltrate in the superficial dermis, and dermal mucinosis • Serological testing: positive ANA, anti-dsDNA, hypocomplementemia	• Biopsy: mild degree of follicular plugging and hyperkeratosis, superficial perivascular and appendageal lymphocytic infiltrates, vacuolisation of the basement membrane, dermal mucinosis, minimal or absent basement membrane thickening • Serological testing: anti-SSA, anti-SSB	Biopsy: follicular plugging, hyperkeratosis, basal layer vacuolar changes, lymphocytic infiltrate near the dermal-epidermal junction, basement membrane thickening, dermal mucinosis

Table 28B // Subtypes of lupus erythematosus

	ACUTE CUTANEOUS LUPUS ERYTHEMATOSUS (ACLE)	**SUBACUTE CUTANEOUS LUPUS ERYTHEMATOSUS (SCLE)**	**CHRONIC CUTANEOUS LUPUS ERYTHEMATOSUS (CCLE)**
Tx	💬 Photoprotection and use of appropriate broad-spectrum sunscreens 🔖 Local corticosteroids, local calcineurin inhibitors, oral glucocorticoids, hydroxychloroquine, immunomodulatory agents (i.e. methotrexate, thalidomide)		
P	Variable		
	90-100% of cases progress to systemic disease	30% of cases progress to systemic disease	5% of cases progress to systemic disease

Table 28C // Subtypes of lupus erythematosus

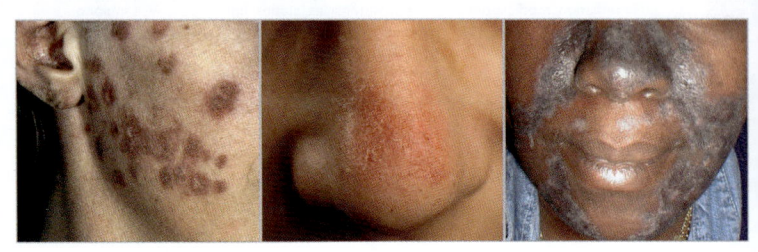

Figure 89 // Chronic discoid lupus erythematosus (CDLE)

Pityriasis lichenoides

	PITYRIASIS LICHENOIDES CHRONICA (PLC)	**PITYRIASIS LICHENOIDES ET VARIOLIFORMIS ACUTA (PLEVA)**
D	PLC is a rare, benign, inflammatory skin condition characterised by the development of red-brown, scaling papules (see Figure 90). The condition is idiopathic.	PLEVA is a rare, benign, inflammatory skin condition that predominantly impacts young adults and chil-dren. It is characterised by an acute eruption of inflammatory papules and papulovesicles that progress to form hemorrhagic or necrotic crusts (see Figure 91).
E	Incidence 50:100,000 per year	
Ae	The pathophysiology of both PLC and PLEVA is poorly understood. The prevailing hypothesis is that these diseases occur as a result of infections or lymphoproliferative disorders.	
R	Certain viral, bacterial, or protozoal infections (e.g. *Toxoplasma gondii*, Epstein-Barr virus, parvovirus B16, HIV)	

Table 29A // Pityriasis lichenoides chronicus and pityriasis lichenoides et varioliformis acuta

	PITYRIASIS LICHENOIDES CHRONICA (PLC)	**PITYRIASIS LICHENOIDES ET VARIOLIFORMIS ACUTA (PLEVA)**
Hx	Gradual onset, different phases of development concurrently present, asymptomatic ⊕, in some cases itching	Acute eruption of skin lesions that resolve within weeks, concurrently new lesions while the old ones resolve → continuous manifestation, itching, burning sensation
PE	P Trunk, buttocks, and proximal extremities A Grouped or diffuse S 4-40 mm S Oval O Well-demarcated N Red-brown E Papules, scales, hyper-/hypopigmented macules, or patches where the papules resolve	P Trunk, proximal extremities, skin flexures A Grouped or diffuse S 3-15 mm S Wedge-shaped O Well-demarcated N Erythematous E Papules and papulovesicles, crusting, hypopigmented macules or patches where the papules resolve, may leave scarring
Dx	Biopsy: parakeratosis, mild spongiosis, minimal lymphocyte exocytosis, minimal vacuolar change and focal, necrotic keratinocytes at the dermoepidermal junction, perivascular and lichenoid (band-like), lymphohistiocytic infiltrate in the superficial dermis, a few extravasated erythrocytes in the papillary dermis	Biopsy: parakeratosis, spongiosis, mild-to-moderate epidermal acanthosis, vacuolar alteration of the basal layer, exocytosis of lymphocytes and erythrocytes into the epidermis, moderately dense, wedgeshaped lymphohistiocytic infiltrate extending from the papillary dermis into the deep reticular dermis
Tx	👁 Considering the mostly benign, self-limiting course of the disease, treatment is not always necessary ✐ • Limited disease: topical corticosteroid monotherapy • Widespread: oral ABx (tetracyclines, macrolides), phototherapy, methotrexate (for severe, refractory disease)	👁 In mild, non-scarring cases, treatment is not always necessary ✐ Oral ABx (tetracyclines, macrolides), phototherapy, methotrexate or other immunosuppressive agents for severe and refractory diseases
P	Self-limiting ⊕	Self-limiting in most cases, may leave scarring
!	PLC associated with cutaneous lymphoma ⊖ → preventive annual skin evaluations recommended. Possible signs of cutaneous lymphoma: prolonged cutaneous inflammatory patches, plaques, or tumour-like nodules.	

Table 29B // Pityriasis lichenoides chronicus and pityriasis lichenoides et varioliformis acuta

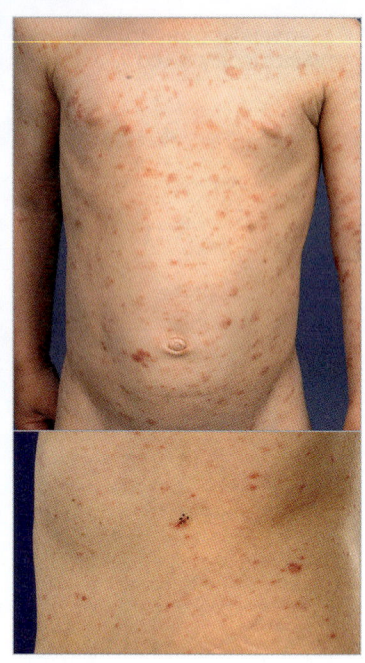

Figure 90 // Pityriasis lichenoides chronica (PLC)

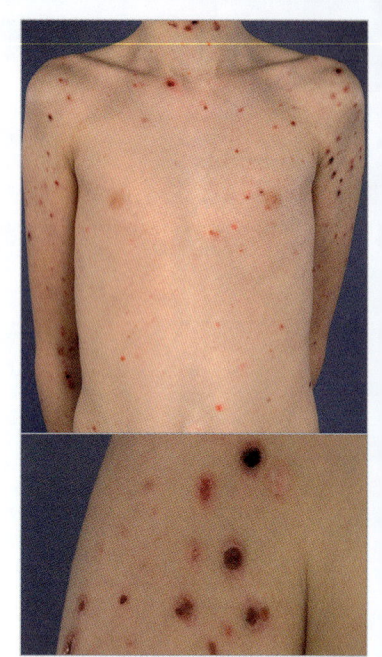

Figure 91 // Pityriasis lichenoides et varioliformis acuta (PLEVA)

Skin tumours

Benign skin tumours

Epidermoid cyst

- (D) An epidermoid cyst, or epidermal inclusion cyst, is a retention cyst with a wall made of epidermis; it is filled mainly with keratin but can also contain pus and bacteria (see Figure 92).
- (E) Most common type of cutaneous cyst. Exact incidence unknown as many do not seek medical care.
- (Ae) Usually arises from an occluded hair follicle, as seen in the centre of the lesion
- (R) ♂>♀, age 30-40
- (Hx) Asymptomatic ⊙, possibly sebum production
- (PE) (P) Scalp, chest, face, neck, scrotum
  - (A) Solitary

- (S) 0.5-2.5 cm
- (S) Convex, often with central punctum
- (O) Well-demarcated
- (N) Skin-coloured to translucent white/yellow
- (E) Nodule

(Dx) No added value

(Tx) • Excision
- In case of inflammation: intralesional injection of triamcinolone acetonide, broad spectrum AB, or incision and drainage

(P) Cyst becomes tender or painful as it grows, may recur if wall is not removed completely

(!) Cyst rupture produces severe inflammatory reaction, multiple cysts can occur in Gardner syndrome or basal cell naevus syndrome (BCNS)

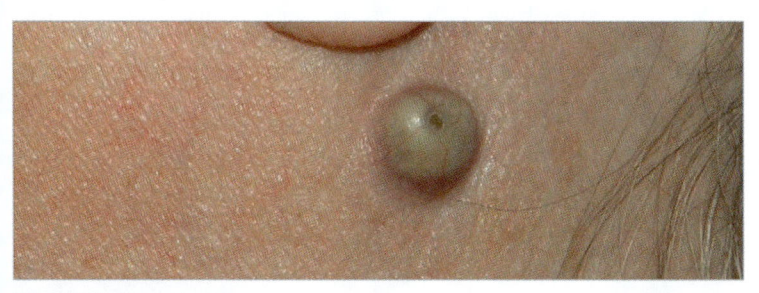

Figure 92 // Epidermoid cyst

Dermatofibroma

(D) A dermatofibroma, or fibrous histiocytoma, is a slow-growing, benign subepidermal nodule (see Figure 93 and 94).

(E) One of the most common cutaneous lesions, incidence largely unknown due to asymptomatic nature (patients do not seek help)

(Ae) Idiopathic, possible association with trauma (esp. insect bites)

(R) ♂:♀ = 1:4, skin trauma

(Hx) Asymptomatic ☺

(PE) (P) Lower and upper extremities
- (A) Solitary or multiple
- (S) 0.1-3.0 cm
- (S) Sunken, indurated lesion, sometimes slightly raised to convex
- (O) Moderately well-demarcated, surrounded by a narrow pigmented margin

(N) Hyperpigmentation or hypopigmentation, pink
(E) Nodule
(Dx) • Dermoscopy: peripheral pseudo pigment network with central scar-like area
  • Biopsy when in doubt: dermal proliferation of uniform fibroblasts, epidermal acanthosis with hyperpigmentation of the basal layer (dirty feet sign)
(Tx) 💬 Generally no treatment needed
  ✏ Consider excision or cryotherapy on cosmetic grounds
(P) Persistence or slow growth
(!) Immunocompromised patients (HIV) and those with autoimmune disorders (e.g. SLE) may present with multiple eruptive dermatofibromas

> 💡 Pinching a fold around the dermatofibroma produces a dimple (dimple sign, see Figure 93) and displaces the epidermis downwards.

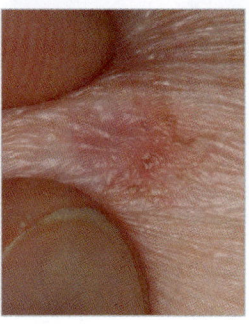

Figure 93 // Dimple sign

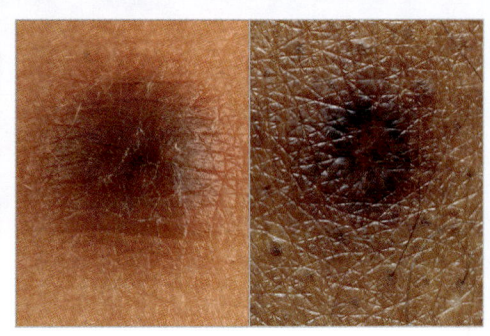

Figure 94A and 94B // Dermatofibroma

Keloid

(D) Keloid is a type of proliferative, sometimes painful and/or itchy scar tissue that grows beyond the boundaries of the original wound (in contrast to hypertrophic scars, which are confined to the boundaries of the original wound; see Figure 95).

(E) Prevalence 0.03-0.2%, prevalence ↑ in darker skin types (Colorimetric scale types 4-5, 4-6%)

(Ae) Impaired wound healing process in damaged tissue

(R) Positive PMHx, adolescence, burns, radiation, wound infection (chronic inflammation), post-acne

(Hx) Asymptomatic ⊕, possibly painful, itching
(PE) (P) Common sites: earlobes, lateral side of the upper arms, shoulder blades
- (A) Solitary or multiple
- (S) Variable, increasing in size
- (S) Variable, based on shape of wound
- (O) Well-demarcated
- (N) Violaceous to skin-coloured
- (E) Shiny plaque that extends beyond the original wound

(Dx) Often not indicated (clinical diagnosis), if in doubt biopsy: chronic dermal inflammation, marked angiogenesis, and keloidal collagen deposits (in contrast to hyperplastic scars which show collagen nodules)

(Tx) Wait-and-see ⊕, consider compression therapy
- Small-to-moderate lesions (<20 cm^2): corticosteroid tape, intralesional corticosteroids, and/or intralesional fluorouracil
- Larger lesions (≥20 cm^2): surgical excision with adjuvant radiation therapy (not in paediatric patients)
- Refractory cases: laser therapy

(P) Lesion reaches maximum size in 12-18 mo, no spontaneous regression

(!) 80-100% of surgically removed keloids recur, follow-up every 3 mo for 18-24 mo

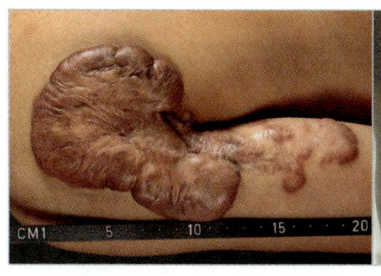

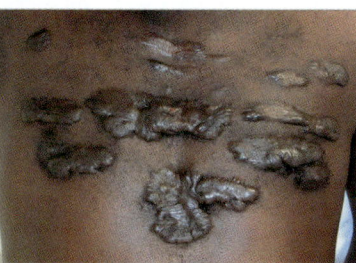

Figure 95 // Keloid

Keratoacanthoma (KA)

(D) KA is a rapidly growing, benign skin tumour emanating from the hair follicle complex (see Figure 96). Clinically and histologically, it is virtually indistinguishable from SCC.

(E) Incidence 100-400:100,000 per year

(Ae) Idiopathic, possible association with UV radiation, HPV infection, skin damage, chemical exposure, or immunosuppression

- (R) Middle age, frequent exposure to sunlight, ♂, fair skin type, trauma (e.g. surgery, laser therapy)
- (Hx) Exposure to sunlight
- (PE) (P) Sun-exposed skin (face or extremities)
  - (A) Solitary
  - (S) 1-2 cm in diameter
  - (S) Convex, raised with a central crater (keratotic plug)
  - (O) Well-demarcated
  - (N) Skin-coloured to red
  - (E) Nodule, crusts, may present with telangiectasias
- (Dx) Radical biopsy to confirm/rule out malignancy: histopathological findings include epidermal hyperplasia with eosinophilic keratinocytes, central invagination with keratotic core, epidermal lipping over the peripheral rim of keratotic core, mixed inflammatory infiltrate in dermis
- (Tx) 💊 Multiple lesions: oral retinoids
  - ✒ Excision with a 5 mm margin, due to close resemblance to SCC
- (P) Characteristic course: rapid growth <6-8 wk, sometimes followed by spontaneous regression within 3-12 mo, often with scarring
- (!) Immunocompromised patients and individuals with Ferguson-Smith syndrome (autosomal dominant disorder) may present with multiple KAs

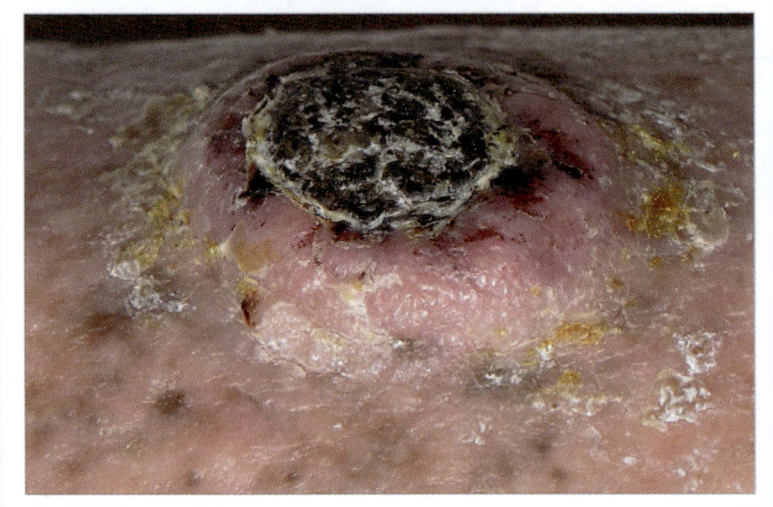

Figure 96 // Keratoacanthoma

Lipoma

- (D) A lipoma is a painless, local accumulation of fat in the subcutis (see Figure 97).
- (E) Prevalence 1%, incidence 210:100,000 per year (underestimated), most common benign soft-tissue neoplasm
- (Ae) Idiopathic, genetic and metabolic components
- (R) DM, hypercholesterolaemia, obesity, ♂>♀, age >40
- (Hx) Asymptomatic ☺
- (PE) (P) Adipose tissue throughout the body, common sites are the neck, proximal extremities, forearms, and buttocks
  - (A) Solitary, multiple lesions (lipomatosis)
  - (S) Few mm to 10 cm
  - (S) Oval, round, or multilobular
  - (O) Moderately to well-demarcated
  - (N) Skin-coloured
  - (E) Flaccid-elastic nodule, separate from underlying and overlying layer
- (Dx) • Histopathological testing or imaging is rarely needed
  - Ultrasound: distinguish from ganglion cyst and rule out malignancy (dedifferentiation → septations and vascularisation). Large lipomas (>11 cm) may warrant an magnetic resonance imaging (MRI) to confirm the diagnosis and rule out liposarcoma with potential neurovascular involvement.
- (Tx) 💬 Generally no treatment needed
  - ✂ Consider excision or liposuction for lipomas in bothersome locations
- (P) Risk of recurrence
- (!) Syndromes such as Gardner syndrome and Richner-Hanhart syndrome can present with multiple lipomas (lipomatosis)

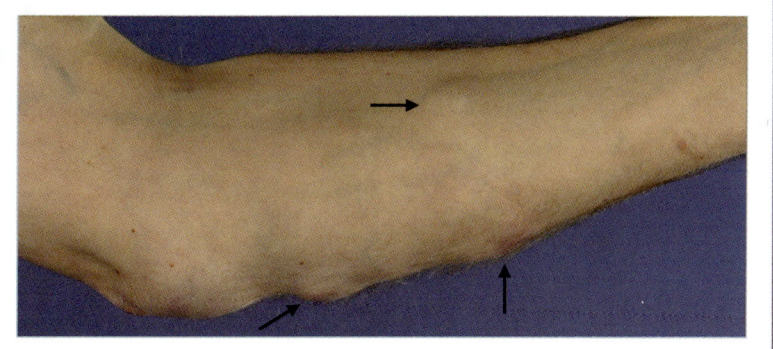

Figure 97 // Lipomas

Seborrhoeic keratosis

- (D) Seborrhoeic keratosis, or senile wart, is a benign papillomatous skin lesion with an oily, verrucous surface (see Figure 98).
- (E) Prevalence ↑ → age ↑, 80-100% in age >50
- (Ae) Exact cause unknown, possible association with activating mutations in fibroblast growth factor receptor (FGFR3), causing epidermal keratinocytes to proliferate
- (R) Advanced age, light skin type, exposure to sunlight
- (Hx) Asymptomatic ⊕, itching ⊖
- (PE) (P) Torso
  - (A) Solitary, sometimes in rows in flexures or in a Christmas-tree pattern on the back
  - (S) Lenticular, several to hundreds in number
  - (S) Round or oval, raised, papillomatous, verrucous
  - (O) Well-demarcated
  - (N) Light to dark brown, black or skin-coloured
  - (E) Papule or plaque
- (Dx) • Dermoscopy: comedo-like openings, milia-like cysts, gyri and sulci, hairpin vessels, fingerprint-like structures, network-like structures
  - If in doubt about diagnosis: PA to rule out malignancy
- (Tx) 💬 Generally no treatment needed
  - 🖊 Liquid nitrogen cryotherapy as first-line treatment on cosmetic grounds. Alternatives include shave excision or electrodesiccation and curettage (ED&C) (for large, thick lesions).
- (P) Increase in number with age, no spontaneous regression
- (!) Leser-Trélat sign is a paraneoplastic phenomenon defined as the abrupt appearance of a large number of seborrhoeic keratosis

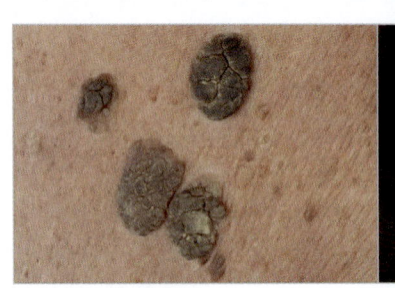

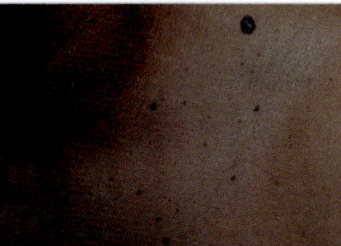

Figure 98A and 98B // Seborrhoeic keratosis

Dermatosis papulosa nigra (DPN)

- **D** DPN is a common benign condition, characterised by small dark coloured papules on the body. The lesions are considered to be a variant of seborrhoeic keratosis.
- **E** 10-30% African American population, prevalence increasing from adolescence
- **Ae** Exact cause unknown, possible association with mutations in FGFR3 and phosphatidylinositol 3-kinase genes
- **R** African descent or other ethnic groups with darkly pigmented skin
- **Hx** Asymptomatic ⊕
- **PE**
  - P Face, neck, upper back, and thorax
  - A Discrete
  - S 1-5 mm, multiple
  - S Round or oval, raised
  - O Well-demarcated
  - N Dark brown to black
  - E Papules
- **Dx** Biopsy to rule out malignancy when in doubt
- **Tx** 🗨 Generally no treatment needed
  - 🔪 Coagulation and curettage, snip removal (for pedunculated lesions), laser therapy
- **P** Increase in number with age, no spontaneous regression
- **I** Due to the risk of hypo- or hyperpigmentation procedures should be done cautiously

---

Benign lichenoid keratosis

- **D** Lichenoid keratosis, or lichen planus-like keratosis, is a common, benign, and often solitary skin lesion. It involves more of a histopathological diagnosis rather than a clinical diagnosis.
- **E** Exact prevalence unknown, considered common
- **Ae** Inflammatory destruction of a pre-existing epidermal lesion (e.g. solar lentigo or seborrhoeic keratosis)
- **R** Pale to fair skin type, adults
- **Hx** Asymptomatic ⊕, itching ⊖
- **PE**
  - P On UV-exposed areas (trunk, upper extremities, face, neck)
  - A Solitary
  - S Generally <1 cm, sometimes ≤2 cm

- (S) Flat, slightly elevated
- (O) Moderately demarcated
- (N) Pink-red (inflammatory phase, grey-brown (pigmented phase)
- (E) Papule or plaque

(Dx)
- Dermoscopy: grey dots uniformly distributed throughout the lesion
- Skin biopsy: band-shaped infiltrate mainly consisting of lymphocytes, histiocytes, sometimes eosinophils or plasma cells, border inflammation with vacuolisation, pigment incontinence, and apoptotic keratinocytes (civatte bodies). Sometimes remnants of lentigo solaris or seborrhoeic keratosis.

(Tx) 👁 Benign, no treatment required
🔪 Cryotherapy (e.g. for cosmetic reasons)

(P) Resolves spontaneously, does not become malignant

(!) May show resemblance to a superficial BCC

Neurofibroma

(D) Neurofibromas are benign peripheral nerve sheath tumours that can manifest as dermal or subcutaneous nodules (see Figure 99). They are categorised into three primary types: localised, diffuse, and plexiform. The plexiform type develops before age 4-5 and is indicative of neurofibromatosis type 1. It is associated with an elevated risk of transformation into malignant sarcoma. Most other neurofibromas arise sporadically and occur in adults.

(E) Incidence of neurofibromatosis type 1 is 100:100,000, type 2 is 3:100:000, ±10% of neurofibromas are associated with neurofibromatosis type 1 or 2

(Ae) Absence of a segment in the NF1 gene → encodes the tumour suppressor protein neurofibromin

(R) Positive FHx

(Hx) Asymptomatic ☺, often cosmetic concern. Some patients may experience irritation, itching, pain, or paresthesia.

(PE)
- (P) Trunk, head, neck, extremities
- (A) Solitary or diffuse
- (S) 2-20 mm
- (S) Oval or round
- (O) Variable, depending on the depth
- (N) Skin-coloured or hyperpigmented
- (E) Papule, nodule, subcutaneous mass, indurated plaque

(Dx) Biopsy required to confirm the diagnosis; in cases of larger lesions additional imaging (computed tomography (CT)/MRI) may be required

- **Tx** 🔪 Surgical excision
- **P** • Local recurrence ⊖
  - Frequently localised lesions with a low risk of progression to malignancy
- **!** • Consider malignant peripheral nerve sheath tumours (MPNST), which arise from peripheral nerves or neurofibromas. They can occur in 50% in association with neurofibromatosis type 1. These tumours are challenging to treat and tend to have a poor prognosis due to their aggressive nature and high rate of recurrence.
  - Watch for other manifestations of neurofibromatosis, e.g. café-au-lait macules, axillary freckling, and Lisch nodules (pigmented iris hamartomas) if multiple neurofibromas are present

> 💡 Neurofibromas exhibit a distinctive **buttonhole sign**, in which the lesion withdraws into the subcutaneous tissue upon palpation and reemerges when pressure is released.

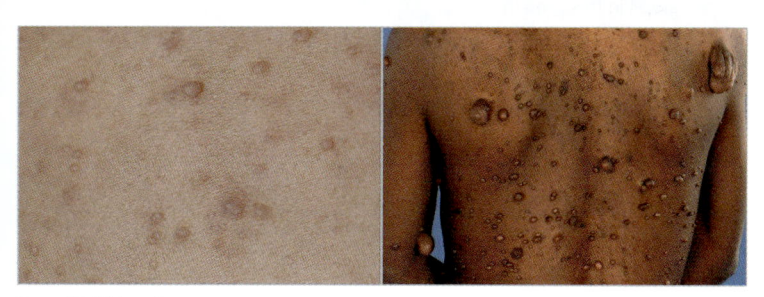

Figure 99 // Neurofibromas

Premalignant skin lesions

Actinic keratosis (AK)

- **D** AK is a common cutaneous lesion that results from the proliferation of atypical epidermal keratinocytes, often appearing as erythematous, scaly papules or plaques on sun-exposed areas of the skin (see Figure 100). This condition is considered premalignant due to its potential progression to SCC.
- **E** Prevalence 14%, incidence 190:100,000 per year
- **Ae** Excessive and cumulative exposure to UV radiation from the sun can lead to pathological changes in the epidermal keratinocytes, resulting in intraepidermal proliferation of dysplastic keratinocytes

- **R** Pale to fair skin, extensive UV/sun exposure, history of sunburn, geographical location (close to Equator, Australia)
- **Hx** Asymptomatic ☺, local tenderness or a stinging sensation in some cases
- **PE**
  - **P** Sun-exposed areas
  - **A** Solitary or multiple
  - **S** Few mm to 2 cm
  - **S** Polymorphic, keratotic
  - **O** Variable demarcation
  - **N** Erythematous or skin-coloured
  - **E** Macule, papule, or plaque, often with scales; a cutaneous horn may be present
- **Dx** Biopsy (deep shave/saucerisation, or punch biopsy) if the lesion >1 cm in diameter, rapidly growing, ulcerated, tender, fails to respond to appropriate therapy, or has underlying induration. If the lesion is too large or scarring is a concern, biopsy only the thickest part of the lesion because SCC most likely develops in this area in AK.
- **Tx**
  - In case of multiple lesions: topical fluorouracil, topical tirbanibulin, imiquimod
  - Liquid nitrogen cryosurgery, photodynamic therapy, shave excision, curettage, carbon dioxide laser
- **P** Progression to SCC in 0.1-3% of cases, most lesions persist as AKs or regress.
- **!**
  - Mostly no progression to SCC
  - The presence of AKs indicates chronic sun damage and therefore ↑ risk of developing SCC and basal cell carcinoma (BCC)

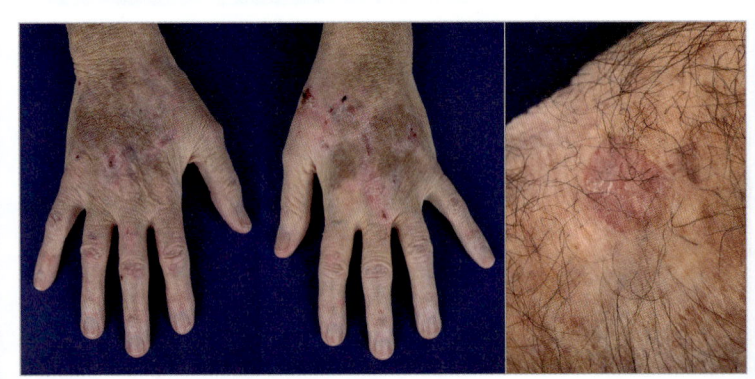

Figure 100 // Actinic keratosis

Bowen's disease

- (D) Bowen's disease (intraepidermal SCC) can be considered an in situ variant of SCC (See Figure 101). Most common in sun-exposed areas, but can also appear elsewhere.
- (E) Incidence 15-174:100,000 per year
- (Ae) Continuous exposure to UV radiation → DNA damage and suppressed immune function → promote clonal expansion of any underlying p53 mutation
- (R) Fair skin, extensive UV/sun exposure, history of sunburn, exposure to carcinogens (e.g. arsenic ingestion through well water, older medications, occupational chemicals), immunosuppression, ionising radiation, thermal skin injury, inflammatory dermatoses
- (Hx) Asymptomatic ↔, gradual enlargement of the lesion over the course of years
- (PE) (P) Head, neck, and extremities (sun-exposed sites)
  - (A) Mostly solitary, sometimes multiple
  - (S) Lenticular to nummular
  - (S) Polymorphic
  - (O) Well-demarcated
  - (N) Erythematous, skin-coloured or pigmented
  - (E) Scaly patch or plaque
- (Dx) Punch biopsy or diagnostic excision if the diagnosis is uncertain
- (Tx) 💊 Topical 5-fluorouracil, imiquimod
  - 🔪 Cryotherapy, curettage with cautery, photodynamic therapy, standard surgical excision, Mohs micrographic surgery, laser, radiotherapy
- (P) Risk of progression to invasive SCC: 3%
- (!) Bowen's disease may serve as a potential indicator for an increased risk of other non-melanoma skin cancers, reported in 33%, BCC typically diagnosed simultaneously with Bowen's disease

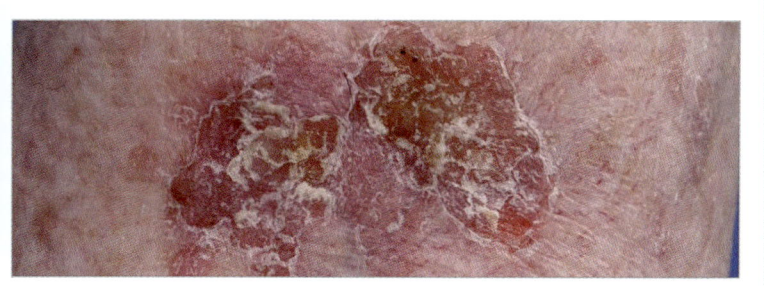

Figure 101 // Bowen's disease (intraepidermal SCC)

Malignant skin tumours

Basal cell carcinoma (BCC)

- (D) BCC is a locally invasive, malignant skin tumour that grows slowly and rarely metastasises (see Figure 102). BCC is the most common malignant tumour and accounts for about 75% of all keratinocyte cancers. Morbidity may be high following infiltration into adjacent tissue; see Table 30 for the different subtypes.
- (E) Average lifetime risk for fair-skinned individuals (Fitzpatrick skin phototype I-II) to develop BCC is approximately 30%. Prevalence in darker skinned patients 4-5%, with higher morbidity due to delay in diagnosis.
- (Ae) UV light → DNA mutations → tumour formation
- (R) Light skin, UV and sun exposure, positive PMHx, ♂, advanced age, immunosuppression, sometimes part of genetic syndromes such as basal cell naevus syndrome, phototherapy (PUVA, PUVB), chronic arsenic exposure
- (Hx) Frequent sun exposure (occupation, gardening), medication (immunosuppressants)
- (PE) (P) Whole body, but typically on sun-exposed areas
  - (A) Solitary
  - (S) Mm to several cm
  - (S) Round or oval, raised margin
  - (O) Well-demarcated
  - (N) Pale to fair skin: gray/pink. Darker skin types: pearly or more commonly pigmented variant.
  - (E) Tumour
- (Dx) • Dermoscopy: pearly lustre, arborising and superficial telangiectasias, multiple erosions, ulceration, ovoid nests, globules, focused dots, leaf-like areas, spoke-wheel areas, concentric structures
  - Histopathological confirmation after excision (diagnostics are also the treatment)
- (Tx) • Superficial BCC: local pharmacological therapy with imiquimod or 5-fluorouracil cream
  - Advanced or metastatic BCC (very rare): vismodegib or sonidegib
  - Superficial BCC: conventional excision, PDT, cryotherapy, laser ablation
  - Nodular, spiky, micronodular BCC: conventional excision or Mohs surgery
- (P) • Depends on growth, site, size, and whether the tumour is primary or recurrent

- Generally favourable: metastasis is very rare and cure rate >95%

! A one-off BCC does not warrant follow-up check-ups. Annual check-ups are enough for patients with multiple tumours or those on immunosuppressants.

> Typical features of BCC are a pearly lustre and telangiectasias upon inspection with a dermatoscope.

> Basal cell naevus syndrome (BCNS), or Gorlin syndrome, is an inherited condition marked by the development of multiple basal cell carcinomas and distinct facial features such as wide-set eyes, a saddle-shaped nose, a prominent forehead (frontal bossing), and a pronounced chin (prognathism).

SUBTYPES	GROWTH PATTERN
Nodular BCC	Well-demarcated
Superficial BCC	Superficial, often multifocal
Infiltrative BCC	Infiltrates the dermis, ill-demarcated borders
Micronodular BCC	Small, rounded nests, aggressive growth
Morpheaform BCC	Ill-demarcated borders, aggressive growth

Table 30 // BCC subtypes and growth patterns

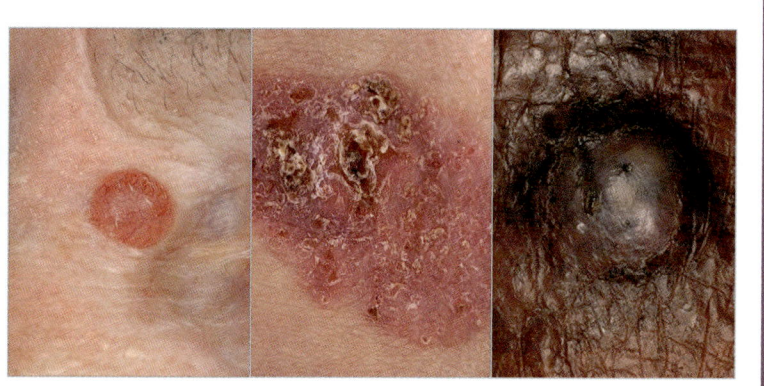

Figure 102A, 102B, and 102C // Basal cell carcinoma, nodular (left and right) and superficial type (middle)

Figure 103 // H zone

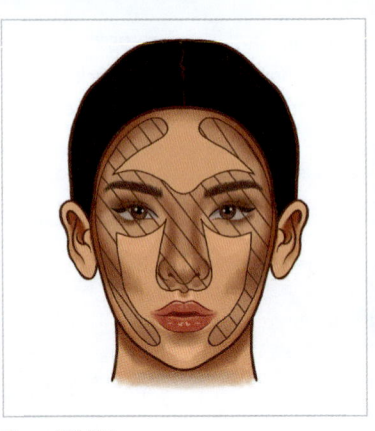

BCCs in the H-zone (see Figure 103) carry a higher risk of deeper tissue invasion and recurrence compared to those in non-H zones. This area may predispose BCCs to a more aggressive course, often associated with ulceration and deeper tissue destruction.

Squamous cell carcinoma (SCC)

- (D) A primary SCC is a malignancy presenting with local invasion, forming from epidermal squamous cells (see Figure 104). Premalignant pathologies are actinic keratosis, leukoplakia, and Bowen's disease. Verrucous carcinoma is a low-grade form of SCC.
- (E) Incidence of cutaneous SCC (cSCC) is ↑, esp. in ♀ 72:100,000 and ♂ >80y 541:100,000 per year
- (Ae) Arises from premalignant pathology: AK → Bowen's disease (= in-situ SCC) → SCC
- (R) ♀: light skin (Fitzpatrick skin phototype I-II), blond or red hair, blue eyes, freckles, exposure to UV/sunlight ☺, ♂, advanced age, smoking, immunosuppression, (premalignant) skin pathology (scars, burns, chronic wounds, lichen sclerosus, AK, Bowen's disease)
- (Hx) Frequent sun exposure (occupation, gardening), medication (immunosuppressants)
- (PE) Suspicion of SCC should prompt palpation of regional lymph nodes for possible metastases:
    - (P) Common sites: head and face, ears, lips, forearms, backs of hands, legs
    - (A) Solitary
    - (S) Variable
    - (S) Jagged, irregular
    - (O) Well-demarcated

- (N) Skin-coloured, red, black
- (E) Nodule, hyperkeratosis, central ulceration
- (Dx) Dermoscopy: erythematous plaque, frequently with central ulceration
  - Histopathology following biopsy or excision: partially absent epithelium, erosion or ulcer, infiltrative epithelial proliferation penetrating the basal membrane
  - Fine needle aspiration cytology of suspected lymph nodes
  - Consider PET CT, CT, or MRI for suspected infiltrative growth or distant metastases, ultrasound-guided biopsy for local lymphadenopathy to diagnose/rule out metastases
- (Tx) Primary cSCC: surgical excision (5 mm clinical margin for low-risk tumours, 1 cm margin for high-risk and recurrent tumours) with postoperative margin assessment or Mohs surgery, adjuvant radiotherapy for high-risk localised SCC or for non-surgical patients/tumours
  - Local radiotherapy or lymph node dissection in case of metastases
  - Metastatic or locally advanced cSCC: anti-PD-1 agents (cemiplimab)
- (P) Prognostic risk factors: >6 mm thickness; perineural invasion; angioinvasion; location on ear, lip, temple, or cheek; moderately, poorly, or undifferentiated carcinoma
  - Low mortality, around 1%
  - The frequency of follow-up visits and diagnostics for subsequent new cSCC depends on underlying risk factors

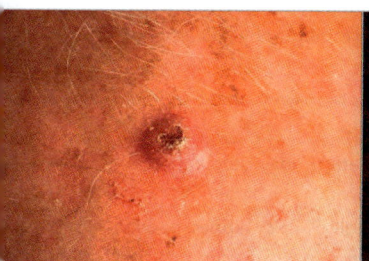

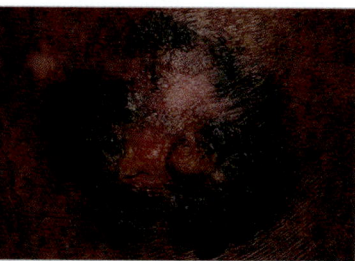

Figure 104A and 104B // Squamous cell carcinoma

Melanoma

(D) Melanomas emanate from melanocytes (pigment-forming cells) and are one of the most aggressive forms of skin cancer. Most melanomas develop over 1-2 years and have a strong tendency to metastasise (see Figure 105).

- (E) Incidence in Europe 10-25:100,000; USA 20-30:100,000; Australia 50-60:100,000 per year
- (Ae) Arises from pre-existing naevi or spontaneously
  - UV light → DNA mutations → tumour formation (esp. in light-skinned individuals)
- (R) Light complexion (Fitzpatrick skin phototype I-II), blond or red hair, blue eyes, freckles, UV or sunlight exposure ☺, positive PMHx, ♀, >100 naevi in total, >5 atypical naevi, actinic damage, and/or lentigines
- (Hx) Positive PMHx, lesion change (e.g. growth), itching, pain, ulcerations, spontaneous bleeding from naevus
- (PE) (P) Whole body
  - (A) Solitary, asymmetrical
  - (S) Often >6 mm
  - (S) Jagged and irregular
  - (O) Well-demarcated
  - (N) >2 colours
  - (E) Macule, ulcerating tumour possible
- (Dx) Dermoscopy: asymmetry, multiple colours, atypical pigment network, irregular brown-black dots/globules/clods, irregular streaks (lines), irregular blotch/hyperpigmented areas, white shiny streaks/lines, and regression structures
  - Histopathology after diagnostic excision (with 2 mm margin): melanoma
  - At advanced stage: cerebral, thoracic, abdominal, and pelvic CT and fluorodeoxyglucose positron emission tomography (FDG-PET)/CT to rule out metastases
  - Suspected metastases: fine-needle biopsy/cytology, sentinel node procedure
- (Tx) Chemotherapy and immunotherapy: may be curative, but mainly palliative for metastases
  - Sentinel node procedure at stage pT1b or higher; patients may qualify for adjuvant therapy based on results
  - Excision: with 1-2 cm margin depending on Breslow depth (Breslow ≤2 mm: 1 cm, Breslow >2 mm: 2 cm), 0.5 cm margin for in-situ melanoma
  - Radiotherapy: both curative and palliative
- (P) >80% heal completely, ±20% develop hematogenous metastases, lymphogenous metastasis possible
- (!) Many melanomas do not present with classic features such as itching, pain

growth, or size and colour change
- Beware of melanoma underdiagnosis in individuals with darker skin types, esp. on hands, feet, and nails
- Early diagnosis is very important given the limited therapeutic options

> Always remove lesions suspicious of melanoma completely: never take a partial biopsy.

> **Hutchinson's sign** is the periungual extension of brown-black pigmentation from longitudinal melanonychia onto the proximal and lateral nail folds, which is an important indicator of subungual melanoma.

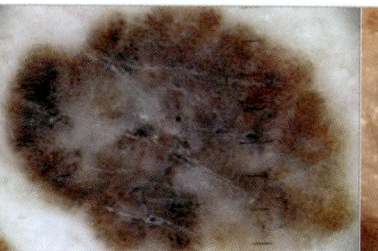

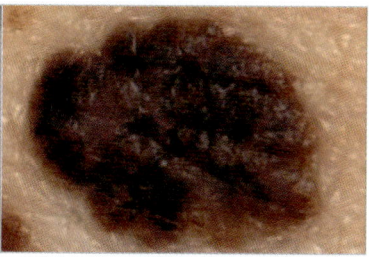

Figure 105A // Melanoma

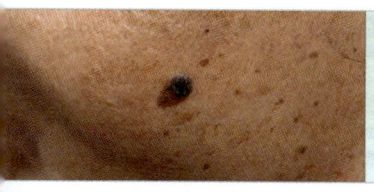

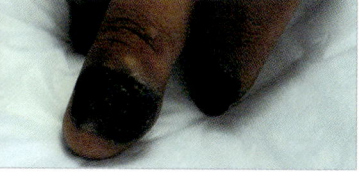

Figure 105B // Melanoma

Lentigo maligna (LM)

(D) LM is a type of melanoma in situ that typically appears on sun-damaged facial and neck skin in older individuals (see Figure 106). LM progresses slowly over many years and has the potential to advance to invasive lentigo maligna melanoma (LMM).

(E) Incidence 5.6:100,000 per year, peak incidence between 65-80y

(Ae) Uncontrolled proliferation of melanocytes → formation of atypical and dysplastic melanocytes in the epidermis

- (R) Age ↑, sun-damaged skin, number of lentigines ↑, number of AK ↑, and history of previous keratinocyte carcinomas
- (Hx) Asymptomatic, asymmetrical, pigmented lesion on severly sun-damaged skin
- (PE) (P) Head or neck
  - (A) Solitary
  - (S) Less than one to several cm
  - (S) Irregular
  - (O) Moderately to well-demarcated
  - (N) From light brown or tan to dark brown, black, pink, red, or white
  - (E) Macula
- (Dx) Excisional biopsy with narrow margins, in some cases deep shave (saucerisation)
- (Tx) 🖉 Topical imiquimod (if surgery is not feasible)
  - 🖋 Excision with 5-10 mm margins, Mohs micrographic surgery, radiation therapy (if surgery is not feasible)
- (P) Progression of LM to LMM in 5%
- (!) LM has a tendency to spread subclinically. Atypical melanocytes frequently extend a significant distance beyond the clinical margin of LM, occasionally involving 'skip' areas. This phenomenon, known as the 'field effect', is responsible for the recurrence of LM at the periphery following an initial, seemingly successful excision.

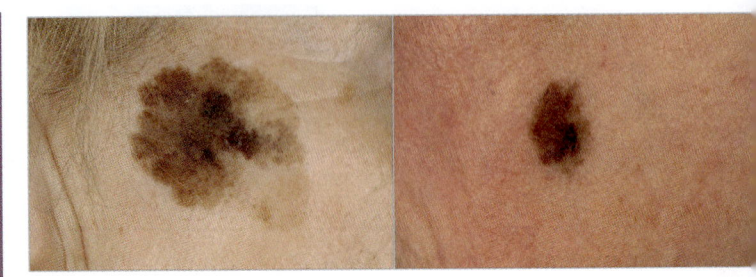

Figure 106 // Lentigo maligna with field effect

Cutaneous T-cell lymphoma (CTCL)

- (D) CTCL is a rare type of non-Hodgkin lymphoma that primarily presents in the skin, with no evidence of extracutaneous disease at the time of diagnosis. The most common type of CTCLs is mycosis fungoides. More rare variants of the disease include Sézary syndrome and primary cutaneous CD30+ lymphoproliferative disorders, such as anaplastic large cell lymphoma and lymphomatoid papulosis (see Figure 107).

- (E) Incidence 1:100,000 per year, peak incidence 55-74y
- (Ae) The pathogenesis of CTCL is thought to involve the dysregulation of specific genes, incl. cancer-testis genes and B lymphoid tyrosine kinase, as well as aberrant signalling through pathways such as JAK3/STAT and NOTCH1
- (R) Cutaneous inflammation (e.g. chronic urticaria, chemical exposure)
- (Hx) Persisting rash, itching ⊖, history of skin diseases
- (PE) (P) Non-sun-exposed areas, e.g. buttocks, thighs, breasts
  - (A) Solitary
  - (S) >5 cm
  - (S) Variable
  - (O) Well-demarcated
  - (N) Erythematous
  - (E) Patches or plaques
- (Dx) Biopsy required to confirm the diagnosis, followed by histopathological and immunophenotype analysis
- (Tx) 🖊 Stage I (limited patches/flat plaques): topical steroids, UVA, UVB, and topical cytostatic agents, e.g. mechlorethamine (nitrogen mustard)
  - 🖊 More advanced stages: local radiotherapy, systemic therapy with IFN-alpha or retinoids, often in combination with UVA; retinoids or total skin electron beam therapy in combination with IFN-alpha
- (P) Variable, depending on the type and stage of the disease
- (!) The common differentials for CTCL include erythroderma like atopic dermatitis, drug eruptions, erythrodermic psoriasis, and lichen planus

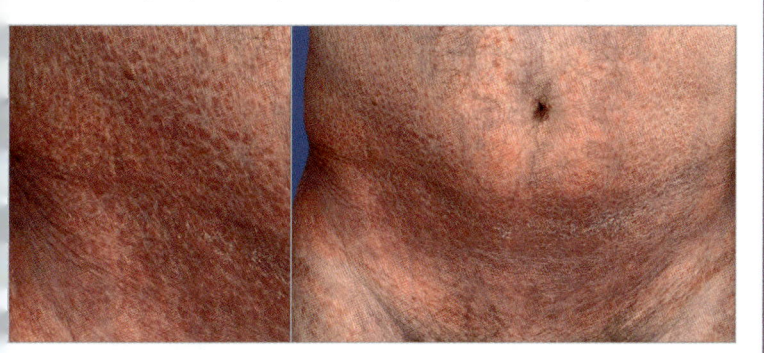

Figure 107 // Cutaneous T-cell lymphoma

Naevi

Acquired melanocytic naevus

- D An acquired melanocytic naevus, also known as a mole or naevocellular naevus, is a benign hyperpigmentation arising from naevus cell proliferation (see Figures 108 and 109). A distinction is made between epidermal naevi, dermal naevi, and compound naevi (see Figures 110 - 113).
- E Common, greatest in number before age 30, followed by a drop-off in number
- Ae Proliferation of altered melanocytes (naevus cells, see Table 31)
- R Hereditary factors, triggers: sunlight, bullous dermatoses, systemic immunosuppression, elevated hormone levels (e.g. pregnancy)
- Hx Asymptomatic ⊕, birthmarks
- PE
  - P Anywhere on the skin
  - A Solitary
  - S Several to multiple, 2-6 mm
  - S Round, oval, or dome-shaped
  - O Well-demarcated
  - N Compound naevus: lighter in colour; dermal naevus: brown, light-brown, or skin-coloured
  - E Compound naevus: papillomatous or verrucous; dermal naevus: papillomatous or papule, may be pedunculated
- Dx
  - Dermoscopy: differentiate from melanoma based on the ABCDE rules (see Figure 17)
  - When in doubt: biopsy/excision to rule out malignancy. Excision is prefered to avoid sample error as malignant transformation may vary within the lesion.
- Tx 🗨 Regular skin checks upon indication (>5 atypical naevi and/or >100 naevi)
  ✏️ Cosmetic indication: shave excision or curretage
- P Dermal naevi pose no risk of malignant progression, large numbers of moles (>100) or atypical moles are a risk factor for developing melanoma
- ! DDx: consider dysplastic naevus or melanoma

Figure 108 // Dermal naevus

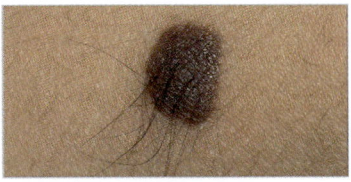

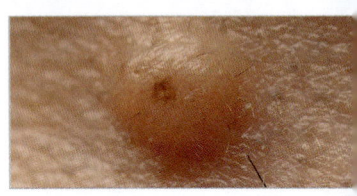

Figure 109 // Naevocellular naevus

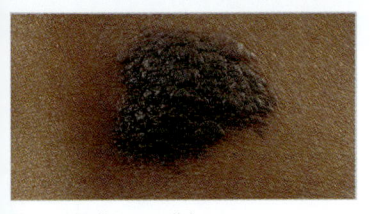

Figure 110 // Naevocellular naevus

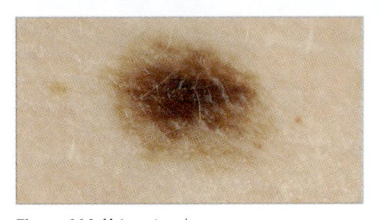

Figure 111 // Junctional naevus

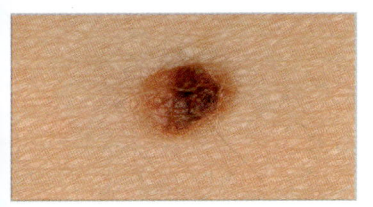

Figure 112 // Epidermal/dermal naevocellular naevus (compound naevus)

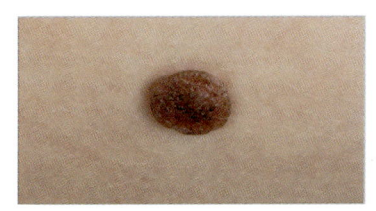

Figure 113 // Papillomatous naevus

Figure 114 // Becker naevus

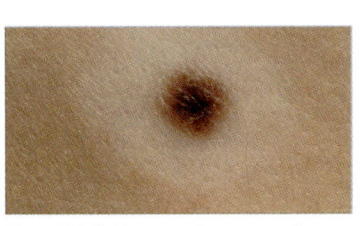

Figure 115 // Halo naevus (Sutton-naevus)

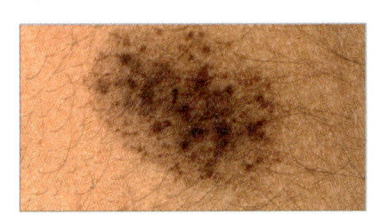

Figure 116 // Sebaceous naevus

Figure 117 // Spilus naevus

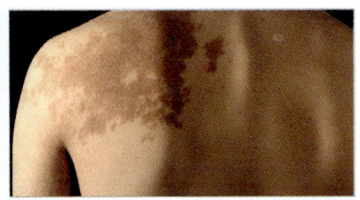

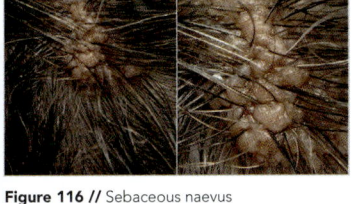

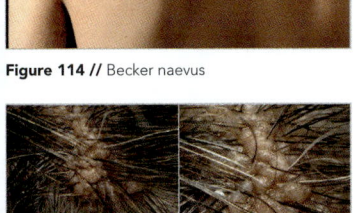

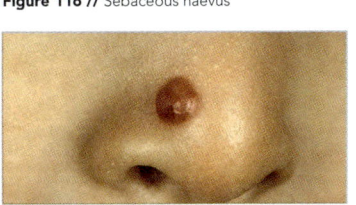

Figure 118 // Spitz naevus

	BECKER NAEVUS	**HALO NAEVUS**
D	Becker naevus, or Becker melanosis, is a common benign cutaneous hamartoma with epidermal or dermal elements (see Figure 114).	Halo naevus, or Sutton's naevus, is a melanocytic naevus surrounded by a round or oval, usually symmetric, halo of depigmentation (see Figure 115).
Ae	Potential role of androgenic stimulation, somatic mutations of beta-actin (ACTB) in pilar muscles	T cell-mediated immune response to naevus antigens, causing regression of the naevus
R	♂>♀	Children, large number of naevi, vitiligo, Turner syndrome
PE	(P) Classically manifests unilaterally on the shoulder and upper trunk (A) Solitary (S) Unilateral, >10 cm (S) Variable (O) Irregular margins (N) Tan to brown (E) Patch or thin plaque	(P) Commonly seen on the back, but could appear anywhere (A) Solitary, sometimes multiple (S) Variable (S) Variable (O) Moderately well-demarcated (N) Brown or pink central naevus, depigmentated halo (E) Macula
Dx	Dermoscopy: prominent pigment network, blotchy hyperpigmentation in the centre, terminal hairs, and parafollicular hyperpigmentation	Dermoscopy: globular and/or homogeneous patterns, minority exhibiting a reticular pattern
Tx	No excision needed. If desired for cosmetic reasons, hyperpigmentation can be treated with laser therapy.	No excision needed

Table 31A // Naevi

NAEVUS SEBACEOUS	NAEVUS SPILUS	SPITZ NAEVUS
Naevus sebaceous is a benign congenital hamartoma characterised by hyperplasia of the epidermis, immature hair follicles, and sebaceous and apocrine glands (pilosebaceous follicular unit), see Figure 116.	Naevus spilus, or speckled lentiginous naevus, is a form of a congenital melanocytic naevi, characterised by a hyperpigmented patch that often develops darker macules and papules in a 'speckled' distribution during puberty (see Figure 117).	Spitz naevus, or Spitz tumour, is a benign, uncommon melanocytic lesion composed of large epithelioid and/or spindled cells, typically presenting during childhood or early adolescence (<12y), see Figure 118.
Postzygotic (sporadic) somatic mutations of the RAS protein family	Localised defect in neural crest melanoblasts	Unknown, potential role for hormonal activation or genetics (≤30% exhibit RAS mutations, 60% exhibit chromosomal rearrangement-induced fusions)
No specific risk factors, affects all genders and ethnicities	No specific risk factors, affects all genders and ethnicities	Pale and fair skin types
(P) Scalp, forehead, face, or neck (A) Solitary (S) One to several cm (S) Oval, round or linear, in older children and adults more elevated or verrucous (O) Well-demarcated (N) Yellow-orange or tan during infancy (E) Plaque	(P) Can appear on any body site, most often the trunk (A) Solitary, sometimes multiple (S) 3-6 cm on average, sometimes up to 60 cm (S) Round, oval, sometimes linear along Blaschko's lines (O) Well-demarcated (N) Tan or light brown (macula), darker brown (speckled lentigines or papules) (E) Macule or patch, with smaller lentigines, macula, or papules	(P) Most commonly located on the lower extremities or face (A) Solitary (S) 1-2 cm (S) Round, dome-shaped (O) Sharply demarcated (N) Pink, red, or brown (E) Papule or plaque
Dermoscopy: yellow or brown globules, whitish-yellow and greyish papillary appearance or homogenous whitish-yellow pattern	Dermoscopy: darker brown reticular or globular pattern on homogenous brown lattice background	Dermoscopy: little to no pigmentation, dotted vascular pattern, starburst pattern, or reticular pattern with peripheral globules
Full thickness excision could be considered based on size and location	No excision needed	- Clinical monitoring every 3-12 mo - Diagnostic excision for atypical appear-ance (asymmetrical, >12y)

BECKER NAEVUS	HALO NAEVUS
Examine clinically for associated soft tissue and bony abnormalities (Becker's naevus syndrome)	In adults, halo naevi rarely represent an immune reaction to a cutaneous melanoma

Table 31B // Naevi

Pigmentation disorders

Café-au-lait macule

- Café-au-lait spots are coffee-coloured macules.
- Prevalence at birth of solitary spots 0.3-0.5% in pale to fair skin, 15-18% in darker skin types
- Prevalence in childhood 13% in pale to fair skin to 27% in darker skin types

Melanin production ↑ in melanocytes and melanin levels ↑ in keratinocytes, cause unknown

Mostly observed in light brown to dark brown skin types

Asymptomatic ☺

- Anywhere on the skin
- Solitary
- 2-5 cm (adults), may be smaller or larger (>20 cm)
- Round or oval
- Well-demarcated, regular borders
- Light to dark brown
- Macule

Multiple lesions (≥6): genetic testing to rule out neurofibromatosis (possible characteristics include neurofibromas and axillary freckling)

- Generally no treatment needed
- Cosmetic indication: partial/total removal using laser therapy (e.g. Q-switched Nd:YAG)

No malignant potential

Consider neurofibromatosis in the presence of multiple (≥6) spots ≥0.5 cm in size

NAEVUS SEBACEOUS	NAEVUS SPILUS	SPITZ NAEVUS
Secondary benign and malignant tumours (e.g. trichoblastoma, syringocystadenoma papilliferum, basal cell carcinoma) rarely occur within sebaceous naevi. Risk of malignancy is almost non-existent in children.	Spilus naevus could occur as part of syndromes, e.g. facial features, anorexia, cachexia, eye and skin abnormalities, neurofibromatosis type 1, Ebstein's anomaly. Very low risk of malignant transformation.	Close histological resemblance to melanoma, prognosis in children is good

Solar lentigo

- D Solar lentigo, also commonly known as solar lentigines, actinic lentigo, liver spots, age spots, or sunspots, is a hyperpigmented macular skin lesion that results from chronic sun exposure (see Figure 119).
- E Incidence increases with age, >90% of patients >50y with pale to fair skin
- Ae UV-induced mutations → activation of melanocytes → enhanced melanin production, and abnormal pigment retention by keratinocytes
- R Chronic sun exposure, older age, pale to fair skin
- Hx Asymptomatic 😊, cosmetic complaints
- PE P Anywhere on the skin
  - A Predominantly multiple, sometimes solitary
  - S Lenticular (3-15 mm)
  - S Round or oval
  - O Regular and well-demarcated borders on skin
  - N Light to dark brown
  - E Macule
- Dx Biopsy if lentigo maligna/LMM is suspected
- Tx No treatment needed
  - 💬 Minimise sun exposure, sunscreen
  - 💊 Topical retinoids, topical hydroquinone (depending on country)
  - 🔪 Cryotherapy, laser therapy (e.g. Q-Switched Nd-YAG), intense pulsed light therapy (IPL), chemical peels
- P No malignancy risk
- ❗ • If misdiagnosed, changes in colour, variability in colour, irregular margins, or development of a papular or nodular component can be signs of malignancy
  - Solar lentigines in hidden areas can be overlooked, make sure to also examine skin folds

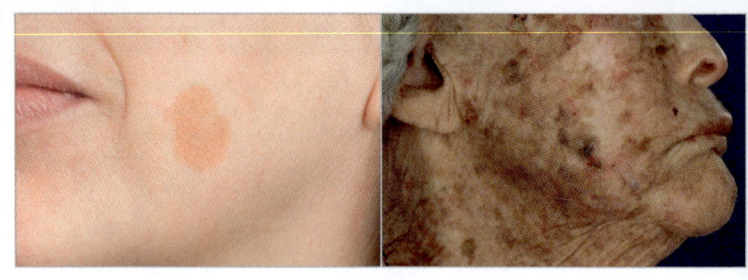

Figure 119 // Solar lentigo

Lentigo simplex

(D) Lentigo simplex is a pigmented lesion that can appear on both the skin and mucous membranes.

(E) Observed worldwide, exact prevalence unknown, first appearance at age 2-3, increases during adolescence and often partially disappears with age ↑

(Ae) Idiopathic, hyperpigmentation caused both by increase of epidermal melanocytes and higher levels of melanin pigment in keratinocytes

(R) None

(Hx) Asymptomatic ☺

(PE) (P) Anywhere on the skin and mucous membranes
- (A) Predominantly multiple, sometimes solitary
- (S) Lenticular (3-15 mm)
- (S) Round or oval
- (O) Regular and well-demarcated borders on skin, irregular pigmentation, fainter/irregular borders on mucous membranes
- (N) Light brown
- (E) Macule

(Dx) No added value

(Tx) 🗨 No treatment needed

✎ For cosmetic indications: chemical peels, cryotherapy, pigment laser (e.g. Q-switched ruby laser), surgical excision

(P) Benign lesion

(!) • Rule out cancerous lesions during physical or histopathological examination
- Generalised lentiginosis may be associated with an underlying syndrome e.g. LEOPARD syndrome or Peutz-Jeghers syndrome

> **Noonan syndrome** with multiple lentigines or **LEOPARD** syndrome is a genetic disease characterised by multiple **L**entigines and café-au-lait spots, **E**lectrocardiographic (ECG) conduction abnormalities, **O**bstructive cardiomyopathy / **O**cular hyperletorism, **P**ulmonar stenosis, **A**bnormal genitalia, **R**etardation of growth, and **D**eafness.

> **Peutz-Jeghers syndrome** (PJS) is a rare genetic disease characterised by hamartomatous gastrointestinal polyps in association with mucocutaneous pigmented macules. This syndrome is associated with an increased cancer risk.

Melasma

- D: Melasma is an acquired, brown pigmentation of the skin in the facial area (see Figure 120). It is often seen in women during pregnancy or using hormonal contraception.
- E: ♀>♂, prevalence 1% (higher prevalent in skin of colour)
- Ae:
  - Exact cause unknown, genetic and hormonal factors involved
  - Melanin production in melanocytes ↑, possibly due to melanocyte-stimulating hormone levels ↑ as a result of elevated oestrogen and progesterone levels during pregnancy
- R: ♀, brown skin type, hormonal contraception, pregnancy, sunlight, medication causing photosensitivity ↑
- Hx: Asymptomatic ☺
- PE:
  - P: Face (forehead, cheeks, temples, periocular, upper lip)
  - A: Solitary or symmetrical
  - S: Variable
  - S: Jagged
  - O: Moderately well-demarcated
  - N: Light to dark brown
  - E: Macule
- Dx: No added value
- Tx:
  - Sun protection (sunscreen SPF 50, avoid sunlight), camouflage cream
  - Consider discontinuing hormonal contraception
  - Monotherapy or combination: hydroquinone 4-5%, non-hydroquinone agents (e.g. corticosteroids (class II), retinoids, azelaic acid, kojic acid, niacinamide), triple therapy (hydroquinone 5%, tretinoin, triamcinolone acetonide). USA: triple combination cream (TCC) (fluocinolone, hy-

droquinone and tretinoin), platelet-rich-plasma (PRP).
- Oral/topical tranexamic acid (off-label)
- Trichloroacetic acid

✏️ Chemical peels, laser therapy (e.g. tixel laser, Q-switched Nd:YAG laser)

(P) Melasma fades or disappears <1y postpartum, less intense in winter

(I) In rare cases, melasma may also occur secondary to ovarian tumours

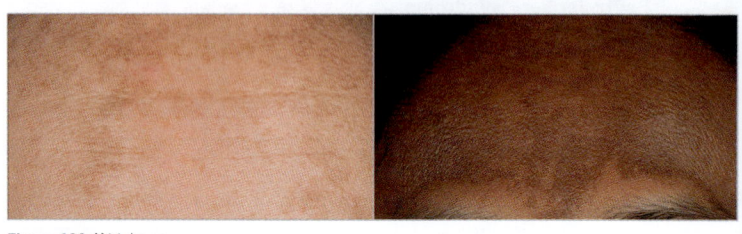

Figure 120 // Melasma

Pityriasis versicolor

(D) Pityriasis versicolor is a yeast infection of the skin (see Figure 121).

(E) Prevalence 30-40% in tropical climates, 1-4% in temperate climates

(Ae) Caused by *Malassezia furfur* (naturally found on human skin); hypopigmentation or hyperpigmentation occurs because *Malassezia* blocks activity of the dopatyrosinase enzyme (blocking the conversion of tyrosine to melanin); transmission unlikely, as it requires highly specific skin conditions

(R) Warm environment, sweat and sebum production ↑, adolescents and adults

(Hx) Itching

(PE) (P) Chest, back, upper arms, face in children
- (A) Multiple, coalescent
- (S) A few mm
- (S) Round or oval
- (O) Moderately to well-demarcated
- (N) Versicolour (= opposite of original skin colour)
- (E) Macular or slightly squamous papules and plaques

(Dx) KOH test if needed: may show budding yeast and have a 'spaghetti and meatballs' appearance

(Tx) 🗨 Hygiene recommendations, e.g. washing towels at 60°C/104°F

💊 • Local antifungal agents e.g. selenium sulfide, ketoconazole cream, terbinafine cream, USA: clotrimazole 1% cream
- Maintenance treatment for scalp (ketoconazole 2% shampoo)

- Systemic: itraconazole, fluconazole
- Prophylaxis: selenium sulfide, ketoconazole 2% shampoo, systemic itraconazole once monthly

P Hypopigmented macules stay visible for a long time after healing and fade after exposure to sunlight, high risk of recurrence

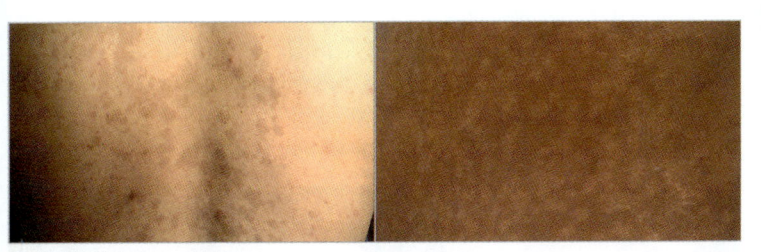

Figure 121 // Pityriasis versicolor

> Supplemental KOH test shows spores and short hyphae, known as 'spaghetti and meatballs'.

> Stretching the skin produces fine scaling in the macule (stretch test).

Vitiligo

D Vitiligo is a benign skin condition associated with well-demarcated depigmented patches (see Figure 122). There are three different morphological types: generalised, segmental, and focal vitiligo.

E Prevalence 0.1-2% in children and adults, 70-80% of adults develop vitiligo <30y

Ae Idiopathic, skin lesions caused by melanocyte destruction, possible autoimmune cause, association with genetic factors

R Age <30, positive FHx (30% familial)

Hx Asymptomatic ☉

PE P Around body orifices (eyes, mouth, genitals, anus), armpits, knees, hands, toes
- A Variable: solitary, segmental or generalised
- S Variable
- S Round, oval, or linear
- O Well-demarcated
- N Depigmentation

- (E) Macule
- (Dx) Wood's lamp to evaluate loss of pigmentation
- (Tx) 💬 Camouflage cream
  - 💊 Topical corticosteroids (class III-IV), topical calcineurin inhibitors, phototherapy, topical JAK inhibitor (ruxolitinib cream 1.5%). If progressing rapidly, oral steroid minipulse
  - 🔪 Consider autologous pigmented skin graft
- (P) Unpredictable condition, progressive, depigmentation is usually permanent and full, spontaneous healing is rare
- (!) Psychological strain on patients can be severe, esp. in dark-skinned patients

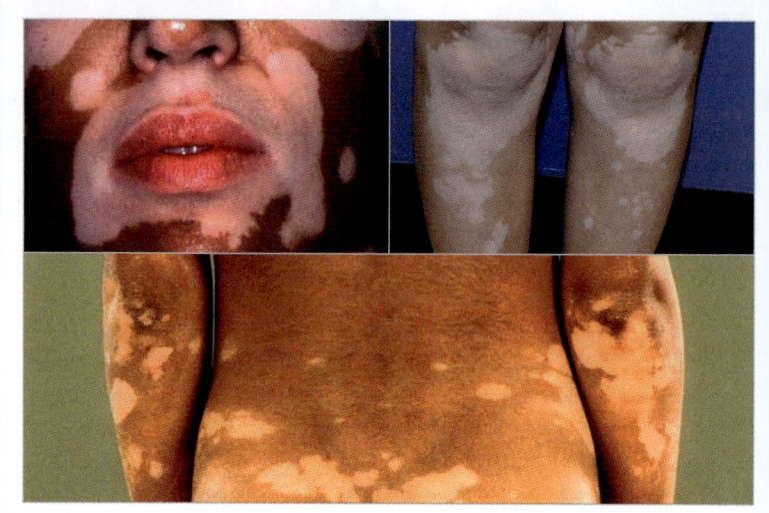

Figure 122A, 122B, and 122C // Vitiligo

Postinflammatory hyperpigmentation (PIH)

- (D) PIH, also known as postinflammatory melanosis or acquired melanosis, is the most common form of hyperpigmentation where the skin develops increased pigmentation as a response to previous inflammation (see Figure 123).
- (E) Exact incidence and prevalence unknown, common
- (Ae) Inflamed skin → release or oxidation of arachidonic acid → prostaglandins and leukotrienes → epidermal melanosis → abnormal distribution of melanin or excess of melanin in epidermis/dermis
- (R) Mostly observed in light brown to dark brown skin types

- **Hx** Preceding inflammatory skin condition, accidental or iatrogenic skin injury
- **PE** **P** Anywhere on the skin
  - **A** Variable: solitary, multiple
  - **S** Variable
  - **S** Variable: round, oval, or linear
  - **O** Well-demarcated
  - **N** Hyperpigmented (e.g. dark brown, gray, or blue-gray)
  - **E** Macule
- **Dx**
  - Biopsy not necessary, only to rule out another cause of the hyperpigmentation
  - Wood's lamp to distinguish primary epidermal melanosis from primary dermal melanosis
- **Tx** 💬 No treatment needed, camouflage
  - 💊 Topical hydroquinone (USA: ≤10% concentration), topical retinoids, hydroquinone-retinoid-corticosteroid triple-agent therapy, azelaic acid
  - 🔪 Chemical peels, laser therapy
- **P** Improves slowly over time
- **!** Be cautious with pharmacological treatment such as topical retinoids, as they can irritate the skin and potentially worsen PIH

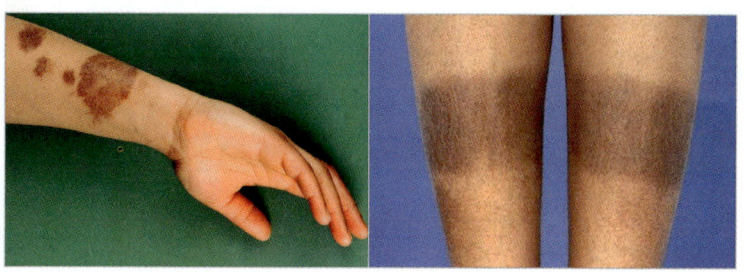

Figure 123 // Postinflammatory hyperpigmentation

Pityriasis alba

- **D** Pityriasis alba is a benign dermatosis characterized by fine scaling and hypopigmentation that primarily affects children and adolescents. It is often regarded as a minor manifestation of atopic dermatitis (see Figure 124).
- **E** Prevalence 5% in children
- **Ae** Exact pathophysiology unknown, associated with melanocytes ↓ in both size and number

- (R) Sun exposure, darker skin types (more prominently visible)
- (Hx) Asymptomatic ⊕, may be itchy
- (PE) (P) Face, upper trunk, upper limbs
  - (A) Solitary, multiple or confluent
  - (S) Variable: 0.5 to a few cm
  - (S) Round, oval, irregular
  - (O) Ill-demarcated
  - (N) Slightly hypopigmented (e.g. pinkish, whitish)
  - (E) Macule or patch, fine scaling
- (Dx) No added value
- (Tx) ● No treatment needed
  - 🔖 Emollients, topical corticosteroid (class I), topical calcineurin inhibitor
- (P) Self-limiting
- (!) • Pityriasis alba can also occur in people who do not have atopic dermatitis
  - Pigmentation variations become more pronounced in the sun, using sunscreen minimises contrast

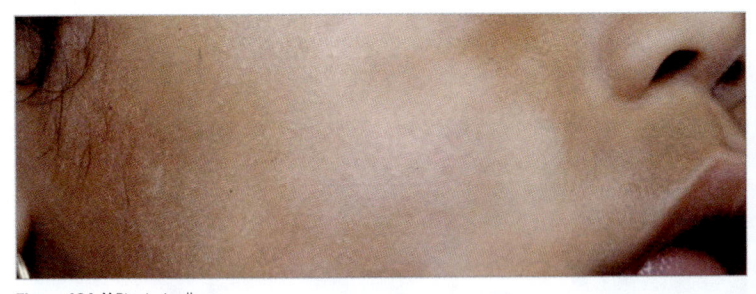

Figure 124 // Pityriasis alba

Acanthosis nigricans

- (D) Acanthosis nigricans is a common condition characterised by hyperpigmentation and hyperkeratosis (thickening) of the skin in the intertriginous areas, causing a velvety, papillomatous skin texture (see Figure 125).
- (E) Prevalence 13.3% of African Americans, 5.5% of Latin Americans, and 34.2% of Native Americans (based on US population data)
- (Ae) Acquired or inherited, associated with insulin resistance → elevated insulin levels → keratinocytes/fibroblast stimulation (IGFR1) → acanthosis nigricans
- (R) Obesity, DM 2
- (Hx) Itchy ⊖, odour ⊖, skin tags

- PE P Neck and axillae, submammary, inguinal region, around the mouth, mucous membranes
  - A Symmetric
  - S Regional
  - S Round, oval
  - O Ill-demarcated
  - N Light brown to dark brown to black
  - E Plaque, papillomatous, skin tags
- Dx
  - Labs: exploratory, incl. glucose, HbA1c, cholesterol, triglycerides, liver function, screening for malignancies if necessary
  - Skin biopsy can be performed to confirm the diagnosis: hyperkeratosis and epidermal papillomatosis
- Tx 💬 Treatment of the underlying cause (e.g. weight loss, diabetes medication)
  - 🔗 Topical retinoids, topical vitamin D analogs, systemic retinoids
  - ✂ Surgical removal of skin tags (e.g. electrocoagulation, cryotherapy)
- P Chronic disorder, responds well when treating the underlying cause
- !
  - Malignant acanthosis nigricans is a rarer form, associated with internal malignancies (e.g. gastric adenocarcinoma). It typically presents with more severe and extensive skin changes compared to the benign form.
  - Associated with obesity, insulin resistance, genetic factors, certain medications (e.g. corticosteroids, oral contraceptives), endocrine disorders (e.g. PCOS)

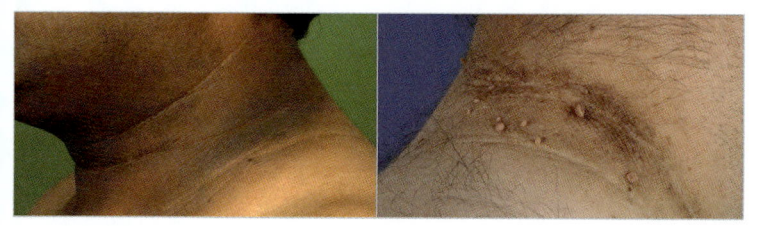

Figure 125 // Acanthosis nigricans

Erythema dyschromicum perstans (EDP)

D EDP, or ashy dermatosis, is a rare, slowly progressing acquired hypermelanosis characterised by the appearance of erythematous macules, which develop into persistent ashy (greyish) or bluish macules, sometimes preceded by a phase with an erythematous macule or border (see Figure 126). It can develop gradually in a symmetric distribution.

- E Exact incidence and prevalence unknown
- Ae Unknown
- R Latin American descent, pale to light beige skin types
- Hx Asymptomatic ⊕
- PE
  - P Trunk, neck, upper extremities, face
  - A Variable: multiple, confluent
  - S Variable size
  - S Variable: oval, circular, irregularly shaped
  - O Moderately-demarcated
  - N Slate-grey to blue-brown
  - E Macules or patches
- Dx Skin biopsy can be performed to confirm diagnosis
- Tx 💬 Difficult to treat, sunscreen, UV light therapy (e.g. PUVA)
  - 🧴 Topical corticosteroids (acute erythematous phase), topical calcineurin inhibitors, topical hydroquinone, oral ABx (e.g. clofazimine, dapsone)
  - ✏️ Laser therapy
- P Slowly progressive and persistent
- ! EPD is difficult to diagnose; shares clinical and histologic features with other entities, e.g. lichen planus pigmentosus, lichenoid drug eruption, infectious diseases (e.g. leprosy), and postinflammatory hyperpigmentation

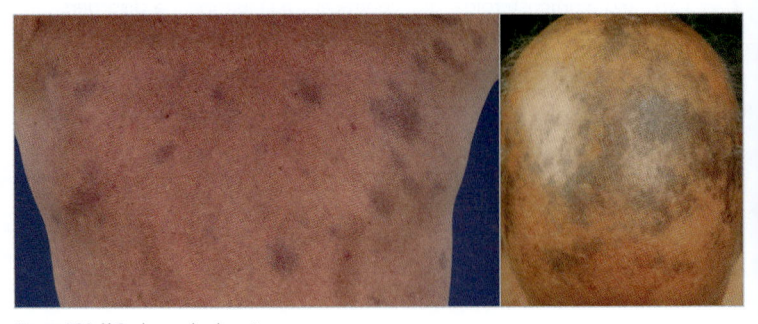

Figure 126 // Erythema dyschromicum perstans

Progressive macular hypomelanosis (PMH)

- D PMH is a common skin disorder characterised by ill-defined, non-scaly hypopigmented macules typically located on the trunk around the midline (see Figure 127).
- E Exact incidence and prevalence unknown

- **Ae** Exact aetiology unknown, association with *Cutibacterium acnes* (or different subtypes of *Cutibacterium* spp.) and smaller/lesser melanised melanosomes → decreased melanin synthesis → hypopigmentation
- **R** ♀, adults and adolescents, darker skin types, tropical environment
- **Hx** Asymptomatic ☺
- **PE**
  - **P** Trunk, upper extremities, neck and head (less common)
    - **A** Diffuse, confluent (in and around the midline)
    - **S** Multiple, nummular
    - **S** Round, oval, irregular
    - **O** Ill-demarcated
    - **N** Hypopigmented
    - **E** Macule
- **Dx** Wood's lamp: punctiform, orange-red, follicular fluorescence in lesional skin, KOH ⊖
- **Tx** 💊 Combination topical ABx (e.g. clindamycin), topical benzoyl peroxide, UV light therapy
- **P** Spontaneous resolution possible
- **!** Treatment is difficult

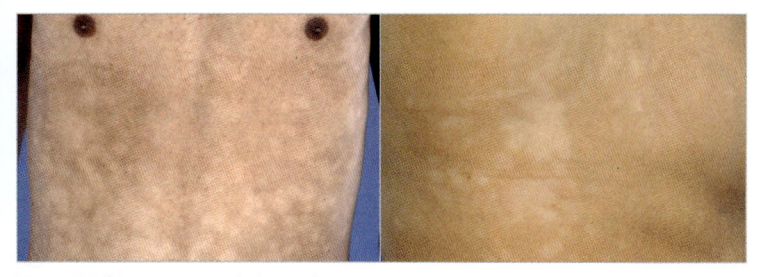

Figure 127 // Progressive macular hypomelanosis

Cutaneous amyloidosis

D Amyloidosis is the abnormal accumulation of amyloid, which are insoluble fibrils formed from beta-pleated sheets of protein, in extracellular tissues. Amyloidosis is classified into cutaneous (localised) amyloidosis and systemic amyloidosis. Cutaneous amyloidosis is characterised by the accumulation of amyloid material in the skin. There are various types, including major forms (e.g. macular, lichen, nodular, and familial primary localised cutaneous amyloidosis ('PLCA')) as well as rare forms (e.g. amyloidosis cutis dyschromica); see Table 32.

	MACULAR CUTANEOUS AMYLOIDOSIS	**LICHEN AMYLOIDOSIS**
D	Macular cutaneous amyloidosis, or interscapular cutaneous amyloidosis, is characterised by a hyperpigmented lichen simplex chronicus-like appearance (see Figure 128).	Lichen amyloidosis, or papular cutaneous amyloidosis, is a severely itching, chronic lichenoid dermatosis, primarily pretibial. The amyloid material originates from keratin and is believed to result from chronic itching and scratching (secondary deposition) (see Figure 129).
E	Exact incidence unknown, uncommon	
Ae	Basal keratinocyte degeneration → cytokeratin release → enzymatic degradation → amyloid k (keratine) formation → extracellular deposition → insoluble sticky fibrils → beta-sheet structure build-up in the skin → clinical manifestations of amyloidosis	
R	Asian, Middle Eastern, or South American descent	
Hx	Itchy ⊕	Itchy ⊕⊕
PE	P Upper back, extensors of extremities A Rippled (pattern) linear streaks S 2-4 mm S Flat, round, oval O Ill-demarcated N Grayish-brown (hyperpigmented) E Macules, laques, papules	P Pretibial A Discrete, multiple (can coalesce) S 2-4 mm S Dome-shaped O Moderately demarcated N Pink to reddish-brown (hyperpigmented) E Papules, plaques (coalesce), scaly
Dx	Skin biopsy (detection of amyloid e.g. PAS staining, Congo Red Staining, Thioflavin T staining)	
Tx	🖉 Emollients, topical antipruritics, topical corticosteroids, topical salicylic acid, oral retinoids (e.g. acitretin)	💬 Discontinue itch-scratch cycle 🖉 Topical antipruritics, systemic antipruritics, topical corticosteroids (under occlusion), intralesional corticosteroid, topical calcineurin inhibitor, topical salicylic acid, oral retinoids (e.g. acitretin), systemic immunomodulators (e.g. ciclosporin) ✎ Light therapy (UVB), laser therapy (e.g. Q-switched Nd:YAG), curettage, electrocoagulation, dermabrasion, excision
!	· Macular amyloidosis and lichen amyloidosis can occur together (biphasic amyloidosis) · Typical anatomical locations for lichen amyloidosis can correlate with areas that can be easily scratched or rubbed	

Table 32 // Macular cutaneous amyloidosis and lichen amyloidosis

> 💡 There is another variant of cutaneous amyloidosis where lichenoid hyperpigmented papules appear between the shoulder blades. This variant is difficult to distinguish from macular cutaneous amyloidosis and can be associated with MEN 2A syndrome (multiple endocrine neoplasia type 2A, Sipple syndrome).

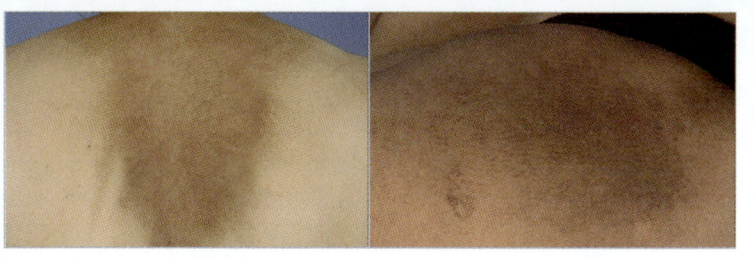

Figure 128 // Macular cutaneous amyloidosis

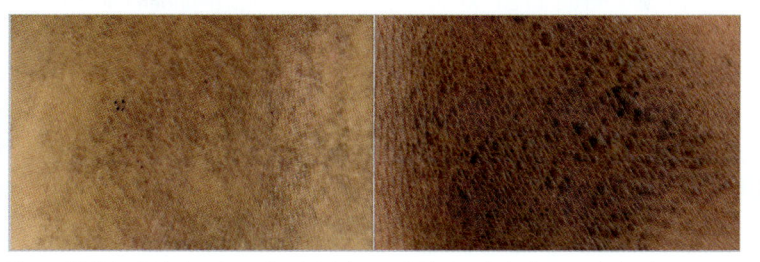

Figure 129 // Amyloidosis cutis papulosa (left: lichen amyloidosis; right: biphasic amyloidosis)

Pressure ulcers

Pressure ulcers

(D) Pressure ulcers, also known as bedsores, are skin injuries caused by pressure or shearing (see Figure 130). Pressure ulcers can be classified into various degrees of severity.

(E) Prevalence 12.7% in acute inpatient care

(Ae) Immobilisation and/or lack of sensation (neuropathy, anaesthesia, paraplegia) → pressure on skin ↑ → tissue damage

(R) • Old age, incontinence, diabetes mellitus, arterial vascular disease, poor nutritional status, bedfast/wheelchair-bound
- Pressure ulcers are classified into different degrees (see Tables 33 and 34):
  - Braden 6-14: high risk of pressure ulcers
  - Braden 15-20: moderate risk of pressure ulcers
  - Braden >21: low risk of pressure ulcers

(Hx) Pain, general malaise, fever (infected pressure ulcers)

(PE) • See Table 34 and Figures 130 and 131
- Common sites: see Figure 132
- T ↑ (infected pressure ulcers)

- **Dx** Infected wound unresponsive to ABx: take wound culture to define targeted therapy
- **Tx** Grade 1-3 pressure sores usually heal after local therapy, grade 4 commonly requires surgical intervention
  - 💬 Prevention: risk assessment (e.g. with Braden score; see Table 33), corresponding preventive measures (frequent position changes, antibedsore mattress, non-medicated cream or ointment, barrier agent in case of incontinence, prophylactic dressings), consult physical therapist
  - Wound treatment: wound cleansing, dressings, debridement of necrotic tissue. USA: topical ABx (if needed), electrical stimulation (adjunctive).
  - Nutritional interventions: adequate protein and fat intake, supplementary oral or tube feeding may be needed, consult dietician, adequate fluid intake. USA: individualised bowel/bladder management, screen nutritional deficiencies.
  - 🔗 Signs of infection: treat infection, pain management
- **P** Quality of life ↓, duration of admission ↑, morbidity ↑, mortality ↑

> 🩺 The typical patient with pressure sores is an immobile elderly person (bedfast or wheelchair-bound) who needs assistance with repositioning or sitting up.

FACTOR	SCORE	FACTOR	SCORE
Sensory perception: the patient's ability to respond to pain and discomfort	1 Completely limited 2 Very limited 3 Slightly limited 4 No impairment	**Mobility:** ability to move and change position	1 Completely immobile 2 Very limited 3 Slightly limited 4 No impairment
Moisture: the degree to which the wound is exposed to moisture from e.g. sweat or urine	1 Constantly moist 2 Very moist 3 Occasionally moist 4 Rarely moist	**Nutrition:** food intake	1 Very poor 2 Inadequate 3 Adequate 4 Excellent
Activity: degree of physical activity	1 Bedfast 2 Chairfast 3 Walks occasionally 4 Walks frequently	**Friction and shear:** degree to which friction and shear are a problem	1 Problem 2 Potential problem 3 No problem 4 N/A

Table 33 // Braden score

GRADE	CHARACTERISTICS
1	Non-blanching erythema of intact skin
2	Partial thickness skin loss or bullae
3	Full thickness skin loss (visible adipose tissue)
4	Full tissue layer loss (muscle and bone visible)

Table 34 // Pressure ulcer grading system

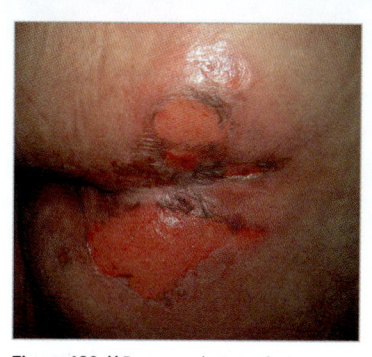

Figure 130 // Pressure ulcer grade 2

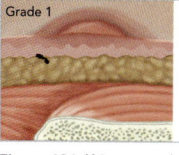

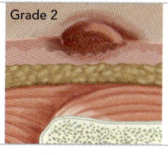

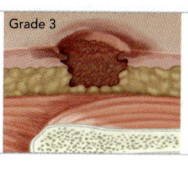

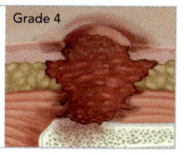

Grade 1 | Grade 2 | Grade 3 | Grade 4

Figure 131 // Pressure ulcer grading system

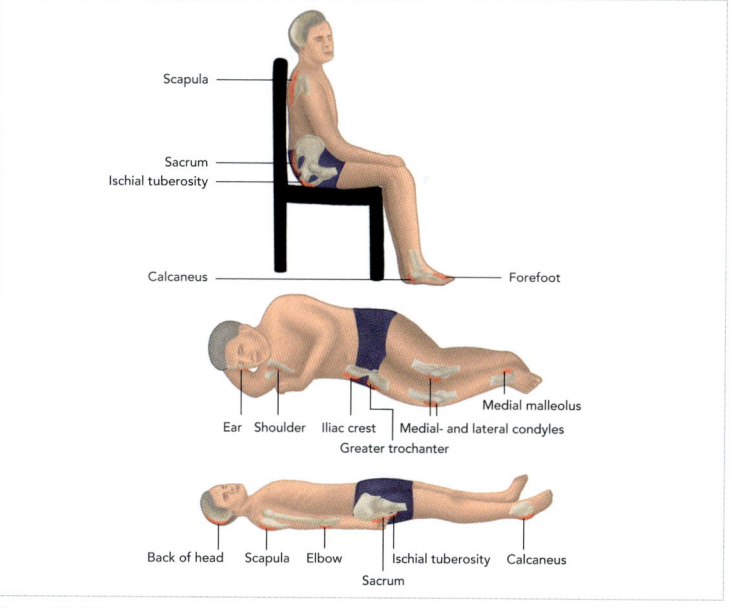

Scapula
Sacrum
Ischial tuberosity
Calcaneus
Forefoot

Ear Shoulder Iliac crest Medial- and lateral condyles Medial malleolus
Greater trochanter

Back of head Scapula Elbow Ischial tuberosity Calcaneus
Sacrum

Figure 132 // Pressure ulcer: common sites

Lymphology

Lymphoedema

- **D** Lymphoedema is tissue swelling caused by the accumulation of lymphatic fluid in the interstitium, resulting from a lymphatic drainage problem with normal capillary filtration (see Figures 133 and 134).
- **E** Prevalence of primary lymphoedema 1:100,000, secondary lymphoedema 100:100,000 per year
- **Ae**
  - Obstruction or malformation of the lymphatic system
  - Primary (congenital or familial) form: e.g. Milroy's disease, Meige's disease
  - Secondary (acquired) form: e.g. obesity, malignancy, radiation, sentinel node procedure, recurrent infection (cellulitis)
- **R** Positive PMHx, malignancies, surgery, trauma, obesity, chronic venous insufficiency, infections, ♀
- **Hx** Swelling, past lymph node dissection (due to malignancy)
- **PE**
  - Oedema on one or both lower legs, incl. feet and toes
  - Square toes
  - Unable to pinch skin at the base of the second toe (Stemmer sign)
  - Skin may be hyperkeratotic or papillomatous
- **Dx** When in doubt about diagnosis: lymphoscintigraphy to distinguish between lymphostatic and non-lymphostatic oedema
- **Tx** 💬 Compression therapy with bandages, pneumatic compression (inflatable sleeves or stockings), manual lymph drainage, and therapeutic compression stockings

  ✏️ Lymphatic bypass procedures, direct excision of lymphoedematous tissues, liposuction
- **P** Pitting oedema on the dorsal surface of the feet, extending to the proximal surface → transformation into non-pitting oedema → induration due to fibrosis
- **!** Oedematous areas are susceptible to ulceration and secondary infections

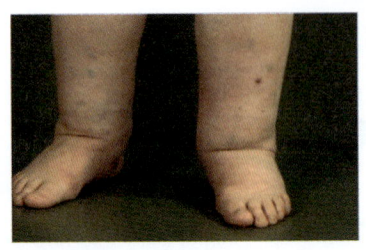

Figure 133 // Lymphoedema legs

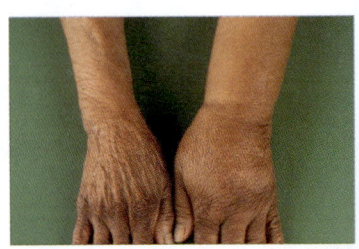

Figure 134 // Lymphoedema

Vascular conditions

Venous skin conditions

Chronic venous insufficiency (CVI)

- D CVI comprises many different venous disorders characterised by impaired blood return in the superficial, perforating, or deep venous system. These include venous dilation, increased vascular permeability, oedema, and chronic release of inflammatory mediators.
- E Present in up to 50% of the population
- Ae • Primary valve insufficiency
  - Secondary valve insufficiency (post-thrombotic syndrome) → venous hypertension → vein, capillary, cutaneous, subcutaneous abnormalities
- R Advanced age, positive PMHx, prolonged standing, high body mass index (BMI), smoking, lower extremity trauma, past DVT, arteriovenous shunt, pregnancy, ♂:♀ = 1:2-3
- Hx Pain, heavy legs, dry skin, muscle cramps, varicose veins, oedema, statis dermatitis
- PE Varicose veins, hyperpigmentation, atrophie blanche, induration, dermatosclerosis and liposclerosis, ulcer (see Table 35 for the CEAP classification of symptoms of chronic venous disorders)
- Dx Duplex ultrasound: identify location of venous insufficiency (superficial, deep, or perforating venous system) and severity of insufficiency
- Tx Ample exercise, weight reduction
  - Compression therapy (graded elastic compression stockings, gauze boots, layered bandaging, and adjustable compression garments)
  - Endovascular laser therapy, laser therapy, radiofrequency ablation (RFA), ultrasound-guided sclerotherapy
- P Chronic condition
- ! For non-healing leg ulcers, consider CVI as underlying cause, oedema management is very important

See the Pocket *Cardiology and Vascular Medicine* for more information on vascular conditions.

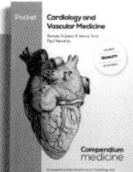

CLINICAL STATUS (C)	AETIOLOGY (Ae)	ANATOMY (A)	PATHOPHYSIO-LOGY (P)
C0: no visible signs of disease	Ec: congenital	As: superficial • S1: Spider/reticular veins • S2: Great saphenous vein - above the knee • S3: Great saphenous vein - below the knee • S4: Small saphenous vein • S5: Other, larger veins	Pr: reflux
C1: telangiectasias or reticular veins	Ep: primary (cause unknown)	Ad: deep • D6: Inferior vena cava • D7: Common iliac vein • D8: Internal iliac vein • D9: External iliac vein • D10: Pelvic veins • D11: Common femoral vein • D12: Deep femoral vein • D13: Superficial femoral vein • D14: Popliteal vein • D15: Tibial vein (anterior, posterior, peroneal) • D16: Gastrocnemius vein, soleal vein, other veins	Po: obstruction
C2: varicose veins	Es: secondary (post-thrombotic, trauma, pregnancy, etc.)	Ap: perforating P17: thigh P18: lower leg	Pr,o: reflux and obstruction
C3: oedema	En: no venous cause identified	An: no venous location identified	Pn: no venous pathology identified
C4a: pigmentation, eczema			
C4b: lipodermatosclerosis, atrophie blanche		N/A	
C5: healed ulcer			
C6: active venous ulcer			
S: symptomatic			
A: asymptomatic			

Table 35 // CEAP classification: classification of symptoms of chronic venous disorders

C2 varicose veins

(D) C2 varicose veins is a disorder of the venous vascular system characterised by permanent blood vessel dilation. Varicose veins present as long, tortuous, and dilated veins of the superficial venous system with a diameter >3 mm (see Figure 135).

(E) Prevalence in Europe: 21%, Asia: 17%, Africa: 5.5%, South America: 22%, Pacific Islands: 19%, annual global incidence: 0.22-2.3%

(Ae) Primary or idiopathic varicose veins usually arise spontaneously and typically appear bilaterally. Secondary varices are usually confined to one extremity and are caused by mechanical obstruction (e.g. tumours of the lesser pelvis, DVT, deep venous anomalies), or arteriovenous fistulae → valvular insufficiency → stasis, reflux, and impaired blood return → venous hypertension and dilated superficial veins (CVI).

(R) ♀, positive PMHx, oral contraceptive use, prolonged standing (standing occupation), obesity, advanced age, ≥2 pregnancies

(Hx) Varicose veins, tired, heavy, or painful legs, nocturnal muscle cramps, itching, restless legs, paraesthesia

(PE) Twisting, nodular veins, hyperpigmented and indurated skin, atrophie blanche (painfull white discolouration with red macule), erythema, palpable arterial pulses, pitting oedema of the lower extremities, ulcers

(Dx) Duplex ultrasound of the venous system, sensitivity 75-100%, specificity 90-100% (venous system reflux and valvular insufficiency)

(Tx) • Education: avoid prolonged standing, elevate leg if possible, weight loss, frequent walks
- Class II compression stockings
- Small and medium varicose veins (with limited deep-system reflux): sclerocompression therapy (SCT), ambulatory phlebectomy
- GSV insufficiency: endovenous laser treatment (EVLT), radiofrequency ablation (RFA) (less suitable than EVLT for varicose veins <12 mm in diameter)
- All types of varicose veins: ultrasound-guided foam sclerotherapy (injection of sclerosing agent mixed with air induces sterile inflammation and vessel obliteration)
- Primary surgery:
  - SSV trunk insufficiency: SSV crossectomy (ligation)
  - GSV trunk insufficiency: endovenous laser/ablation treatment
- Convolutectomy with crossectomy: removal of superficial varicose trib-

- utaries after crossectomy
  - Subfascial endoscopic perforator surgery (SEPS): perforator vein ligation
- P • Compression stockings are symptomatic, surgical intervention is usually required in the long term due to poor adherence
  - Recurrence rate after SCT >90% (after 10y)
  - Recurrence rate after ultrasound-guided foam sclerotherapy 1-51%, often multiple treatments required
- ! Watch out for venous leg ulcer, risk of thrombophlebitis ↑, variceal haemorrhage

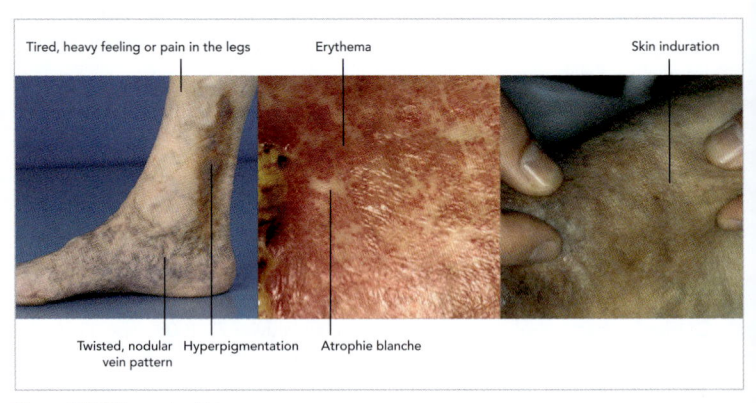

Figure 135 // Venous insufficiency

> 💡 Cosmetic complaints are not a surgical indication for varicosis. Surgical indications are bleeding, pain, ulcers, and superficial thrombophlebitis, or a serious impact on quality of life (beyond cosmetic concerns).

Venous leg ulcer

- D A venous leg ulcer is a skin defect of the lower leg, typically on the medial side, extending into the subcutis or deeper structures. It takes more than two weeks to heal and/or shows no signs of healing within two weeks of starting treatment (see Table 36). Venous leg ulcers are characterised by jagged margins without undermining (see Figure 136).
- E Prevalence of active ulceration 0.3%, lifetime prevalence 1%, <60y ⊖

- **Ae** CVI → venous and capillary pressure ↑ → capillary bed defects and cutaneous and subcutaneous changes
- **R** DM, heart failure, oedema of the lower extremities, hypertension, rheumatoid arthritis (RA), immobility, varicose veins, prolonged standing, other skin conditions
- **Hx** Nocturnal pain, muscle cramps, signs of infection
- **PE** Inspect ulcer (see Table 36)
- **Dx**
  - Ankle-Brachial Index (ABI) (≥0.9): to rule out arterial ulcer
  - Duplex ultrasound of the venous system of the lower extremities: venous insufficiency
  - Take biopsies if an ulcer responds poorly to therapy or has atypical features
- **Tx** 💬 • General wound management: provide a moist wound environment, control excess exudate
    - Ambulatory compression therapy: bandaging
  - 👁 Walking and functional exercise, train calf muscles
  - 💊 In signs of infection: ABx
  - 🔪 Necrosectomy
- **P** Long recovery period, healing process typically progressing steadily after 3 wk of compression therapy, high recurrence rate (10% per year after compression therapy)
- **!** Watch out for infection

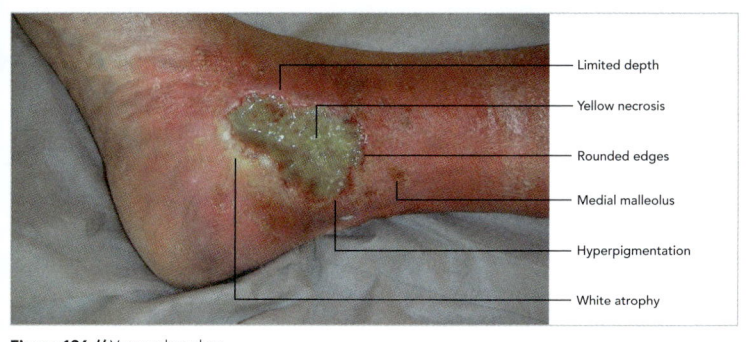

Figure 136 // Venous leg ulcer

> 💡 **Venous leg ulcer:** the GSV is found on the medial side of the leg, and GSV insufficiency therefore causes long-term defects on the medial side of the ankle/lower leg.

CHARACTERISTICS	VENOUS LEG ULCER	ARTERIAL LEG ULCER
Percentage of all leg ulcers	80%	20%
Pain	⊖	⊕⊕
ABI	= (≥0.9)	<0.9
Palpable arterial pulses in leg/foot	=	↓
Skin temperature	=	↓
Wound margins	Jagged	Sharp
Wound bed	Grannulation tissue, exsudate ⊕⊕	Necrosis, exsudate ⊖
Oedema	⊕⊕	⊖
Location	Around medial malleolus, low on lower legs	Lateral side of tibia, forefoot, toes
Depth	Limited	Profound necrosis
Dermal cyanosis	⊖	⊕
Symptoms	Foul odour ⊕, nocturnal pain, muscle cramps, elevating leg → pain ↓, varicose veins, hyperpigmentation, atrophy blanche and induration, heavy/tired legs when standing still (decreases when walking), itching	Often more painful than venous ulcers, nocturnal pain (allow leg to hang down → pain ↓), cold, blue-white foot

Table 36 // Characteristics venous leg ulcer and arterial leg ulcer

Arterial skin conditions

Arterial leg ulcer (Fontaine IV)

- D An arterial leg ulcer is a dermal defect of the lower leg that usually develops on the lateral sides of the leg due to arterial insufficiency (see Figure 137).
- E 5-20% of lower extremity ulcers
- Ae Arterial insufficiency
- R Atherosclerosis, DM, hypertension, smoking
- Hx History of trauma, dysregulated DM, positive PMHx for cardiovascular disease (CVD)
- PE Inspect ulcer (see Table 36)

- **Dx** • ABI <0.9, exercise test: ABI drops by >0.15 or toe pressure <30 mmHg
  - Duplex ultrasound: affected artery and degree of stenosis
- **Tx** • Treat underlying disease (hypertension, DM)
  - Wound treatment, e.g. with bandage or vacuum-assisted closure (VAC)
  - Antiplatelet and statin
  - Percutaneous transluminal angioplasty (PTA) with balloon dilation and potentially intravascular stent
  - Arterial bypass
  - Debridement, necrosectomy, skin grafting
- **P** Prolonged healing process
- **!** Watch out for Martorell's ulcer

> **Martorell's ulcer** can occur in patients with long-standing hypertension and is the cause of ±1% of ulcers on the lower leg. Patients present with a painful, erythematous, bullous lesion, which turns blue-purple and eventually ulcerates. The peripheral vascular resistance increases and ABI remains the same. Therapy consists of anticoagulation and analgesia, local wound management, and blood pressure regulation.

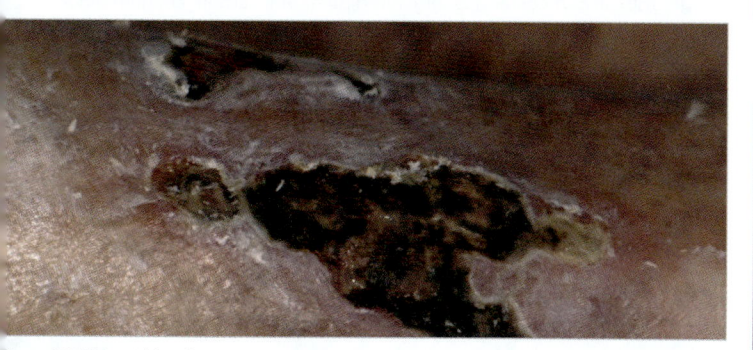

figure 137 // Arterial leg ulcer

Pernio

Pernio, also known as perniosis or chilblains, is an abnormal reaction of the microvasculature to cold. The most common sites involved are the fingers and toes; occasionally blistering, ulceration, or secondary infection may occur (see figure 138). Symptoms commonly begin in early winter and resolve by spring as cold exposure decreases.

- **E** Exact incidence and prevalence unknown, vary with climate
- **Ae** Exact aetiology unknown, possibly genetic predisposition, association with cold-induced vasoconstriction/vasospasm → hypoxaemia → inflammatory response
- **R** ♀, young-middle aged, exposure to cold, damp environments
- **Hx** Acute eruption 12-24h after cold exposure, pain ☺, swollen ☺, red ☺, itchy ☺, burning ☺, improvement with elimination of cold exposure
- **PE**
  - **P** Fingers, hands, toes, feet, heels, lower legs, thighs (horse riders' perniones), tip of nose, ear edges
  - **A** Symmetric, discreet, confluent
  - **S** Single or multiple, a few mm to a few cm
  - **S** Round, oval, irregular
  - **O** Moderately demarcated
  - **N** Erythematous, purple, bluish, skin discolouration
  - **E** Papules, patches, plaques, ulceration
- **Dx** Based on clinical presentation
- **Tx** 🗨 Minimise cold exposure (e.g. properly insulated clothing, gloves, footwear), discontinue smoking

  💊 Topical corticosteroids, oral nifedipine, oral calcium channel blockers
- **P** Acute pernio resolves within a few weeks, but can also have a chronic or recurrent course
- **!**
  - Pernio has been associated with other systemic diseases (e.g. lupus erythematosus, COVID-19)
  - A clinically identical presentation with more severe ulcerations can be seen in patients with SLE and is considered a separate entity known as chilblain lupus erythematosus

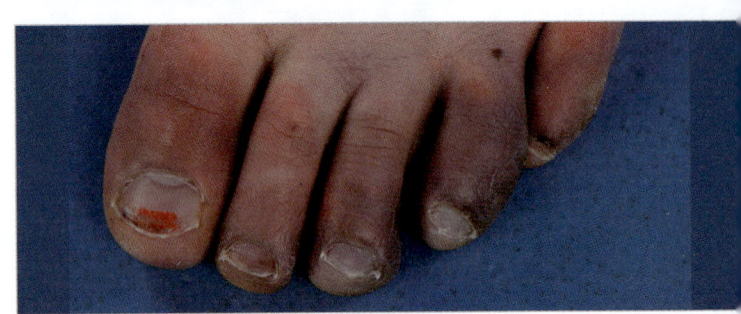

Figure 138 // Chilblains

Cherry angioma

D Cherry angiomas, also known as angioma senilis or Campbell de Morgan spots, are common benign skin growths characterised by the proliferation of capillaries. They typically appear as small, bright red, flat or dome-shaped lesions on the trunk and extremities (see Figure 139).

E Increase with age, esp. >40y, pale to fair skin types

Ae Exact aetiology unknown, possible association with oncogenic mutations in GNAQ and GNA11

R Middle aged, older adults

Hx Asymptomatic ☺

PE **P** Anywhere on the skin (except mucous membranes)
- **A** Solitary, multiple, to dozens
- **S** 1-6 mm
- **S** Flat, dome-shaped
- **O** Well-defined
- **N** Bright red, pink to dark red, purple
- **E** Papule

Dx Dermoscopy: red, purple, or blue-black lagoons (lobular pattern)

Tx 🗨 No treatment necessary

✂ Cryotherapy, laser therapy, electrocoagulation, shave excision, punch biopsy or excision

P No malignant potential

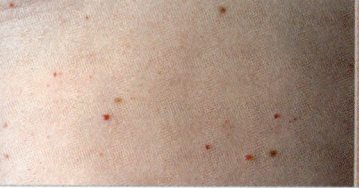

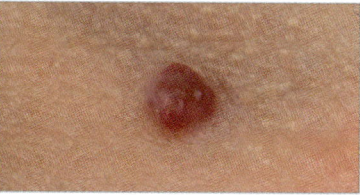

Figure 139 // Cherry angioma

Pyogenic granuloma

D Pyogenic granuloma or lobular capillary hemangioma is a benign vascular tumour of the skin or mucous membranes characterised by rapid growth, friable surface, and bleeds easily. It is relatively common in children and young adults and starts as a small, red papule that grows rapidly over weeks to months and then stabilises (see Figure 140).

- (E) Prevalence 0.5% of all skin nodules in children with peak incidence at 20-30y, 2-3% in pregnancies (intraoral)
- (Ae) Exact aetiology unknown, possibly associated with hyperplastic and neovascular responses to an angiogenic stimulus with imbalance of promoters and inhibitors
- (R) Trauma, pregnancy, immunosuppressive medication
- (Hx) Bleeding ⊖, ulceration ⊕
- (PE) (P) Trunk, extremities, fingers, head and neck (children)
    - (A) Solitary (sometimes multiple)
    - (S) A few mm to a few cm
    - (S) Round, lobulated, dome-shaped, pedunculated
    - (O) Well-demarcated
    - (N) Bright/dark red, purple
    - (E) Papule, nodule, tumour, ulceration
- (Dx) No added value

  Dermoscopy: pink, homogenous papule with a white collarette of scale, white, intersecting lines
- (Tx) 💊 Topical beta blockers, topical corticosteroids (high potency), topical imiquimod, topical phenol, intralesional injection (e.g. bleomycin, corticosteroids)

  ✏️ Surgical excision, shave excision, curettage, laser therapy, cryotherapy, chemical cauterization (e.g. silver nitrate)
- (P) Varying recurrence rate 0-15%, depending on location of lesion and treatment
- (!) • Pyogenic granuloma can be triggered by medication (e.g. ciclosporin, high-dose retinoids, oncological therapies, antiretroviral, monoclonal medications, epidermal growth factor receptor inhibitors)
  - Pyogenic granuloma can also arise in an existing capillary vascular malformation (e.g. port wine birthmark, naevus simplex)

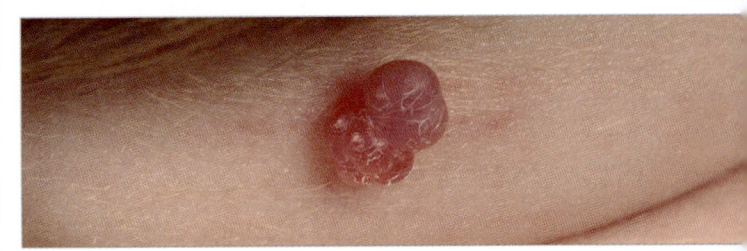

Figure 140 // Pyogenic granuloma

Sexually transmitted infections (STIs)

Chlamydia

- D Chlamydia is a urogenital bacterial STI caused by *Chlamydia trachomatis*.
- E Incidence ♀ 4% and ♂ 2.5%, in Europe 182:100,000, USA 496:100,000 per year, esp. during reproductive age, peak prevalence 15-24y
- Ae *Chlamydia trachomatis*: intracellular Gram-negative bacteria, incubation period 1-3 wk
- R Multiple sexual partners, unprotected intercourse, PMHx: chlamydia infection, age <25
- Hx • Asymptomatic (♀ 60-70%, ♂ 50%)
  - ♀: discharge ↑, burning sensation/pain during urination, abnormal vaginal bleeding, lower abdominal pain
  - ♂: watery discharge or dysuria
- PE • Asymptomatic ☉, abdominal tenderness and rebound tenderness on palpation, muscular defence
  - Speculum exam: cervicitis
  - Vaginal exam: adnexal and cervical motion tenderness pain (indications of salpingitis/pelvic inflammatory disease (PID))
- Dx • Nucleic Acid Amplification Test (NAAT) on first-catch urine sample, ♀ intracervical or ♂ urethral swab (also perform gonorrhoea test, given increased risk of co-infection), or rectal if anal sex, anal symptoms, or anal intercourse
  - Labs: chlamydia antibody titre (CAT) positive
- Tx ● Contact tracing (all sexual partners over the past 6 mo)
  - 💊 ABx: azithromycin, doxycycline (first choice in case of rectal chlamydia). Alternatives (e.g. if allergic): amoxicillin, erythromycin.
- P Frequent re-infection if left untreated: 20% chance of complications, incl. chronic pelvic pain, subfertility/infertility, ectopic pregnancy, Fitz-Hugh-Curtis syndrome (perihepatitis) with PID
- ! • Pregnancy: risk of prelabour rupture of membranes (PROM) and premature birth
  - Possible vertical transmission to foetus with risk of neonatal conjunctivitis and pneumonia
  - Asymptomatic chlamydia infections are no longer considered to cause long-term sequelae like PID and tubal factor infertility. For this reason, in some countries chlamydia is no longer routinely tested in asymptomatic individuals.

> 🔔 Be aware of a possible chlamydia infection, if a female patient has frequent breakthrough bleeding.

> 🔔 *Chlamydia trachomatis* is an intracellular bacteria, so remember to rub thoroughly when collecting the culture sample.

Gonorrhoea

- **D** Gonorrhoea, or 'the clap', is a bacterial STI caused by *Neisseria gonorrhoeae* (see Figure 141).
- **E** Incidence: USA 200:100,000, Europe 32:100,000 per year
- **Ae** *Neisseria gonorrhoeae (gonococcus)*, intracellular Gram-negative diplococcus, incubation period 2-14d
- **R** Chlamydia infection, multiple sexual partners, unprotected intercourse, anal intercourse, prostitution, ♂:♀ = 4:1
- **Hx** Asymptomatic ⊕, abdominal pain, dysuria, fever ⊖, pharyngitis ⊖, ♀ vaginal discharge ↑ (30-60%), ♂ urethritis (with purulent discharge) or proctitis
- **PE** Speculum exam: red, irritated cervix, cervicitis
- **Dx**
  - Labs: CAT due to risk of chlamydia/gonorrhoea co-infection ↑
  - Urine: PCR on first-catch urine sample
  - Culture: ♀ intracervical or ♂ urethral swab, rectal culture if anal sex, anal symptoms, or anal intercourse
  - Oral culture if unsafe oral sex
- **Tx** 💬 Contact tracing (all sexual partners over the past 60d)
  - 💊 Single-dose IM ceftriaxone
- **P** Untreated: risk of subfertility/infertility, ectopic pregnancy, Fitz-Hugh-Curtis syndrome with PID (perihepatitis)
- **!** Many women are asymptomatic, resulting in delayed treatment

Figure 141 // Gonorrhoea

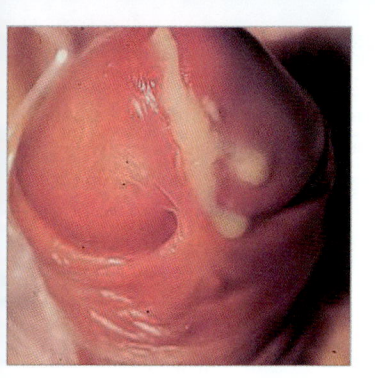

> 🔔 Neonates may be exposed to vertical transmission, possibly causing neonatal conjunctivitis.

Genital herpes

- D Genital herpes is an HSV infection in the genital region (see Figure 142). There are two types of HSV: HSV-1 and HSV-2.
- E Prevalence Americas 11-24%, Europe 3-11%, Asia 7-10%, Africa 25-44%
- Ae HSV-2 (80%), HSV-1 (20%)
- R Decreased immunity, increased risk of infection and exacerbation, multiple sexual partners, unprotected intercourse
- Hx Irritation, burning sensation, pain, fever
- PE
  - P Genital area
  - A Grouped
  - S Miliar
  - S Round
  - O Well-demarcated
  - N Red
  - E Vesicles and ulcerations
  - Primary infection: regional lymph node swelling, urethritis symptoms, vaginal discharge (♀)
  - After 6-7d: clear fluid-filled blisters that burst open, followed by ulcers
  - Location: glans, foreskin, and shaft of the penis (♂), vulva, perineum, or cervix (♀), skin pathology around the anus or proctitis (anal intercourse)
- Dx Labs: PCR on ulcer swab
- Tx Supportive measures: bathing in water
  - Analgesia for pain relief
  - Antivirals (aciclovir, famciclovir, valaciclovir) for 7-10d, extend treatment duration if patient develops new lesions

- (P) Recurrence ☉: >1 in 90%, >10 in 20%, HSV-2 infection poses greater recurrence risk, absence of visible ulcerations does not rule out infection
- Lesions heal in 7-28d without scarring, during recurrences, herpetiform blisters appear that produce non-indurated painful ulcers

(!) Extragenital complications: aseptic meningitis, urinary retention (lumbar radiculopathy: Elsberg's syndrome), skin pathology elsewhere on the body

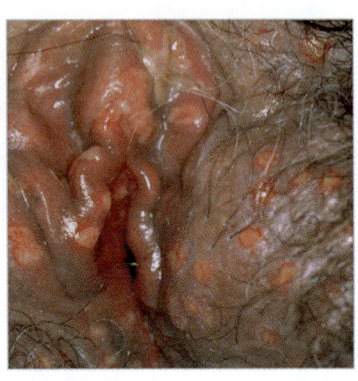

> 🔔 **Kiss of death**: HSV infections in neonates can be fatal. This is why patients with infectious HSV should be advised to not have physical contact with neonates (kissing/hugging) while they have symptoms.

Figure 142 // Genital herpes

Condylomata acuminata

- (D) Condylomata acuminata, or anogenital warts, are caused by human papilloma virus (HPV), a DNA virus with over 100 serotypes. It is a sexually transmitted disease of the mucous membranes in the anogenital region (see Figure 143).
- (E) Annual incidence: global 195:100,000, in Europe 130-160:100,000 per year
- (Ae) HPV types 6 and 11, incubation period: 1-8 mo
- (R) Multiple sexual partners, unprotected intercourse, ♂, smoking, oropharyngeal HPV, immunocompromised patients, anal intercourse
- (Hx) Itching, irritation, discharge with urethral and vaginal infection
- (PE) (P) Anogenital area, cervix, urethra
  - (A) Solitary or multiple
  - (S) Miliar to lenticular
  - (S) Verrucous, papillomatous
  - (O) Well-demarcated
  - (N) Skin-coloured, violaceous, or brown
  - (E) Papula
- (Dx) • Clinical diagnosis, additional diagnostics not needed

- Biopsy if in doubt: histology and/or HPV test. Histology shows typical koilocytes that may harbour viruses, usually accompanied by hypergranulosis.
- Cytology on smear test: cervical intraepithelial neoplasia (CIN)
- Colposcopy with 3-5% acetic acid staining and lugol: atypical and damaged cells stain white

(Tx) Prevention: condom use (does not provide full protection though, virus may still be transmitted near the base of the condom)

Genital warts: podophyllotoxin, imiquimod, sinecatechins

Excision, electrocoagulation, cryotherapy, curettage, laser surgery, trichloroacetic acid

(P) Spontaneous remission in 20% after 3 mo and 90% after 2y

(!) Risk of developing carcinoma in oncogenic serotypes after 10-15y

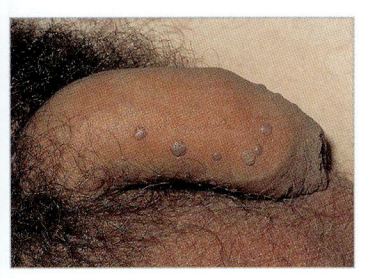

Figure 143 // Condylomata acuminata

> Immunocompromised patients may develop very large and difficult-to-treat genital warts, known as giant condylomata acuminata of Buschke-Löwenstein.

Pediculosis capitis

(D) Head lice infestations are caused by *Pediculus humanus capitis*, an ectoparasite that feeds on human blood.

(E) Incidence varies by region: Europe 0.5%, Africa and Americas up to 60%, more common in school-aged children

(Ae) Transmission: direct head-to-head contact (person-to-person), fomites

(R) Infection risk: close contacts in classrooms and day care facilities

(Hx) Itching

(PE) Excoriations on scalp, neck, and/or postauricular skin, secondary infections, cervical lymph node enlargement. Direct visualisation of a louse, nymph, or nit on the hair shaft or scalp.

(Dx) Not indicated

(Tx) Topical treatment with permethrin 1% or ivermectin shampoo

(P) Education: teach children to not share combs, brushes or hats

- Incubation period: 8-9 days
- Examination of household members must be included

Pediculosis pubis (phthiriasis pubis)

Pubic lice infestations are caused by *Phthirus pubis*, a blood-sucking louse that feeds on human blood. Pubic lice are found in the pubic area and can spread to other areas with body hair by scratching (armpits, chest hair, eyebrows, eyelashes).

Annual incidence in adult populations: 2%

- Transmission: physical intimacy (person to person), sharing clothes
- Incubation period: >5d
- Nymphs and mature lice feed on blood → allergic reaction to bites → itching
- Infection risk: multiple sexual partners, travellers (sleeping on used sheets)
- More severe course: corticosteroids → lice count ↑

Itching ☺, secondary bacterial skin infections ⊖

Lice on skin or at the base of unshaven pubic hair, excoriations, impetigo

Microscopy or magnifying glass: detect lice (see Figures 144 and 145), nits

💬 Removal of nits from the hair, e.g. by combing or using fine tweezers

💊 Topical treatment (e.g. permethrin cream, pyrethrins with piperonyl butoxide) to all suspected infested regions

- Treatment most effective way to control nymphs and mature lice
- Frequent use of pediculicides results in persistent itching

Pediculosis pubis is usually sexually transmitted → deploy diagnostics for other STIs

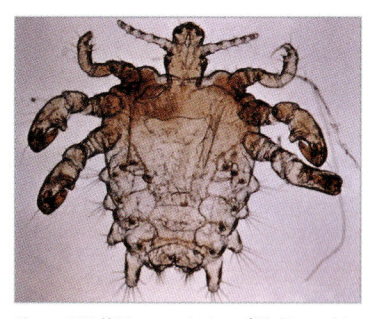

Figure 144 // *Microscopic view of Phthirus pubis*

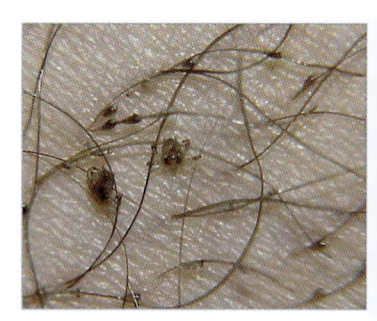

Figure 145 // *Pediculosis pubis*

Scabies

- (D) Scabies is a highly contagious infestation of the epidermis by the *Sarcoptes scabiei* mite. The mite burrows into and lives in the area between the stratum corneum and stratum granulosum. Transmission occurs through prolonged or frequent direct contact. The mites can also be spread by fomites (inanimate objects).
- (E) Prevalence 4.2-71%
- (Ae) Intense itching due to an allergic reaction to enzyme production, faeces and parasitic antigens
- (R) Poor hygiene, multiple sexual partners, residential care facilities, immune disorder
- (Hx) Severely itchy lesion, esp. at night, 2-6 wk incubation period
- (PE) (P) Interdigital space, flexor surfaces of wrists, lateral border of the foot, head is unaffected in adults, ♂ penis, ♀ around the nipples (see Figure 148)
  - (A) Grouped, symmetrical
  - (S) Several to dozens of lesions (see Figure 146)
  - (S) Round, raised, sometimes linear (burrows)
  - (O) Highly variable
  - (N) Skin-coloured to red
  - (E) Papules, papulovesicles, crusts, and scratch marks
- (Dx) • Dermoscopy: larger mites can resemble small dark triangles (V shape, delta sign, see Figure 147)
  - KOH test: detect mites or nits
- (Tx) 🗨 Wash clothing, bedding and towels at 50°C/122°F, also treat partners or roommates
  - 💊 Apply permethrin to whole body or take oral ivermectin, repeat both after one week
- (P) Complete eradication very likely with adequate treatment
- (!) Scabies crustosa or Norwegian scabies is a very severe, highly contagious form of scabies that occurs esp. in immunocompromised or elderly people in care facilities and is characterised mainly by hyperkeratosis, papules, and nodules, esp. on the extremities

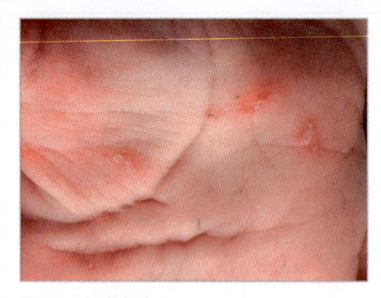

Figure 146 // Scabies

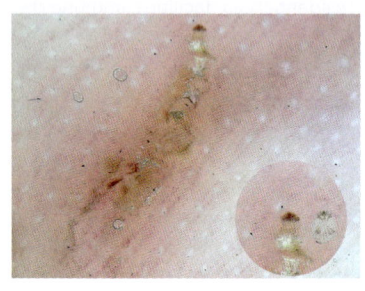

Figure 147 // Delta sign in scabies

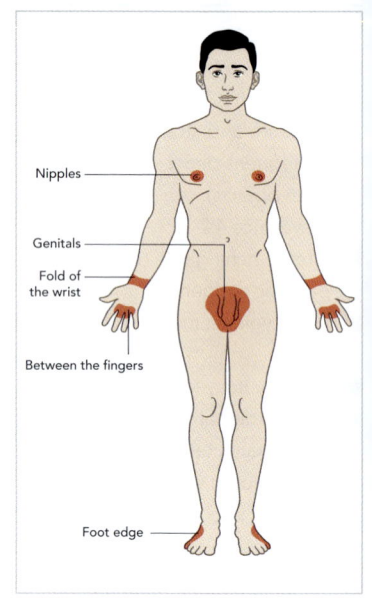

Figure 148 // Scabies: common sites

Syphilis

- Ⓓ Syphilis is a bacterial STI caused by *Treponema pallidum ssp. pallidum*. It has two stages: early syphilis, with an infection duration <1 year (contagious) and late syphilis, with an infection duration >1 year (non-contagious). Syphilis can be systemic and often occurs in combination with HIV.
- Ⓔ ♂:♀ = 9:1, incidence of active syphilis in Africa 420:100,000, the Americas 650:100,000, Eastern Mediterranean 110:100,000, Europe 30:100,000, Southeast Asia 40:100,000, Western Pacific 130:100,000 per year
- Ⓐe *Treponema pallidum ssp. pallidum*, a spirochete that invades the skin through small lesions produced during sexual activity or pre-existing lesions
- Ⓡ Anal intercourse, prostitution, persons from STI-endemic areas, multiple sexual partners, unprotected intercourse
- Ⓗx Painless skin lesions, ulcer, fever, general malaise, weight ↓, muscle and joint pain
- Ⓟe • Early syphilis:
  - Ⓟ At contact site (genitals, cervix, anal, mouth)
  - Ⓐ Solitary

- (S) Miliar to lenticular
- (S) Round or oval
- (O) Well-demarcated
- (N) Red
- (E) Macule, papule, later ulcer (painless)
- Secondary syphilis: many different manifestations, incl. palmar and plantar roseola (red macules), non-itching exanthema on extremities and trunk, condylomata lata, syphilitic alopecia (noncicatricial alopecia), ulcers over the body
- Neurological exam: to rule out neurosyphilis
- Vitals: T ↑

(Dx)
- Labs: antibodies positive (treponema pallidum particle agglutination (TPPA) and/or enzyme immunoassay (EIA))
- Darkfield microscopy: direct fluorescent antibody (DFA) visible on exudate from suspicious lesions
- Eye exam: possible reduced vision in ocular syphilis
- Rarely indicated: cardiac ultrasound in cardiovascular syphilis (thoracic aortic dilation, aortic valve insufficiency) and/or lumbar puncture in neurosyphilis (lymphocytic pleiocytosis, protein ↑)

(Tx)
- Standard treatment for early syphilis: one-off IM benzathine benzylpenicillin injection. Late syphilis: IM benzathine benzylpenicillin injection on day 1, 8, and 15.
- 2nd choice for patients with a penicillin allergy: doxycycline, erythromycin, or azithromycin

(P) Good after adequate treatment, follow-up anti-treponemal therapy with 2y of serological screening and consider lumbar puncture, electrocardiogram, and chest X-ray after 1y

(!)
- Possibility of transplacental transmission with risk of premature childbirth and foetal bone, kidney, and skin abnormalities, previous infection does not confer immunity
- Test for co-infection with HIV, treatment with benzathine benzylpenicillin can spark Jarisch-Herxheimer reaction due to endotoxins released by dead spirochetes

> 🔔 Syphilitic skin abnormalities may resemble other skin pathology. This is why syphilis is also known as 'the great pretender'.

> **Stages of syphilis** (see Figure 149):
> - 1st stage (primary syphilis): after ±3 wk, a papule (painless, firm, round, or oval ulcer (hard chancre); see Figure 150) develops at the site of infection → heals in 3-6 wk.
> - 2nd stage (secondary syphilis): usually occurs 3-10 wk after the hard chancre, following haematogenous spread and bacterial proliferation. General symptoms (e.g. fever, general malaise, weight ↓, muscle and joint pain) and skin symptoms (e.g. erythematosquamous plaques) develop in this stage. Symptoms often spread to the palms. Syphilis is also accompanied by condylomata lata, flat, shiny, red-to-grey papules or plaques localised mainly in the anogenital region. These lesions contain many spirochetes and are therefore highly contagious.
> - Early latent syphilis: after 3-12 wk, 2nd stage symptoms may disappear spontaneously, may recur after <1y.
> - Late latent phase: the immune system response has eliminated most bacteria from the body. Skin abnormalities disappear, but ±66% remain in this latent phase and clearance of all bacteria is unlikely. Granulomatous nodules and nodular/ulcerative gummata, neurosyphilis and cardiovascular syphilis may occur at this stage.

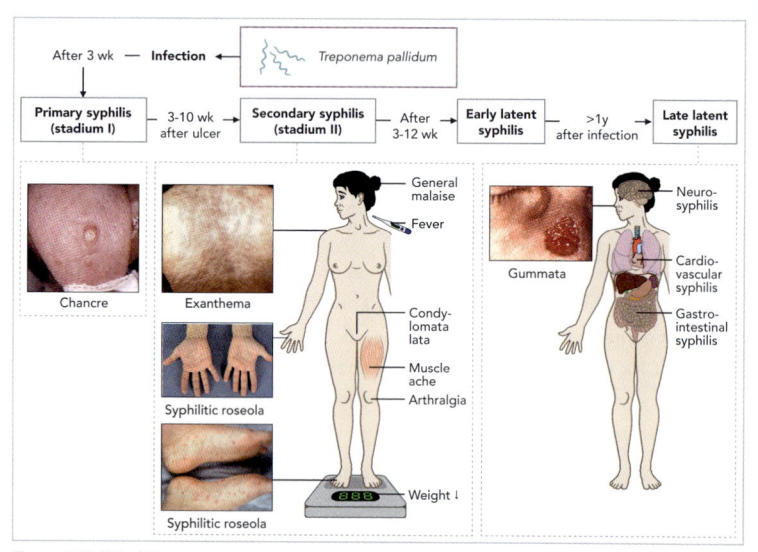

Figure 149 // Syphilis: stages

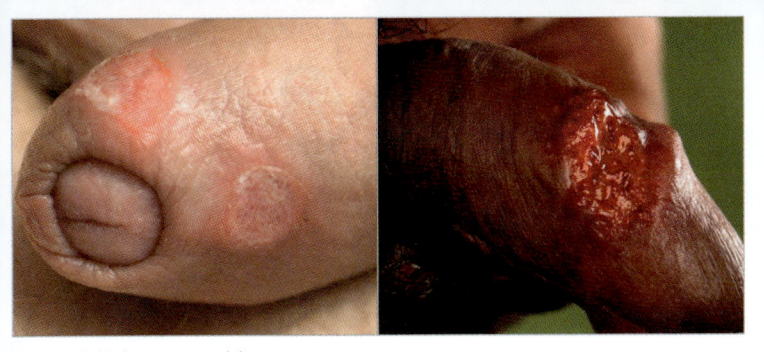

Figure 150 // Ulceration in syphilis

Trichomoniasis

- D Trichomoniasis is a vaginal infection caused by the *Trichomonas vaginalis* parasite (see Figure 151)
- E Prevalence in Australia 8.4-48%, South America 2.6-20%, Asia 7.8-8.5%, USA 2.5-26.2%, Europe 1.5%
- Ae *Trichomonas vaginalis*: protozoa, flagellar locomotion, colonises vagina and urethra
- R Prostitution, individuals from STI-endemic areas, multiple sexual partners, unprotected intercourse
- Hx Asymptomatic (50-85%), ♂: occasional urethritis, prostatitis, or epididymitis; ♀: malodorous green, foamy vaginal discharge
- PE Speculum exam: strawberry cervix (erythematous papules on cervix/vaginal wall with pinpoint haemorrhages), discharge (visible trichomonads in 10-30%)
- Dx • Labs: PCR on vaginal swab (to rule out other STIs)
  - Microscopy: vaginal discharge, pH ↑
- Tx 🖉 Metronidazole
- P • ♀: asymptomatic infection (long-term parasite carriage)
  - ♂: heals spontaneously
  - Rare complications: prostatitis, balanitis, epididymitis, infertility
- ! • Greater risk of prematurity, dysmaturity, prelabour rupture of membranes (PROM) in pregnant women
  - Also treat the patient's partner

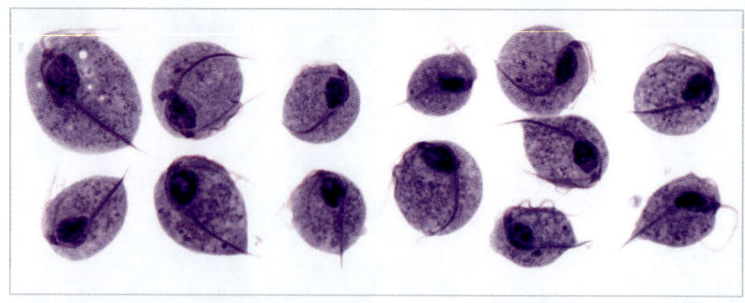

Figure 151 // *Trichomonas vaginalis*

Lymphogranuloma venereum (LGV)

- D LGV is a bacterial STI caused by *Chlamydia trachomatis* with two distinct variants: anorectal LGV and inguinal LGV.
- E Annual incidence of 3,000 reported cases in Europe, incidence unknown in USA, not nationally reportable
- Ae *Chlamydia trachomatis*, serotypes L1, L2, and L3, an intracellular Gram-negative bacterium, incubation period: 2-12 wk
- R Anal intercourse
- Hx STI risk assessment, anal/unprotected/frequent intercourse or intercourse with persons from endemic areas
- PE • Stage 1:
  - P Genitals
  - A Solitary
  - S Miliar to lenticular
  - S Round or oval
  - O Well-demarcated
  - N Red
  - E Papulovesicle, papule, ulcer
  - Stage 1: lesions disappear after a few days
  - Stage 2: painful lymph node swelling in the groin that may fluctuate and develop into an abscess (buboes; see Figure 152), swelling rupture may produce fistulas
  - Stage 3: genito-anorectal syndrome with proctocolitis accompanied by symptoms such as anal discharge, itching, constipation, cramps, or diarrhoea
- Dx PCR for *Chlamydia trachomatis*, followed by serovar test (to determine type of bacteria)

- Tx 💊 Doxycycline, followed by control PCR
- P Treatable, severe infections may present with chronic anal and perianal inflammation (abscesses and fistulas) that may require surgical intervention
- ! Chronic inflammation with fistula and abscess formation, risk of recurrence

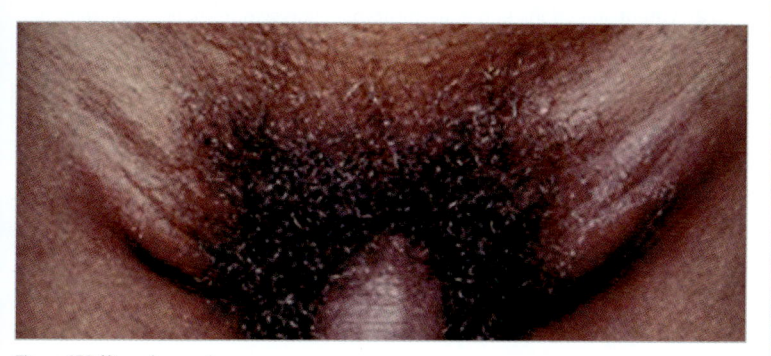

Figure 152 // Lymphogranuloma venereum

Human immunodeficiency virus (HIV) infection and acquired immunodeficiency syndrome (AIDS)

- D HIV infection is caused by the human immunodeficiency virus (HIV), a retrovirus with two genotypes (HIV-1, HIV-2). When untreated, this infection leads to a decrease in CD4+ T lymphocytes and progressive suppression of cellular immunity ensues. AIDS is defined as HIV infection complicated by opportunistic infection.
- E Global incidence 15-49y is 0.7%, incidence in Africa 3.2%
- Ae • Transmission: blood-to-blood contact, sexual contact (esp. anogenital contact), mother to child (vertical, breast milk)
  - Incubation period: 2-4 wk
  - HIV infects host cells (T lymphocytes, macrophages, dendritic cells) that express a CD4 receptor and a second chemokine receptor (CCR5 or CXCR4)
  - HIV is a retrovirus: adhesion to and penetration of host cell → single-stranded RNA is converted into DNA by reverse transcriptase enzyme → fusion with host-cell genome by integrase enzyme → production of viral protein by protease enzyme (see Figure 153)
- R Infection risk: anal intercourse, persons with multiple sexual partners, IV drug users, children of HIV-positive mothers

Hx Three phases (see Figure 154):
  1. Acute retroviral syndrome (acute HIV): 50-70% of people infected with HIV (typical: presents as infectious mononucleosis with fever, general malaise, sore throat, rash)
  2. Latent infection: either asymptomatic or symptomatic (e.g. weight ↓, swallowing symptoms, white patches in mouth, skin pathology, dysuria, genital skin pathology)
  3. AIDS: advanced stage of HIV infection; typical: presence of AIDS-defining conditions (conditions that occur in immunocompromised patients)

PE
  1. T ↑, lymphadenopathy, maculopapular rash
  2. Weight ↓, oropharyngeal candidiasis, herpes zoster, various STIs
  3. AIDS-defining conditions (e.g. infections, malignancies, neurological disease)

Dx
- Labs: CD4+ T lymphocytes ↓, Hb ↓, platelets ↓
- HIV antigen and antibody test
- Immunoblot: to detect specific antibodies against HIV-1 and HIV-2 infection
- PCR: detect viral RNA, determine viral load

Tx
- Lifetime antiretroviral combination therapy (cART). First-line cART: usually two nucleoside analogue reverse transcriptase inhibitors (NRTIs) with a non-nucleoside reverse transcriptase inhibitor (NNRTI) or a protease inhibitor.
- Pre-exposure prophylaxis (PrEP): HIV chemoprophylaxis
- Post-exposure prophylaxis (PEP): after possible high-risk exposure

P Variable interval between infection and progression to AIDS without cART: 1-15y

> **Window phase:** it usually takes 2-6 wk for antibodies to form after HIV infection. During this immediate post-infection period until seroconversion – the window phase – antibody-based HIV tests (serology) do not yet return positive results.

> **Different definitions of AIDS:**
> - The presence of one or more AIDS-defining conditions regardless of CD4 cell count.
> - The presence of one or more AIDS-defining disorders and/or a CD4 cell count <200/mm^3.

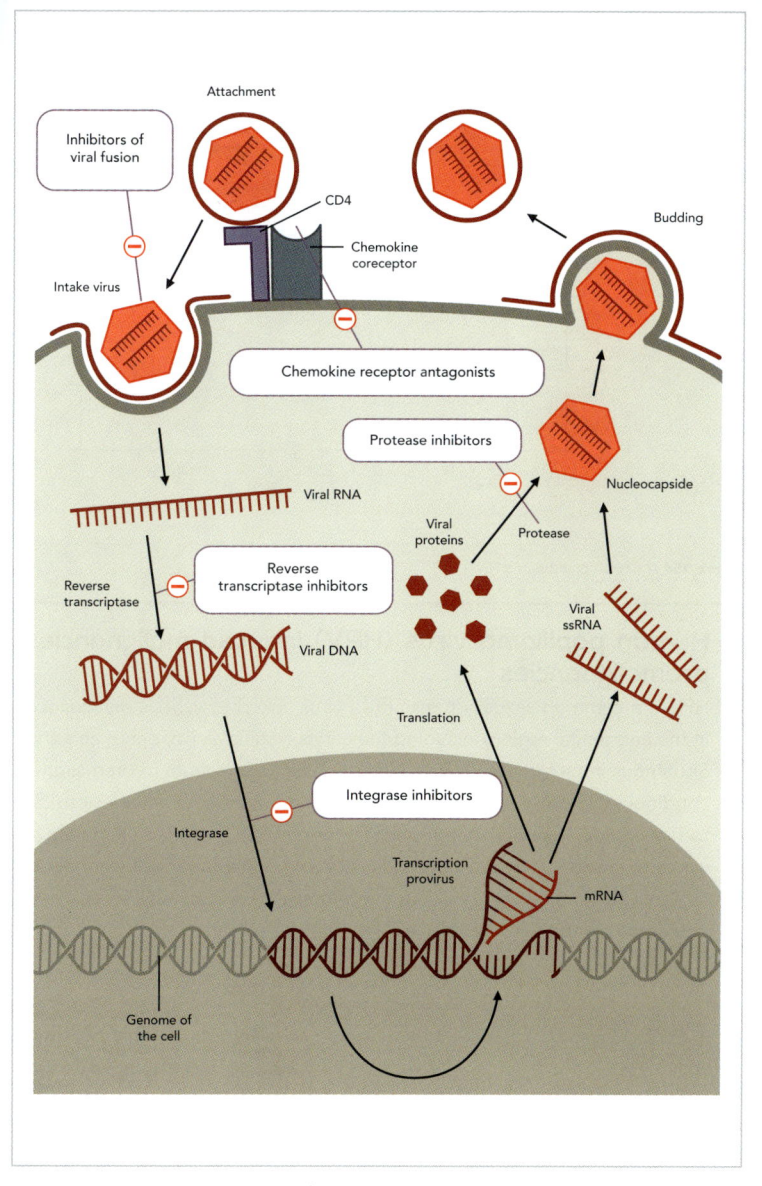

Figure 153 // HIV replication and targets of antiretroviral drugs

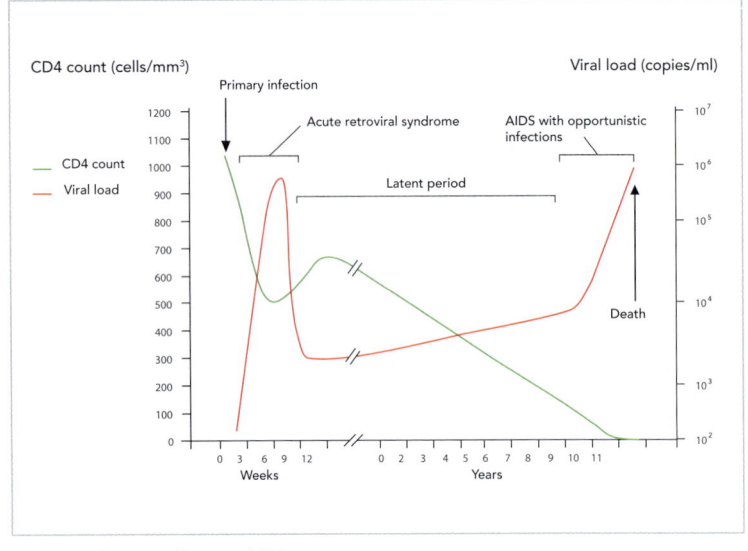

Figure 154 // Course of untreated HIV

Human papilloma virus (HPV) induced malignancies/premalignancies

D HPV is a common sexually transmitted virus linked to various malignancies in the anogenital region, including the cervix, vagina, vulva, penis, and anus. Squamous intraepithelial lesions (SIL) represent a spectrum of premalignant conditions that progress from low-grade squamous intraepithelial lesion (LSIL) to high-grade squamous intraepithelial lesion (HSIL) and can ultimately advance to invasive cancer. The classification of neoplasia varies by anogenital region: CIN for the cervix, vulvar intraep-ithelial neoplasia (VIN) for the vulva, and anal intraepithelial neoplasia (AIN) for the anal canal.

For more information on CIN and VIN, see the pocket *Obstetrics and Gynaecology*.

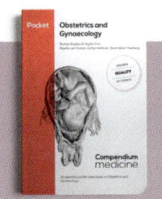

Anal intraepithelial neoplasia (AIN)

- **D** AIN is a precursor to anal carcinoma. It is classified based on the severity of squamous epithelial changes into low-grade AIN (LSIL-AIN 1) and high-grade AIN (HSIL-AIN 2 and HSIL-AIN 3); see Table 37. These manifestations are commonly detected at the anal transition zone (ATZ; see Figure 155).
- **E** Prevalence of HSIL is 22.4% in anal intercourse living with HIV and 6% in HPV type 16+ women. Incidence anal carcinoma 89:100,000 per year
- **Ae** High-risk HPV type 16
- **R** Anal HPV infection, living with HIV, history of gynaecological (pre-)cancers, immunosuppression, anal intercourse, multiple sexual partners, smoking
- **Hx** Asymptomatic ☺, condylomata may occur with itching and bleeding. Alarm symptoms for anal cancer: pain, bleeding, perceived lump, tenesmus.
- **PE** • Assessment of lymphadenopathy
  - P Intra-anal, esp. close to the squamo-columnar junction; perianal
  - A Often multifocal, circumscribed
  - S Varying
  - S Varying
  - O Well-demarcated
  - N Acetowhite (white discolouration after staining with acetic acid)
  - E Hyperkeratotic, plaque, thickened surface, velvety surface, punctate lesions, erosions, mosaic pattern, metaplastic changes
- **Dx** High-resolution anoscopy (HRA), biopsy if suspicion for squamous intraepithelial lesions (SIL)
- **Tx** • Prevention through vaccination prior to sexual initiation
  - Screening of high-risk individuals (e.g. anal intercourse living with HIV, history of vulvar cancer, immunosuppression for solid-organ transplant) between ages 30-65 every 5y: Papanicolaou (PAP) smear/HPV co-test or HPV test
  - LSIL: wait-and-see and annual HRA check up (incl. high-risk patients), cryotherapy in case of symptomatic condylomata
  - 🖉 HSIL: topical imiquimod, topical fluorouracil, topical trichloroacetic acid
  - ⚕ HSIL: electrocoagulation, laser ablation, surgical resection
- **P** Prognosis depending on type and severity, LSIL may spontaneously regress, 14% of HSIL progresses to anal carcinoma <5y in high-risk patients
- **!** • High recurrence rate → regular check-ups after treatment
  - Other HPV-induced premalignancies, such as penile intraepithelial neoplasia (PeIN) and vaginal intraepithelial neoplasia (VaIN), are rarer but can also result from HPV infection

	CLASSIFICATION	**AIN**	**SEVERITY OF CELLULAR PROLIFERATION**
Low-grade intraepithelial neoplasia (LGAIN)	LSIL	AIN-1	Not directly a precursor to anal cancer, but may occur in patients at high risk for HSIL in anal or other anogenital areas
High-grade intraepithelial neoplasia (HGAIN)	HSIL	AIN-2	Premalignant with the potential to develop into invasive anal cancer
		AIN-3	

Table 37 // Classification of AIN

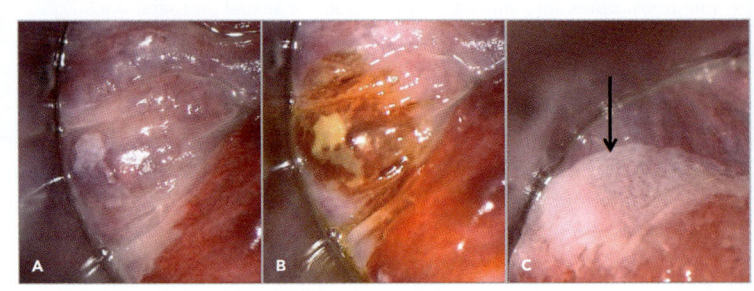

Figure 155 // Anal intraepithelial neoplasia (AIN)
A: AIN-1 with acetic acid **B:** AIN-1 with lugol **C:** AIN-2

> VIN is the precursor of vulvar carcinoma and is classified into two entities that differ in terms of pathophysiology, background, prognosis, and management:
> - Vulvar HSIL (previously VIN-2/3) is the most common form of VIN and is associated with HPV infection;
> - Patients with vHSIL have a cancer risk of 9.7% after 10y follow-up;
> - HPV-independent VIN (often clinically referred to as differentiated VIN/dVIN) is a premalignant lesion not related to HPV and may develop on an existing vulvar lesion (e.g. lichen sclerosus). Patients with dVIN have a cancer risk of 50.0% after 10y of follow-up;
> - VIN is treated with topical imiquimod, laser ablation or surgical resection.

Bacterial infections

	CELLULITIS	**ERYSIPELAS**
D	*Streptococcus pyogenes* or *Staphylococcus aureus* infection affecting the deep dermis and subcutis (see Figure 156).	Infection caused by *Streptococcus pyogenes*, affecting dermis and lymphatic vessels.
E	Incidence 555:100,000 per year	Incidence 20-2,500:100,000 per year
Ae	<td colspan="2"><ul><li>Microorganism invades dermis through a breach in the skin</li><li>Hematogenous spread</li><li>Entry point e.g. between toes due to tinea pedis</li></ul></td>	
R	DM, peripheral vascular disease, IV drug use, immunodeficiency, lymphoedema, alcohol abuse	Childhood, ♂, advanced age, impaired resistance, lymphoedema, chronic leg ulcers
Hx	<td colspan="2">Fever, chills, general malaise, swollen regional lymph nodes, tender/oedematous/warm skin</td>	
	<td colspan="2">T ↑</td>	
PE	(P) Head and neck area in children, limbs in adults (A) Solitary (S) Several, size depends on progression of infection, regional (S) Variable (O) Ill-demarcated, non-raised margin (N) Red (E) Erythematous macule, severe infection may present with vesicles, pustules, bullae	(P) Lower legs and face (A) Solitary (S) Several, size depends on progression of infection, regional (S) Variable (O) Well-demarcated, raised margin (N) Red (E) Erythematous plaque, severe infections may present with vesicles, bullae or haemorrhagic necrosis
Dx	<td colspan="2">No added value</td>	
Tx	<td colspan="2">ABx targeting beta-hemolytic *Streptococcus* and *Staphylococcus aureus*, oral or parenteral (systemic signs of toxicity, rapid, extensive erythema)</td>	
P	Risk of recurrence, complications rare (glomerulonephritis, subacute bacterial endocarditis, lymphoedema)	Frequent recurrences, complications very rare (subcutaneous abscesses, glomerulonephritis, sepsis)
!	<td colspan="2">Consider necrotising fasciitis in case of extreme pain, therapy resistance, or incipient necrosis</td>	

Table 38 // Bacterial skin infections

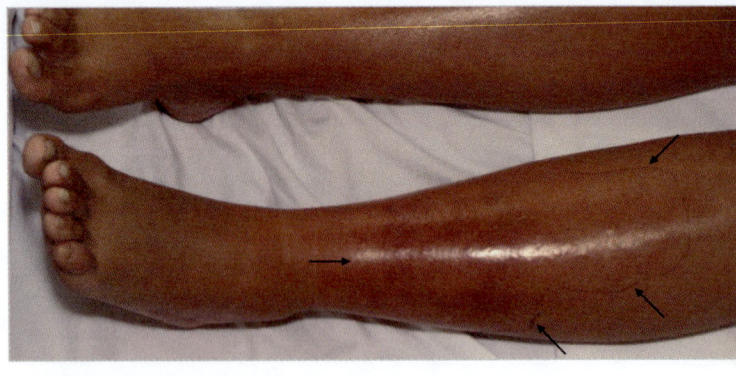

Figure 156 // Cellulitis on the lower/left leg

Erythrasma

- **D** Erythrasma is a skin infection caused by *Corynebacterium minutissimum*, characterised by well-demarcated reddish-brown and slightly scaly lesions in the skin folds, esp. in the groin, armpits, and between the toes (see Figure 157). Often accompanied by pitted keratolysis of the feet and hyperhidrosis in the armpits and on the feet.
- **E** Prevalence 20%
- **Ae** *Corynebacterium minutissimum*
- **R** Hot, humid environment, poor hygiene, DM, impaired resistance, excessive sweating
- **Hx** Asymptomatic ⊕, itching ⊖
- **PE** **P** Between the toes, in the armpits, groin, intergluteal cleft, inframammary fold, navel
  - **A** Solitary
  - **S** Several cm to dozens of cm
  - **S** Variable
  - **O** Well-demarcated
  - **N** Violaceous or brown
  - **E** Erythematous macule with scaling and fissures
- **Dx** Wood's lamp: coral-red fluorescence
- **Tx** 💬 Good local hygiene
  - 🔗 Topical ABx, e.g. local erythromycin lotion
- **P** Risk of chronic skin infection

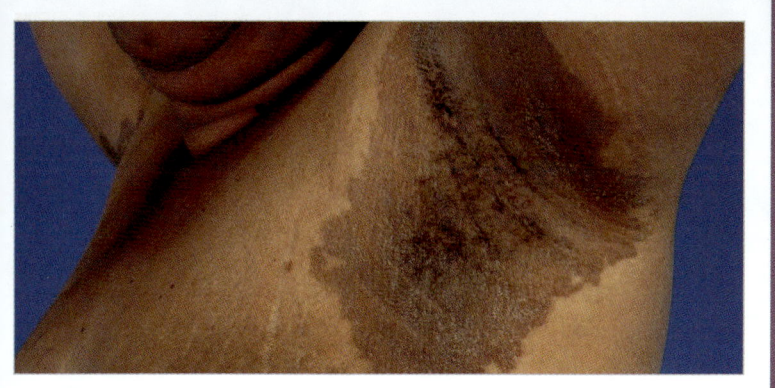

Figure 157 // Erythrasma

Necrotising fasciitis

- D) Necrotising fasciitis is a rare form of cellulitis usually caused by group A *Streptococcus* (e.g. *Streptococcus pyogenes*), a mixed infection, or in some cases (e.g. immunocompromised patients) a fungal infection. It is a fulminant infection, characterised by necrosis of all skin layers, fascia, and muscle.
- E) Incidence: 0.3-15:100,000 per year
- Ae) *Streptococcus pyogenes*, mixed infection, or fungal infection
- R) DM, obesity, impaired immune system, liver disease, drug abuse
- Hx) Very painful, sometimes crepitus upon palpation (due to gas in underlying tissues, esp. in *Clostridium* spp. infection)
- PE)
  - P) Mainly limbs but can occur everywhere
  - A) Solitary
  - S) Regional, rapidly increasing in size
  - S) Variable
  - O) Ill-demarcated erythema initially, well-demarcated bullae, and ulcerations later
  - N) Red, lesions quickly turn grey-blue with blistering and black necrosis
  - E) Erythematous macules with bullae, necrosis, and ulcerations
- Dx)
  - Clinical suspicion warrants immediate surgical exploration, consider CT for regions that are hard to assess or do not improve after necrosectomy
  - X-ray: subcutaneous gas/emphysema in *Clostridium* spp.
- Tx) Immediate combination of broad-spectrum, high-dose IV ABx in consultation with microbiologist, analgesia for pain management, IV immunoglobulin for streptococcal toxic shock syndrome

- Excision of all affected soft tissue, removal of non-vital skin and surgical debridement when necessary with daily dressing
- 25% mortality
- Always consider necrotising fasciitis in cases of extremely painful cellulitis unresponsive to ABx
- Treatment differs in case of a fungal infection

Viral infections

Oral herpes

- Oral herpes, also herpes labialis or cold sore, is a viral infection on the lips or in the mouth caused by the herpes simplex virus (HSV) (see Figure 158).
- Incidence of recurrent herpes labialis 160:100,000 per year, in Europe 67%, seropositivity in USA 48%
- HSV, HSV-1 ⊙, HSV-2 ⊖, transmission through saliva, orogenital or oro-anal contact
- Fever and sunlight exposure are triggering factors
- Primary infection usually in children aged 1-5y
  - Most common clinical presentation of primary HSV-1 infection: herpetic gingivostomatitis
  - After the 2-12d incubation period: fever, general malaise, salivation, pain when eating or drinking, halitosis
  - Recurrence on and around the lips (oral herpes): itching or burning and blisters on or around the lips
- P On and around the lips, in the mouth
  - A Herpetiform, coalescent
  - S Several mm
  - S Round
  - O Well-demarcated
  - N White and red
  - E Vesicles, later erosions, papules, and crusts
- No added value
- Antiseptics, adequate hydration, analgesics
- Topical or systemic aciclovir, valaciclovir, or famciclovir
- Recovery within 7-10d
- High risk of recurrences (4-5x/y), recurrences become less common after age 35

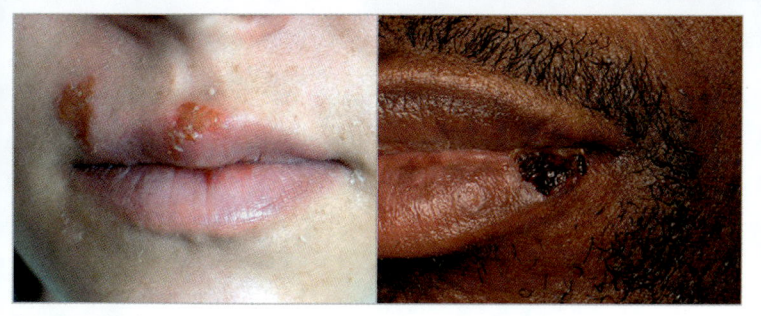

Figure 158 // Oral herpes

Herpes zoster

- **D** Herpes zoster, or shingles, is a painful skin condition caused by reactivation of the latent Varicella zoster virus (VZV, HHV-3) (see Figure 159).
- **E** Incidence: Europe 300:100,000, USA 290:100,000 per year
- **Ae** · Reactivation of latent VZV, another herpes virus
  · Acquired in childhood (chickenpox), followed by nesting in the sensory ganglia of the spinal cord or brain (see Figure 160)
- **R** ♀, advanced age, reactivation triggered by e.g. stress, fever, tissue damage, or immune system suppression
- **Hx** Onset characterised by pain, itching, tingling, hyperaesthesia, fever
- **PE** **P** One or several dermatomes, unilateral, torso and face
  - **A** Herpetiform, coalescent
  - **S** Multiple, several mm to cm (larger than in herpes simplex), segmental
  - **S** Round, polycyclic
  - **O** Well-demarcated
  - **N** Red
  - **E** Haemorrhagic, pustular, or erosive vesicles and bullae on an oedematous substrate → crusts
- **Dx** No added value
- **Tx** · Antivirals (e.g. aciclovir), preferably start <72h of onset of rash
  · Immunocompromised patients: IV aciclovir
  · Reduce risk of postherpetic neuralgia: e.g. amitriptyline or carbamazepine
  · Local analgesia: capsaicin cream, systemic analgesia: paracetamol or tramadol
- **P** Heals spontaneously in immunocompetent patients, worse prognosis with

more pain and complications in elderly and immunocompromised patients
- Postherpetic neuralgia (persistent nerve pain), blindness in herpes zoster of the optic nerve (herpes zoster ophthalmicus)

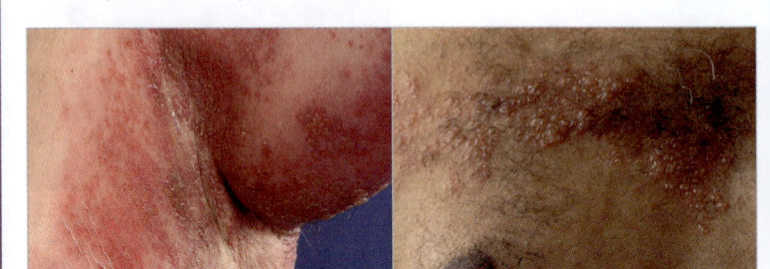

Figure 159 // Herpes zoster

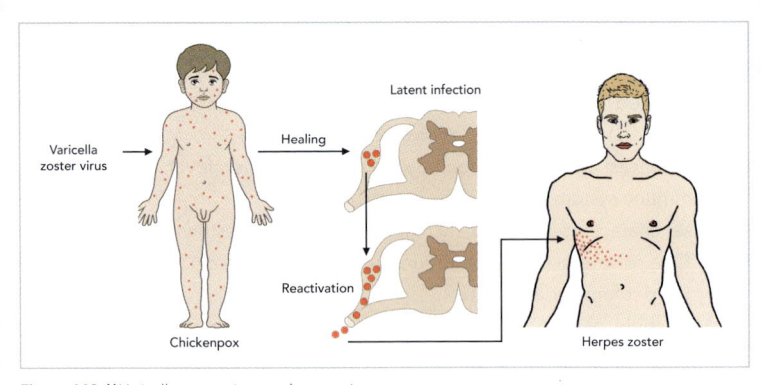

Figure 160 // Varicella zoster virus: pathogenesis

Molluscum contagiosum

- (D) Molluscum contagiosum is a viral skin infection caused by Molluscum contagiosum virus (MCV) (see Figure 161).
- (E) Annual incidence 1,200-1,400:100,000 per year (in children aged 0-14y)
- (Ae) Caused by a poxvirus (molluscum contagiosum virus), transmitted by direct skin-to-skin contact
- (R) Young age
- (Hx) Itching, pain, signs of inflammation, contact with infected people, signs of immunosuppression, dermatitis
- (PE) (P) Torso, skin folds, and genital region

- (A) Grouped
- (S) Several, 2-5 mm
- (S) Round or oval
- (O) Well-demarcated
- (N) Pearly white to skin-coloured, red when body initiates immune response and healing process
- (E) Firm papules with central umbilication, area surrounding lesions may be eczematous
- (Dx) No added value
- (Tx) 💬 Generally no treatment needed, advise against scratching to prevent spread of infection
  - 💊 Treatment can be considered in some cases (e.g. lesions in the genital area, underlying atopic disease), using topical treatments: podophyllotoxin, potassium hydroxide, benzoyl peroxide, silver nitrate, and cantharidin
  - 🔪 Curettage or cryotherapy are not recommended (no evidence of efficacy)
- (P) Heals spontaneously within 6 mo-1y
- (!) Consider impaired immunity in case of extensive or large lesions

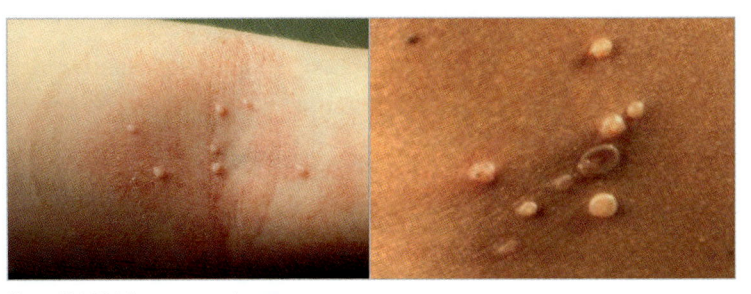

Figure 161 // Molluscum contagiosum

Verruca vulgaris

- (D) Verruca vulgaris, or a wart, is caused by infection with HPV (see Figures 162 and 163).
- (E) Prevalence 1-12%
- (Ae) Caused by HPV, a DNA virus, transmission via direct contact with an infected person or indirect contact (e.g. in shower room)
- (R) Childhood, individuals working in the meat and fish processing industry
- (Hx) Sites and number of warts, course (since when, growth in size or quantity over

time), pain, irritation, cosmetic concerns
- PE
  - P Fingers, backs of hands, elbows, knees
    - A Solitary, grouped, or coalescent
    - S Often multiple, ranging from mm to cm
    - S Flat or convex
    - O Moderately to well-demarcated
    - N White-yellow to brown
    - E Verrucous papules and plaques
- Dx No added value
- Tx 💬 Generally no treatment needed
  - 💊 Salicylic acid preparations. Alternatives: imiquimod or 5-fluorouracil cream and bleomycin.
  - 🔪 Cryotherapy, electrocoagulation, pulsed dye laser
- P 60% of warts go into spontaneous remission after 2y in immunocompetent individuals
- ❗ Consider impaired immune system in case of protracted or rapidly spreading warts

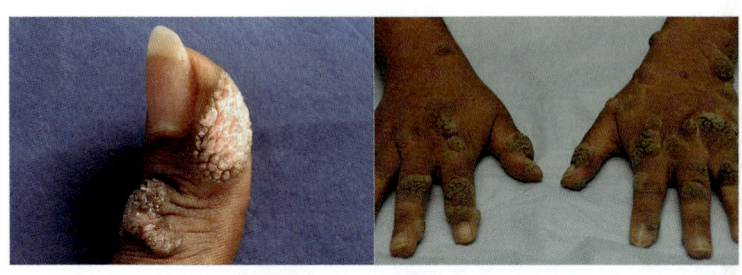

Figure 162A and 162B // Verruca vulgaris

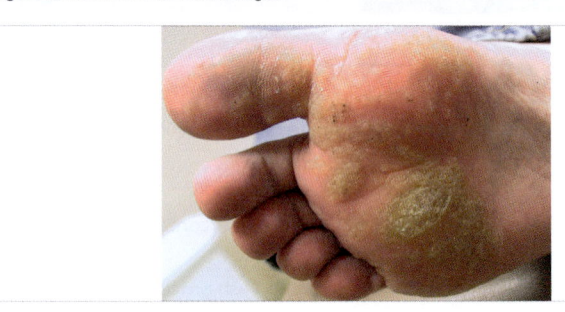

Figure 163 // Verruca vulgaris on the sole of the foot (verruca plantaris)

Kaposi sarcoma (KS)

KS is an angioproliferative disorder characterised by the abnormal growth of blood vessels, leading to tumours that can affect the skin, mouth, lymph nodes, and internal organs. It is considered a low-grade malignant vascular tumour and can be classified into four types based on the clinical circumstances in which it develops: classic, endemic, iatrogenic, and AIDS-associated. The clinical presentation can vary from minimal mucocutaneous involvement to extensive multiorgan involvement, and KS is one of the most common cancers among patients with HIV (see Figure 164 and Table 39).

> There is discussion on whether there may be a 5th group: anal intercourse without HIV infection. In classic, non-HIV-related Kaposi sarcoma, 28% of cases are found among anal intercourse not living with HIV, suggesting human herpesvirus 8 (HHV-8) transmission independent of HIV status. This group presents with milder disease and more genital lesions, with transmission likely via sexual or oro-oral contact.

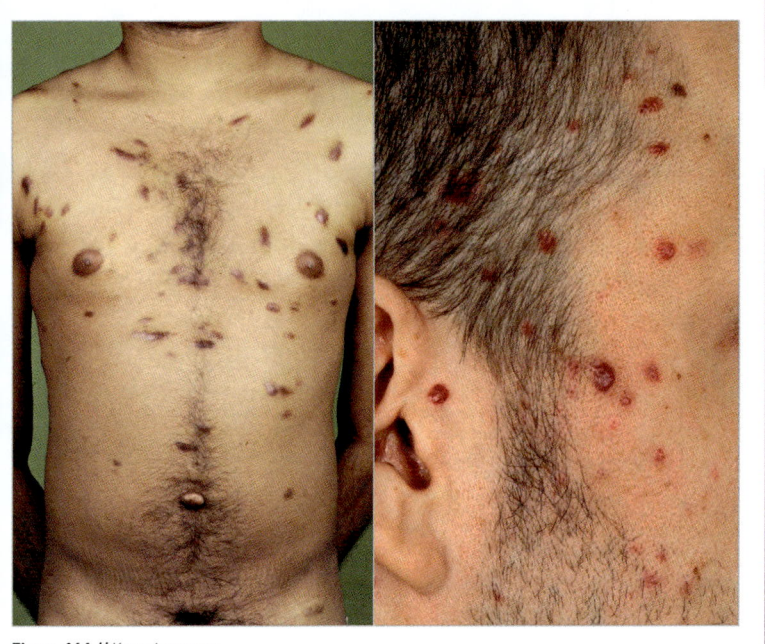

Figure 164 // Kaposi sarcoma

	CLASSIC KS (SPORADIC)	**IATROGENIC KS (IMMUNOCOMPROMISED)**
D	The classic variant of KS is characterised by slowly progressive lesions, and it is not related to AIDS or immunosuppression. This variant is much rarer than the other types.	Iatrogenic KS, or transplant-related KS, is typically seen in people after solid organ transplantation, as it is associated with immunosuppressive drug therapy in transplant patients.
E	Incidence 0.39:100,000 per year in general population worldwide	
Hx	Asymptomatic ⊖	
Ae	Human herpesvirus 8 (HHV-8) → transmitted saliva → Kaposi sarcoma-associated herpesvirus (KSHV)	
R	♂, >60y, Mediterranean descent	Exogenous immunosuppression, solid organ transplant, >50y
PE	Oval, erythematous macules, papules, and plaques that can develop into purple-black nodules and tumours, varying from a few mm to a few cm	
	Distal extremities: lower legs, feet	Clinically similar to classic KS, can be more locally aggressive: lower extremity lymphoedema in adults
Dx	• Biopsy to confirm diagnosis: spindle cell proliferation, angiogenesis, and inflammation across all subtypes. The disease histologically progresses following a patch, plaque, and nodular stage. • Ultrasound, chest X-ray, or CT scan: screening for internal involvement only in case of symptoms (e.g. pulmonary symptoms, GI symptoms, lymphadenopathy) • Stool test for occult blood (e.g. GI involvement), if positive → endoscopy • Bronchoscopy in case pulmonary lesions on chest X-ray/chest CT	
Tx	💬 Symptom management, prevention progression, tumour reduction to alleviate oedema, treatment not necessary in immunocompetent patients with stable disease 💊 • Intralesional injection (e.g. vinblastine, bleomycin), topical retinoid • AIDS-related subtype: initiate combined antiretroviral therapy (ART) 🔪 Cryotherapy, surgical excision, electrocoagulation, laser therapy (e.g. CO$_2$ laser), radiation therapy (local or total body)	
P	• Rarely aggressive and disseminated, slow course • Involvement of visceral organs ⊖	• Often in remission after reducing or discontinuing immunosuppressive therapy • Involvement of visceral organs ⊕
!	Classic KS is associated with other malignancies (e.g. non-Hodgkin lymphoma)	No increased risk of KS in patients with congenital immunodeficiency

Table 39 // Kaposi sarcoma subtypes

ENDEMIC KS (AFRICAN)	AIDS ASSOCIATED KS
Endemic KS is that reported in HIV-negative individuals, particularly in sub-Saharan Africa.	Most common and aggressive form of KS. Morbidity and mortality have significantly decreased since (active ART) immune restoration.
Incidence 0.39:100,000 per year in general population worldwide
colspan="2" Asymptomatic ⊕
Human herpesvirus 8 (HHV-8) → transmitted saliva → Kaposi sarcoma-associated herpesvirus (KSHV)
♂:♀ = 1:1, African descent (sub-Saharan Africa), 20-40y	AIDS patients (low CD4 cell count)
Oval, erythematous macules, papules, and plaques that can develop into purple-black nodules and tumours, varying from a few mm to a few cm
• Distal lower extremities, could be disseminated • Internal organs involved in a subset of adult patients	Localised or disseminated
• Biopsy to confirm diagnosis: spindle cell proliferation, angiogenesis, and inflammation across all subtypes. The disease histologically progresses following a patch, plaque, and nodular stage. • Ultrasound, chest X-ray, or CT scan: screening for internal involvement only in case of symptoms (e.g. pulmonary symptoms, GI symptoms, lymphadenopathy) • Stool test for occult blood (e.g. GI involvement), if positive → endoscopy • Bronchoscopy in case pulmonary lesions on chest X-ray/chest CT
💬 Symptom management, prevention progression, tumour reduction to alleviate oedema, treatment not necessary in immunocompetent patients with stable disease 💊 • Intralesional injection (e.g. vinblastine, bleomycin), topical retinoid   • AIDS-related subtype: initiate combined antiretroviral therapy (ART) 🔪 Cryotherapy, surgical excision, electrocoagulation, laser therapy (e.g. CO_2 laser), radiation therapy (local or total body)
• Indolent to locally invasive in adults, aggressive in children, fatal course • Involvement of visceral organs and lymph nodes ⊕	• Indolent or aggressive, can regress with effective HIV treatment, at times fatal outcome • Involvement of visceral organs ⊕ (esp. in patients with poor HIV control)
Several factors (e.g. malaria, malnutrition) compromise the immune system and can increase the risk of KSHV infection	• KS can still occur even with a good CD4 count • The presence of visible KS can be stigmatising due to its association with AIDS, which can lead to social discrimination

Dermatomycoses

> 💡 Mycids can occur in all mycoses. A mycid (id reaction, autoeczematisation) is a type IV hypersensitivity reaction caused by a mycosis elsewhere on the skin. It is characterised by erythematovesicular or erythematosquamous lesions, esp. on palms and fingers. Mycid reactions are treated by treating the triggering mycosis.

> 💡 Deep mycosis are systemic fungal infections often caused by opportunistic fungi. These infections can be life-threatening, esp. in patients with compromised immune systems. Common types of deep mycosis include candidiasis, aspergillosis, and cryptococcosis. Systemic mycoses may present with a range of skin changes, incl. papules, nodules, and purpuric lesions.

Onychomycosis

- (D) Onychomycosis, or tinea unguium, is a fungal infection of the nail (see Figure 165).
- (E) Prevalence 3-22%, up to 90% in elderly patients
- (Ae) Caused by *Trichophyton* species, usually *Trichophyton rubrum* or *Trichophyton mentagrophytes*, associated with tinea pedis or tinea manuum
- (R) ♂, DM, immunosuppression, impaired perfusion, damaged nails (mechanical or psoriasis)
- (Hx) White or yellow discolouration of the nail, progressing from distal to proximal
- (PE) • Nail
  - Yellow-brown, thickened, and brittle nail if nail bed is affected
- (Dx) • Culture to test for resistance or distinguish dermatophyte or *Candida*
  - KOH test or microscopic exam of nail specimen with PAS staining to rule out onychomycosis
  - Mycological culture or PCR test
- (Tx) 🗨 Wear well-fitting breathable shoes. Keep feet dry, change socks daily. Wear shower flip flops when using communal showers.
  - 💊 • Topical (in mild-to-moderate cases): ciclopirox, amorolfine, or terbinafine nail polish (6-12 mo)
  - Systemic (in moderate-to-severe cases): terbinafine, itraconazole, or fluconazole
- (P) • Harmless defect, but chronic course may eventually affect all nails

- Fingernails are more responsive to therapy than toenails, which take longer to respond due to their slower growth rate
- Watch out for a mycid reaction
- Prevent re-infection by applying an antimycotic powder to shoes and socks

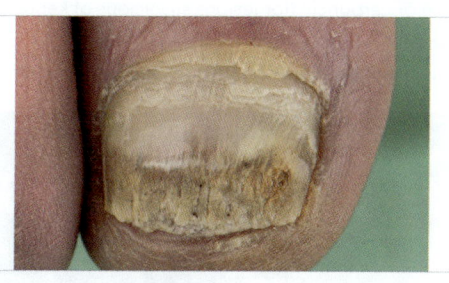

Figure 165 // Onychomycosis of the toenail

Tinea capitis

Tinea capitis, or trichomycosis, is a fungal infection of the scalp and/or head hair (see Figure 166). There are three types of tinea capitis: endothrix (in the hair, most common), ectothrix (around the hair), and kerion (prominent inflammation).

Esp. in young children, more common in warm and humid regions

- Ectothrix: *Microsporum audouinii, Microsporum canis*
- Endothrix: *Trichophyton tonsurans, Trichophyton soudanense, Trichophyton violaceum*
- Kerion: *Trichophyton mentagrophytes, Trichophyton verrucosum*

Contact with infected people, animals, or pets, young age

Itching, baldness (alopecia) ⊖

Hair on scalp:

- Ectothrix: bald patches with scaling/broken hairs, sometimes inflammatory
- Endothrix: black dots visible, because of broken hairs
- Kerion: inflammation with plaque, crusts, and abscesses, hair loss, fever, lymphadenopathy

- Wood's lamp: *Microsporum canis* and *Microsporum audouinii* produce a greenish yellow colour, *Trichophyton* species do not respond
- KOH test to confirm presence of spores in (endothrix) or on (ectothrix) the hair
- Mycological culture or PCR test

- Tx • Terbinafine, griseofulvin, itraconazole, or fluconazole
  - Adjust as necessary following culture or PCR findings
- P Superficial infections heal spontaneously after years, risk of permanent hair loss (cicatricial alopecia) with suboptimal treatment of kerion, recurrence is rare
- ! • DDx: furuncle or carbuncle (for lesions suspicious of kerion)
  - Topical treatment fails to effectively infiltrate the hair follicles, but can be used as adjunctive treatment alongside systemic medication

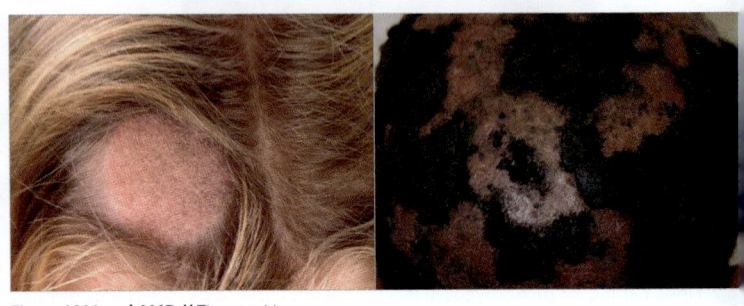

Figure 166A and 166B // Tinea capitis

Tinea corporis

- D Tinea corporis, or ringworm, is a superficial fungal infection on the skin of the torso and extremities (see Figure 167).
- E Incidence of mycoses 310:100,000 per year, incl. tinea corporis
- Ae • All dermatophytes, most common: *Trichophyton rubrum*, *Trichophyton mentagrophytes*, *Epidermophyton floccosum*
  - Transmission by direct contact
- R Heat, humidity, contact with infected people, pets and other animals
- Hx Lesion may itch or burn
- PE P Torso or limbs
  - A Solitary or multiple/grouped, later coalescent
  - S Variable, ranging from small to very large, regional
  - S Round, later oval or annular due to central healing
  - O Well-demarcated, raised margin with scaling
  - N Red, brown, or grey
  - E Erythematosquamous lesion, peripheral scaling with occasional vesicles or pustules
- Dx KOH test on a sample taken from active lesional margins to confirm funga hyphae

- **Tx** 🔹 Topical antifungal treatment (azoles, allylamines, butenafine, ciclopirox, tolnaftate, amorolfine), oral drugs (terbinafine itraconazole, griseofulvin, and fluconazole)
- **P** Favourable due to good response to therapy, most recurrences are triggered by re-wearing own clothes
- **!** Regular recurrences → possibly impaired immune system function ⊖

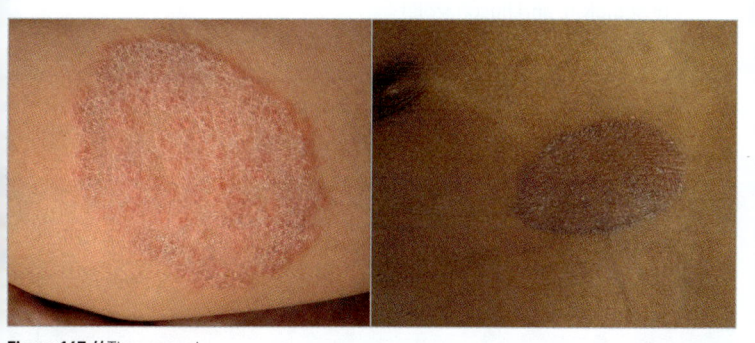

Figure 167 // Tinea corporis

Tinea pedis

- **D** Tinea pedis, or athlete's foot, is a superficial fungal infection of the foot. There are two types: tinea pedis plantaris (soles of the feet) and tinea pedis interdigitalis (between the toes) (see Figure 168).
- **E** Prevalence 3%
- **Ae** *Trichophyton rubrum* ⊙
- **R** Moist environment (swimming, sports), poor foot hygiene, non-breathable footwear, young age
- **Hx** Slightly itchy, burning lesion
- **PE** **P** Sole or between toes (esp. the 4th and 5th toes), often begins between toes and spreads to sole
  - **A** Regional, coalescent after spread
  - **S** Variable
  - **S** Round
  - **O** Well-demarcated, onset on sole is generally characterised by peripheral activity (vesicles or pustules)
  - **N** Red
  - **E** Erythematosquamous lesion, may present with swelling, weeping erosions, and fissures

- Dx: KOH test of specimen taken from the active edge of the lesion: to detect fungal hyphae
- Tx: 💬 Wear well-fitting breathable shoes. Keep feet dry, change socks daily. Wear shower flip flops when using communal showers.
  - 💊 Topical antifungal treatment (azoles, allylamines, butenafine, ciclopirox, tolnaftate, amorolfine), oral antifungal drugs (terbinafine, itraconazole, griseofulvin, and fluconazole)
- P: High risk of recurrences, rarely cured without treatment
- !
  - Always apply miconazole nitrate powder to footwear to prevent re-infection
  - Advise patients to regularly rotate footwear
  - Increased risk of erysipelas due to skin defects

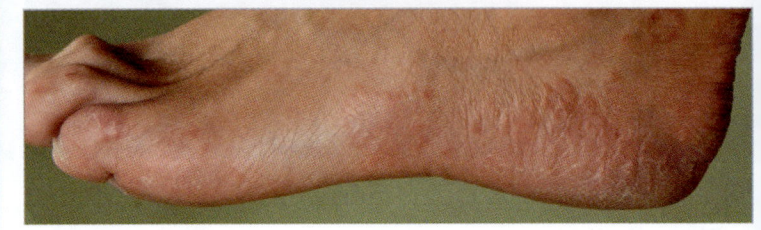

Figure 168 // Tinea pedis

Trichosis

> 💡 The psychological impact of hair conditions must not be underestimated, patients may need psychological counselling.

Alopecia areata

- D: Alopecia areata is a patchy, non-cicatricial form of alopecia suspected to be a hair-specific autoimmune disease (see Figure 169).
- E: Prevalence 0.12% in adults, 0.03% in children, lifetime risk approx. 2%
- Ae:
  - Idiopathic, potentially an autoimmune disorder
  - Normal hair follicle keratinocytes generally do not express major histocompatibility complex (MHC) antigens
  - Interaction between cytotoxic T lymphocytes and hair matrix cells through expression of HLA (human MHC)
- R: Positive FHx, young adults, atopy, Down syndrome, age 20-50
- Hx: Bald spots on the head/beard region

- **PE**
  - **P** Scalp, beard region, eyebrows, eyelashes
  - **A** Solitary
  - **S** Few mm to generalised spread
  - **S** Round to polygonal
  - **O** Well-demarcated
  - **N** Normal skin colour, peripheral hairs may show depigmentation
  - **E** Exclamation mark hairs (short hairs that get increasingly narrow near the scalp; see Figure 170), scalp appears normal, intact hair follicles
- **Dx** When in doubt between alopecia areata and tinea capitis: mycological testing
- **Tx** 💬 Difficult to treat, camouflage therapy (hairpiece or wig), wait-and-see (up to 80% spontaneous remission <1y)
  - 💊 • Limited patchy hair loss: topical corticosteroids (class II-IV), intralesional corticosteroids, topical minoxidil 5% (limited evidence and only for patients with limited alopecia areata)
    - Extensive patchy hair loss or alopecia universalis: contact immunotherapy (e.g. diphenylcyclopropenone (DPCP)), wig/hairpiece
    - Systemic: corticosteroids, ciclosporin, methotrexate, azathioprine, JAK1/2 inhibitor (e.g. baricitinib), JAK3/TEC inhibitor (e.g. ritlecitinib)
- **P** Favourable spontaneous course if lesions are small and solitary, worse prognosis with onset of alopecia at younger age, frequent recurrences, complaints >1y, positive FHx, nail problems, ophiasis type, patient with constitutional dermatitis)
- ⚠ Alopecia areata is associated with vitiligo, autoimmune thyroid disorders, pernicious anaemia, and systemic lupus erythematosus. Other forms of alopecia are alopecia totalis (complete loss of hair on the scalp), alopecia universalis (complete loss of all body hair), ophiasis, and alopecia areata incognita.

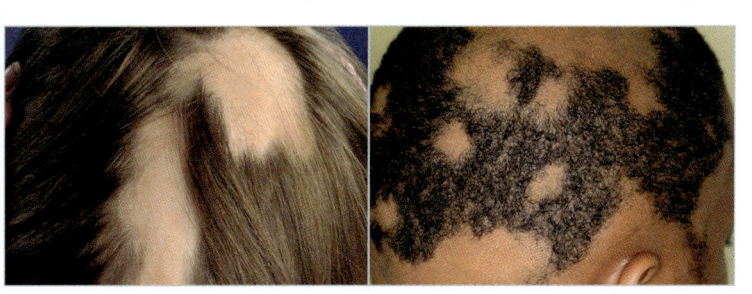

Figure 169A and 169B // Alopecia areata

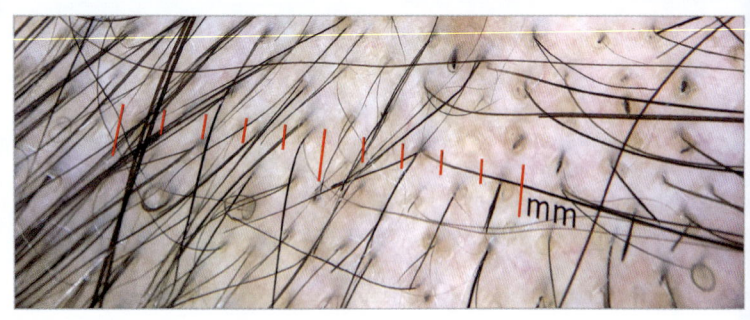

Figure 170 // Exclamation mark hair

Androgenetic alopecia

- (D) Androgenetic alopecia, or pattern hair loss (male or female), is a condition characterised by the progressive loss of terminal hairs of the scalp in a distinctive distribution, caused by an excessive response to androgens. Androgenetic alopecia affects both males and females (see Figure 171).
- (E) Affects approx. 50% of males and females, incidence aligning with age (i.e. 50% by 50y and 80% by 70y in males with pale to fair skin)
- (Ae) Heightened androgenic milieu in the scalp (elevated dihydrotestosterone (DHT) production, heightened levels of 5-alpha reductase, and increased abundance of androgen receptors) → increased androgen receptor activation → progressive shortening of the growth (anagen) phase → follicular miniaturisation and characteristic pattern of hair thinning and hair loss
- (R) Pale to fair skin, familial predisposition
- (Hx) Gradual hair loss
- (PE) Terminal hair loss typically begins in the temporal scalp, midfrontal scalp, or vertex area of the scalp in males. In females, the hair thinning appears more diffuse. No signs of skin abnormalities on the scalp and no scarring are common. May be accompanied by nail abnormalities.
- (Dx) Trichoscopy: hair diameter diversity, perifollicular pigmentation/peripilar signs, and yellow dots
- (Tx) 🗨 Education on disease course and prognosis
  - 💊 • Topical minoxidil 5% solution, oral 5-alpha reductase inhibitor finasteride
    - In women, oral antiandrogens like spironolactone are often used to treat pattern baldness
  - ✏️ Hair transplantation

- P Several factors, incl. early onset, gender, surface area involvement, FHx, treatment choices, therapy compliance, and lifestyle factors, can influence the prognosis of androgenetic alopecia
- ! Potential correlation between pattern baldness and cardiovascular diseases in males and polycystic ovarian disease in females

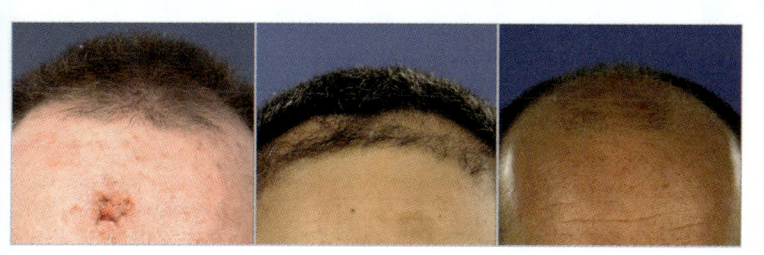

Figure 171 // Androgenetic alopecia

Cicatricial alopecia

- D Cicatricial alopecia, also known as alopecia atrophicans or scarring alopecia, is characterised by patchy hair loss accompanied by scarring of the scalp (see Figure 172). It is a collective name for several diagnoses characterised by scarring (see Table 40).
- E Exact incidence and prevalence unknown
- Ae • Primary form: inflammatory reaction directed against the hair follicle
  - Secondary form: non-specific processes affecting the hair follicle (e.g. burns, ionising radiation, cutaneous malignancies)
- R Inflammatory dermatoses, burns, radiation, malignancies
- Hx Bald spots and scarring of the scalp
- PE Single or several bald patches on a smooth, shiny, and thin-skinned scalp, absence of follicle openings is essential for diagnosis
- Dx Biopsy: identify underlying pathology
- Tx 💬 Sun protection, vitamin D suppletion, smoking cessation (discoid lupus erythematosus), avoid chemical straighteners, tension-free hairstyling (central centrifugal), avoid hair care products causing inflammation
  - 💊 • Topical corticosteroids (class III-IV), topical calcineurin inhibitors, intralesional corticosteroids, minoxidil 5% (off-label)
    - Systemic: hydroxychloroquine, ciclosporin, methotrexate, glucocorticosteroids, retinoids (follicular hyperkeratosis), tetracyclines
- P Hair growth cannot be restored

	LICHEN PLANOPILARIS (LPP)	**FRONTAL FIBROSING ALOPECIA (FFA)**
D	A form of lichen planus characterised by perifollicular erythema, follicular hyperkeratosis, and permanent hair loss (follicular form lichen planus; see Figure 173).	A form of cicatricial alopecia characterised by symmetric, progressive recession of the fronto-temporal hairline (or occipital scalp), with bilateral eyebrow hair loss (Hertoghe's sign; see Figure 174).
E	Uncommon, exact incidence and prevalence unknown	
E	Prevalence 8% of all types of alopecia	Prevalence 11% of all types of alopecia, occipital FFA 7-32% of FFA patients
R	25-70y	♀, adult-onset, postmenopausal, 50-70y
PE	P Crown (vertex) A Diffuse or focal (starts in centre spreading laterally), perifollicular S A few mm, dozens S Round O Moderately demarcated N Red-brown or purple erythema E Hyperkeratotic papules	P Frontal hairline (or occipital) A Regional (band-like patches) or perifollicular S A few mm, dozens S Round O Well-demarcated N Red E Erythematosquamous papules or hypopigmented (band-like) macule
	• Difficult to treat, once hair follicle is lost damage is irreversible • Most beneficial treatment within active disease	
Tx	✏ Topical or intralesional corticosteroids, systemic corticosteroids, hydroxychloroquine, ciclosporin	✏ • Preferably combination topical and oral treatment • Topical corticosteroids, topical calcineurin inhibitors, intralesional corticosteroids, minoxidil 5%, oral 5-alpha reductase inhibitors (5-ARIs), hydroxychloroquine, oral retinoids, oral ABx (tetracyclines), methotrexate ✂ Hair transplantation
!	• Eyebrow, axillary, and pubic hair loss possible • 20-50% of patients also have typical lichen planus lesions • LPP is divided into 3 variants: classic LPP, FFA, and Graham-Little-Piccardi-Lasseur syndrome (Graham-Little syndrome; GLPLS)	• Papules can also appear on the face • The disease progresses at an average rate of 0.9 mm per month until only a tuft of hair remains on the top of the head (clown alopecia)

Table 40 // Cicatricial alopecia subtypes

DISSECTING CELLULITIS OF THE SCALP (DCS)	**FOLLICULITIS DECALVANS (FD)**
Also known as perifolliculitis capitis abscedens et suffodiens, or Hoffman's disease; scalp disorder caused by severe inflammation of the hair follicles. It is characterised by abscesses, pus-filled cavities, and fistulas forming beneath the skin (see Figure 175).	Form of cicatricial alopecia characterised by the presence of pustules, originating from the hair follicles. The presence of tufts is a classic feature (multiple hairs emerging from a single opening; see Figure 176).
Uncommon, exact incidence and prevalence unknown	
Prevalence 1% of all types of alopecia	Prevalence 3% of all types of alopecia
♂, African descent, 20-40y	Unknown
(P) Scalp (A) Discrete or confluent (S) Nummular, single, or multiple (S) Round (O) Moderately demarcated (N) Skin-coloured to red (E) Pustules, small and large nodules, abscesses, fistulas, scarring	(P) Scalp, beard area, neck, face (A) Discrete or confluent (S) Mm to a few cm (S) Varying (O) Moderately demarcated (N) Erythematous, yellowish (E) Pustules, crusts, tufting, scarring, bald patches
• Difficult to treat, once hair follicle is lost damage is irreversible • Most beneficial treatment within active disease	
● Reduce inflammation, reduce follicular occlusion, and prevent and treat secondary infection ⚕ Oral ABx (tetracyclines), oral retinoids, TNF inhibitor ✂ If necessary: incision & drainage, intralesional corticosteroids, surgical excision	● Bacterial cultures of pustules and sensitivity testing (e.g *Staphylococcus aureus*) ⚕ Local antiseptics, topical/oral ABx, oral retinoids, topical or intralesional corticosteroids, systemic corticosteroids ✂ Hair transplantation, laser therapy
• Can occur in combination with acne conglobata, hidradenitis suppurativa, and pilonidal sinus (acne tetrad) • Can be associated with joint complaints (e.g. arthritis), keratitis-ichthyosis-deafness (KID) syndrome, or sternoclavicular hyperostosis	-

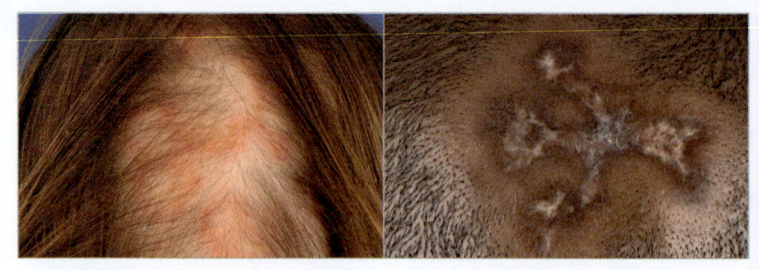

Figure 172 // Cicatricial alopecia

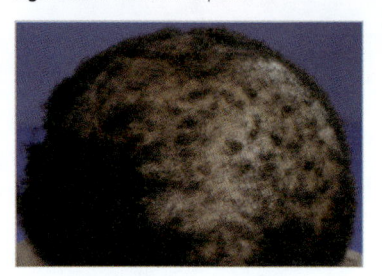

Figure 173 // Classic lichen planopilaris

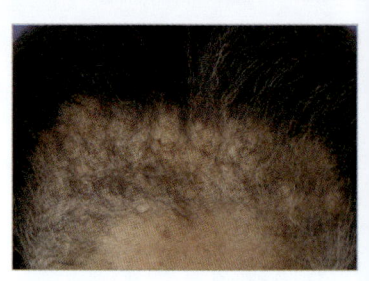

Figure 174 // Frontal bossing alopecia

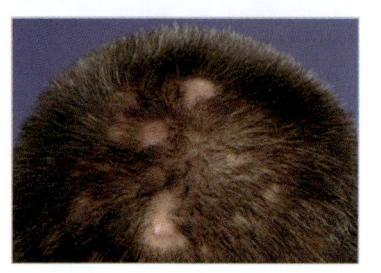

Figure 175 // Perifolliculitis capitis abscedens et suffodiens (dissecting folliculitis)

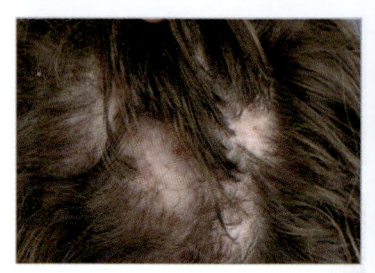

Figure 176 // Folliculitis decalvans

Telogen effluvium

- Telogen effluvium is a form of diffuse, nonscarring, often acute hair loss caused by an abnormal shift in follicular cycling, leading to the premature shedding of hair (see Figure 177).
- Unknown prevalence, considered quite common
- Metabolic stress, hormonal changes, or medications (e.g. beta blockers, retinoids, anticoagulants, carbamazepine) → disturbed balance of growth factors, neuroendocrine signals and cytokine involvement in follicular home-

ostasis → premature catagen induction or prolongation, accelerating the transition of hairs into telogen phase → extrusion from the follicle causing notable shedding

- (R) ♀>♂, childbirth, emotional stress, nutritional changes (e.g. rapid weight loss, caloric restriction, nutritional deficiencies), hypothyroidism
- (Hx) Relatively abrupt-onset hair shedding, usually without other symptoms, ask for potential causative events up to 6 mo prior to shedding
- (PE) Reduced in scalp hair density, often without visible abnormalities of the skin. Hair shafts typically appear normal.
- (Dx)
  - Hair pull test: positive
  - Trichoscopy: empty follicles and many upright regrowing hairs of normal thickness
  - Wood's light examination: seborrheic dermatitis is associated with telogen effluvium
- (Tx) 💬 Education, identification, and removal of the underlying cause
  - 💊 Topical minoxidil has been proposed, yet efficacy remains unclear
- (P) Self-limiting, often good prognosis for hair density recovery

> 🔔 The hair pull test aids in the recognition of active hair shedding. Grasp 50-60 hair fibres close to the skin surface and gently tug the hairs from the proximal to distal ends. Extraction of >5 telogen hair fibres in a single pull or >15 telogen hairs in three pulls indicates active telogen effluvium.

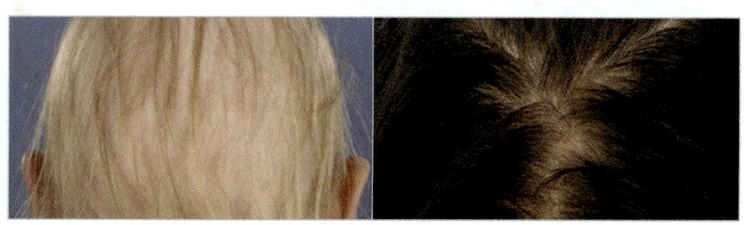

Figure 177 // Telogen effluvium

Hirsutism

- (D) Hirsutism is a form of excessive male-pattern hair growth in women with several different variants.
- (E) Prevalence 5-10% ♀ of reproductive age
- (Ae) Testosterone level ↑, hair follicle sensitivity to androgens ↑ or local conversion

- (R) Obesity, polycystic ovarian syndrome (PCOS), Cushing's syndrome, androgen-producing tumours, medication (e.g. steroids or androgens)
- (Hx) Excessive male-pattern hair growth in women
- (PE) Presence of terminal hairs, esp. on the upper lip, chin, neck, chest, abdomen, back, and inner thighs. The severity of excess hair growth is highly variable. Other signs of hyperandrogenism are androgenetic alopecia, amenorrhoea, vocal deepening, and clitoral hypertrophy.
- (Dx) Suspected hormonal disorders: blood test, consult gynaecologist (PCOS test) or internist/endocrinologist
- (Tx) Treat underlying cause, lifestyle changes (if there is obesity and PCOS)
    - Try to use treatment for >6 mo: OC to suppress ovarian androgen production, spironolactone, cyproterone acetate (postmenopausal women), eflornithine cream (facial hair)
    - Excess hair removal or bleaching with laser therapy, regular photo-epilation, laser therapy e.g. electrolysis (light hairs), Nd:YAG or diode laser (dark hairs)
- (P) Depends on underlying cause
- (!) • Refer patients to a gynaecologist or endocrinologist
    • Hirsutism may cause severe psychosocial problems

Central centrifugal cicatricial alopecia (CCCA)

- (D) CCCA a form of scarring alopecia, characterised by permanent hair loss on the vertex or crown of the scalp (see Figure 178).
- (E) Most common type of cicatricial alopecia among women of African descent, reported prevalence 2-7%
- (Ae) Largely unknown, potentially caused by premature desquamation of the inner root sheath → mechanical irritation of hair shaft pressing against the outer root sheath as well as allowing external factors (e.g. chemicals, bacteria) to enter the follicular unit → inflammatory response and follicular rupture
- (R) Potential influence of scalp infections (esp. frequent), autoimmune diseases, DM 2, or genetic factors. Hair care practices, e.g. use of chemical relaxers or hot combs, are often thought to contribute, though evidence is lacking.
- (Hx) Progressive hair loss usually starting at the vertex of the scalp, progressing centrifugally and symmetrically, sometimes mild burning or itching
- (PE) Often starting as a subtle patch of partial hair thinning on the vertex, over time the severity of the hair loss increases and the area widens in centrifugal

fashion. Loss of follicular ostia between residual hair shafts, hyperpigmentation, perifollicular erythema, and tufted hairs may be present.

- Dx • Trichoscopy: loss of follicular ostia, white peripilar halo, islands of unaffected hairs with polytrichia within affected areas
  - Skin biopsy and histology: premature desquamation of the inner root sheath and inflammation
- Tx • Minimise hair grooming
  - Mild CCCA: topical high-potency corticosteroid
  - Severe or refractory CCCA: combination therapy of topical high potency corticosteroid with ABx (tetracyclines), intralesional corticosteroid injections, Plaquenil, Dapsone
- P Poor prognosis in patients with advanced disease, only slight potential for hair regrowth due to scarring

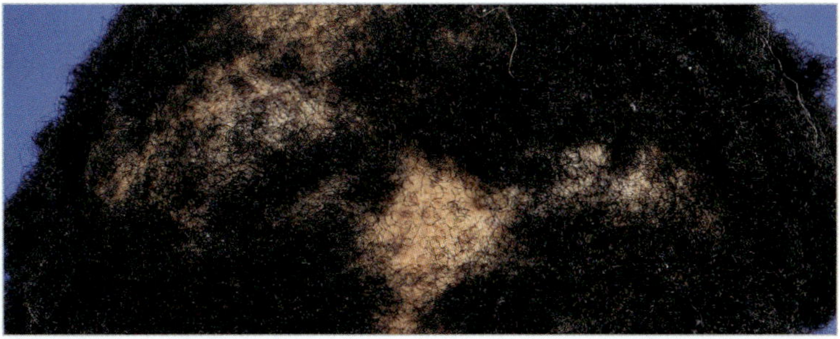

Figure 178 // Central centrifugal cicatricial alopecia (CCCA)

Traction alopecia

- D Traction alopecia is a form of hair loss that results from prolonged or repetitive tension on hair (see Figure 179).
- E Most frequent in females with Afro-textured hair with a prevalence of 9-30%
- Ae Repetitive or chronic tension on the hair affecting the dermal papilla, causing reduction of the hair follicle
- R Individuals with hairstyles that produce a continuous pulling force on the hair roots, e.g. tight braids or ponytails, bun hairstyles (often worn by ballerinas), hair extensions, hair pins, knotting of the beard hair
- Hx Onset of hair loss in temporal regions, preauricular, above the ears or other regions of the scalp, particularly where 'corn row' patterns are adopted
- PE Reduced hair density and length, often along the marginal hairline (frontal,

temporal, and occipital regions), sometimes with alopecic patches. The characteristic finding of retention of hair follicles of lesser diameter along the marginal hairline is called the fringe sign. Earlier stages are often characterised by perifollicular erythema, inflammatory papules, or pustules in sites of traction on hair.

- **Dx** Trichoscopy: hair cast, reduction in hair follicle density, absence of follicular openings, and presence of large number of freely mobile hair casts at the periphery of the patch
- **Tx**
  - Discontinue traction hairstyles
  - Signs of inflammation: topical corticosteroids
  - Augment hair growth: topical minoxidil
- **P** Traction alopecia is reversible in early disease, whereas chronic disease is scarring and permanent

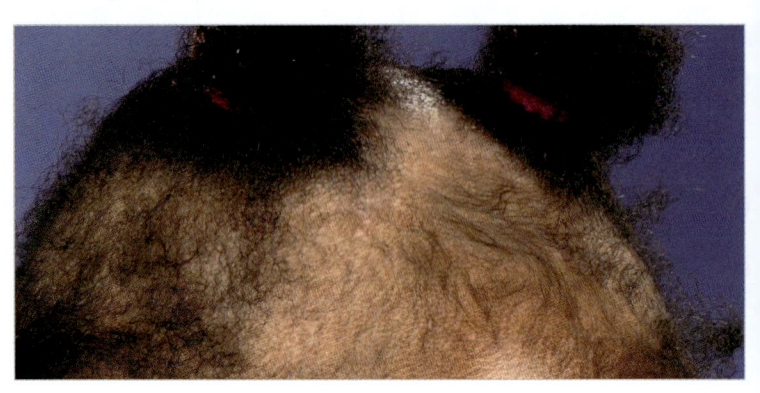

Figure 179 // Alopecia mechanica (traction alopecia)

Hyperhidrosis

- **D** Hyperhidrosis is a disorder characterised by excessive sweating beyond the purpose of homeostatic temperature regulation, due to the overstimulation of cholinergic receptors on eccrine glands. Primary hyperhidrosis typically presents early in life with a more localised expression. Secondary hyperhidrosis typically presents due to adverse events of medication or due to systemic disorders.
- **E** Prevalence 1-5% in the general population, most common at 20-60y
- **Ae** Impaired negative feedback to hypothalamus → hyperactivity of the sympathetic nervous system → excessive release of acetylcholine from nerve end-

ings → excessive sweating
- Primary hyperhidrosis: unknown aetiology, potential role of genetic factors
- Secondary hyperhidrosis: medication (dopamine agonists, SSRIs, antipsychotics, insulin), systemic disorders (diabetes mellitus, hyperthyroidism, TB), neurological disorders, tumours (e.g. pheochromocytoma, lymphoma)

(R) Medication (see Ae), systemic disorders, chronic excessive alcohol consumption, postmenopausal women

(Hx) Excessive sweating, usually in areas with high eccrine gland density (e.g. palms, soles, face, head, axillae)

(PE) Focal (mainly palms, soles, face, neck, axillae) or generalised, visible, excessive sweating

(Dx) If a secondary cause is suspected, consider laboratory tests incl. complete blood count, basic metabolic panel, thyroid-stimulating hormone, sedimentation rate, antinuclear antibody, haemoglobin A1C; chest X-ray (in case of suspected TB infection)

(Tx) Topical antiperspirants (e.g. aluminium chloride hexahydrate 20%), topical glycopyrronium (esp. for axillary hyperhidrosis). In generalised forms oral glycopyrronium or oxybutynin oral (off-label).

Iontophoresis, botulinum toxin injections

(P) Recurrence of hyperhidrosis is common with all currently available treatment options

(!) Hyperhidrosis may have a significant impact on quality of life, with social embarrassment, emotional distress, and work or school-related disability being important factors

Paediatrics

> Measles and rubella are notifiable diseases, which means that healthcare providers must report any suspected, probable, or confirmed cases to the public health services (<24h).

> Childhood diseases are highly **contagious**: every non-immunised child with measles or chickenpox infects 13 and 16-26 new patients, respectively. By comparison, a flu patient infects an average of 1.5 new patients.

	MEASLES (morbilli)	**SCARLET FEVER** (scarlatina)	**RUBELLA** (German measles or three-day measles)
D	Highly contagious viral infection, spreads via airborne transmission (see Figure 180).	Toxin-mediated disease *Streptococcus pyogenes*, spreads via airborne and cutaneous transmission.	Highly contagious viral infection, spreads via airborne and cutaneous transmission (see Figure 183).
E	Rising incidence worldwide 0-9.2:100,000 cases in Europe	Exact incidence unknown, relatively rare, not documented	Incidence 100,000 infants per year worldwide
Ae	Morbillivirus	*Streptococcus pyogenes* (group A *Streptococcus*)	Rubella virus
R	Unvaccinated children, esp. in clusters and resource-limited settings (partly due to breaks in the cold chain, e.g., poor refrigeration or storage of vaccines, reducing effectiveness)	Viral lower RTI, impaired immune system, residents of impoverished areas	Unvaccinated people without group immunity
I*	7-21d	5-7d	14-21d
Hx	Prodromal phase (3-5d): fever up to 40°C/104°F, conjunctivitis, cough, cold	Prodromal phase (4-5d): fever, sore throat, tonsillitis, vomiting	• Prodromal phase (1-2d): absent or very mild symptoms • Malaise ⊖, subfebrile ⊖, cold ⊖, lymphadenopathy ⊖
PE	• 2d before onset of exanthema: white Koplik spots on buccal mucosa (see Figure 181) • Exanthema (3-5d) (see Figure 134): facial onset followed by generalised centrifugal expansion, lenticular-nummular, macular, discrete, coalescent (torso and face)	Exanthema (3-5d): generalised bright red exanthema, esp. in flexures, perioral area unaffected, miliar, follicular, maculopapular, coalescent, red, swollen tonsils and bright red tongue with elevated papillae (raspberry tongue, see Figure 182)	Exanthema (1-3d): slightly erythematous, facial onset, generalised centrifugal expansion, lenticular-macular, discrete, minimal coalescence (torso) (see Figure 183)
Dx	• Clinical diagnosis • Serology: IgM/IgG antibodies	Bacterial throat culture	Serology: IgM antibodies, consider supplementary PCR (throat swab or urine)

Table 41A // Exanthematous childhood diseases
I* = incubation period

ERYTHEMA INFECTIOSUM (5th disease)	EXANTHEMA SUBITUM (6th disease, roseola infantum)	CHICKENPOX (varicella)
Viral infection that spreads via airborne and vertical transmission (see Figure 185).	Viral infection, transmitted through saliva, placenta, blood transfusion, and organ donation (see Figure 186).	Highly contagious viral infection that spreads via airborne, droplet, and placental transmission (see Figure 187).
Seroprevalence increases with age, 50-80% of adults have measurable parvovirus B19-specific IgG antibodies	Peak prevalence 7-13 mo, 90% of cases are children <2y	Incidence 1,300-1,600:100,000 per year, highest incidence children 1-9y, >90% of people become infected before adolescence
Human parvovirus B19	Human herpesvirus type 6 (HHV-6)	Varicella zoster virus
Children in primary school/day care centres and relatives, crèche staff, medical staff	Impaired immune system	Immunologically naive individuals to VZV
7-21d	7-14d	10-21d
Prodromal phase (1-2d): may present with mild inflammation of mucous membranes	Prodromal phase (3-4d): high fever (39.0-40.5°C/ 102-105°F)	Prodromal phase (1-2d): fever, muscle pain, anorexia, headaches, cold
Exanthema (5-10d): mild, slightly erythematous rash beginning on the cheeks (butterfly rash, slapped cheek; see Figure 184), widespread expansion (esp. extremities and buttocks), initially macular and well-demarcated, later coalescent and annular (lace-like exanthema, see Figure 185)	Exanthema (2-4d), in 5% of children: slightly erythematous rash beginning on torso, possible centrifugal expansion, lenticular-macular, discrete, minimal coalescence (see Figure 186)	Exanthema (1-2 wk): vesicles, scalp also affected in classical presentation, centripetal distribution, erythematous, lesions in different stages: macule → papule → vesicle → (pustule) → crust → may present with or without scarring (see Figure 187)
Serology: IgM/IgG antibodies	No added value, clinical diagnosis	No added value, clinical diagnosis, can be confirmed with a PCR on vesicular fluid or serology in atypical cases

	MEASLES (morbilli)	**SCARLET FEVER** (scarlatina)	**RUBELLA** (German measles or three-day measles)
Tx	💬 Symptomatic 🔧 Supportive care: antipyretics, fluids, treat bacterial superinfection		
	💬 Prevention through vaccination (measles, mumps, and rubella (MMR)) 🔧 Vitamin A supplementation	💬 No vaccine available 🔧 Severe course: AB e.g. penicillin (first choice), amoxicillin, clindamycin	💬 Prevention through vaccination (MMR)
P	Generally favourable course, very severe complications ⊖	Mild course, severe course presents with peeling skin on hands and feet	Mild course, severe complications ⊖
!	• Complications: pneumonia, encephalitis, subacute sclerosing panencephalitis (SSPE) (lethal) • Infectious from prodromal phase until ±5d after appearance of exanthema	• Complications: sepsis, acute rheumatoid arthritis, post-streptococcal reactive arthritis (PSRA), glomerulonephritis, pneumonia, meningitis • Infectious as long as patient carries streptococci	• Complications: encephalitis and Guillain-Barré syndrome. During pregnancy: congenital rubella syndrome. • Contagious from 10d before to 7d after appearance of exanthema

Table 41B // Exanthematous childhood diseases
I* = incubation period

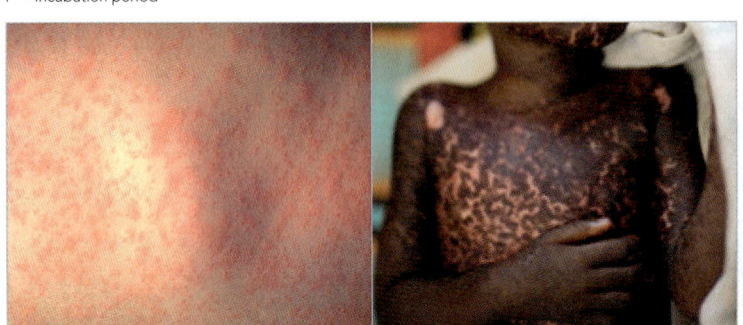

Figure 180A and 180B // Exanthema in measles

ERYTHEMA INFECTIOSUM (5th disease)	**EXANTHEMA SUBITUM** (6th disease, roseola infantum)	**CHICKENPOX** (varicella)
💬 Symptomatic 💊 Supportive care: antipyretics, drinking fluids, good hygiene, pain management, keep fingernails short (varicella)		
💬 No vaccine available		💬 Prevention through vaccination in certain countries, e.g. USA, Canada, Australia, South Korea. As of 2019, worldwide prevention in 18% of countries, in 6% of countries for risk groups only. 💊 • Antiviral therapy (aciclovir IV, valaciclovir) in high-risk patients • Antihistamines, non-aspirin NSAIDs (e.g. acetaminophen)
Good, complications ⊖	HHV-6 remains latent without clinical ramifications	• Favourable course, remains latent • without clinical ramifications
• Joint pain ⊖ • Primary infection during pregnancy: risk of hydrops fetalis and intrauterine foetal demise • Contagious from 1 wk after infection until appearance of exanthema	• Complications: febrile convulsions • May be reactivated following immunodeficiency	• Complications: varicella pneumonia (adults), superinfections due to skin flora (impetigo, cellulitis), acute cerebellar ataxia, encephalitis • Contagious from 48h before the appearance of skin pathology • May be reactivated as herpes zoster • No aspirin for children with chickenpox, watch out for Reye's syndrome

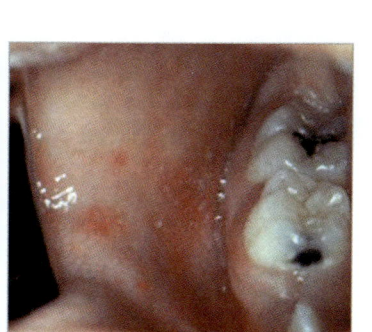

Figure 181 // Koplik spots

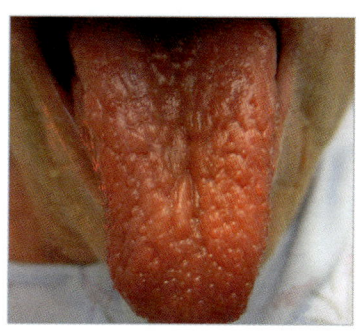

Figure 182 // Raspberry tongue

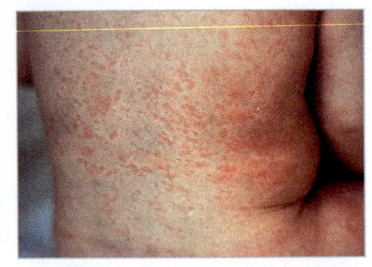

Figure 183 // Exanthema in rubella

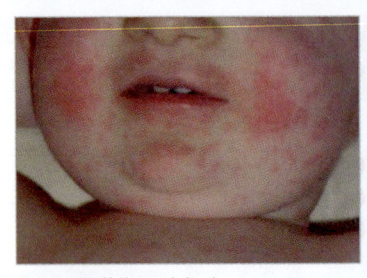

Figure 184 // Slapped cheeks

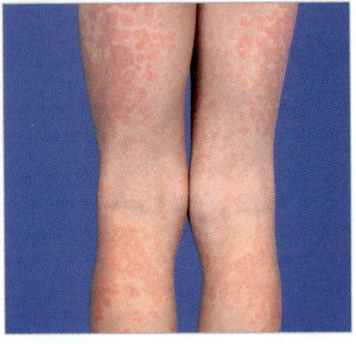

Figure 185 // Lace-like exanthema in erythema infectiosum

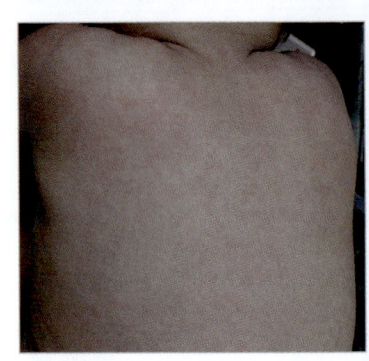

Figure 186 // Exanthema in exanthema subitum

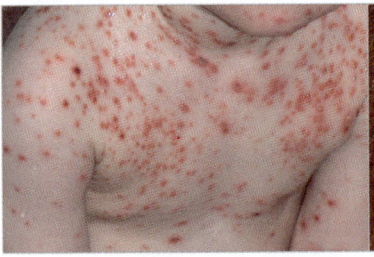

Figure 187 // Vesicles in chickenpox

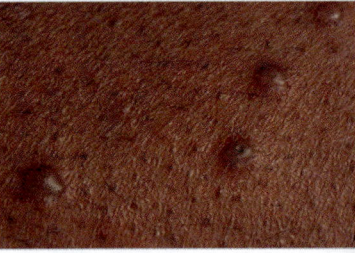

Haemangioma (strawberry naevus)

D Haemangioma, also called infantile haemangioma or strawberry naevus, is a benign proliferation of endothelial tissue and the most common tumour in the neonatal period (see Figure 188). A distinction is made between superficial, deep and mixed haemangiomas.

- **E** Prevalence 1-3% in first days of life, 10% >1y
- **Ae** Idiopathic, often appears soon after birth; various hypotheses, e.g. link to endothelial cell precursors, placental cells that have entered foetal circulation, or extrinsic factors such as hypoxia
- **R** ♀:♂ = 2-5:1, premature birth, low birth weight
- **Hx** Asymptomatic, red tangle of blood vessels
- **PE**
  - **P** Head and neck region, torso, extremities, anogenital area
  - **A** Solitary
  - **S** Highly variable, from one to dozens of cm
  - **S** Jagged, round, or oval
  - **O** Well-demarcated
  - **N** Bright red to purple-red
  - **E** Plaque or tumour with telangiectasias
- **Dx** Imaging may be useful to assess lesion depth or to differentiate between haemangioma and vascular malformation
- **Tx** 💬 Generally no treatment needed, wait-and-see with regular check-ups
  - 💊
    - For complications such as ulcerations or threat to surrounding structures: beta blockers (systemic or local), intralesional or systemic corticosteroids (rapidly growing), ABx if needed (ulcerative)
    - Premature: systemic > local beta blockers (penetration ↑)
    - USA: propranolol hydrochloride (e.g. hemangeol)
  - 🔪 Surgical excision
- **P** Erythematous plaque with telangiectasias, followed by a growth phase (usually until 9-12 mo) and finally an involution phase (until 10y)
- **!** Visual disturbances secondary to a periocular haemangioma require referral to an ophthalmologist

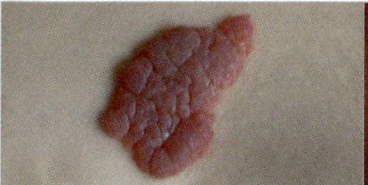

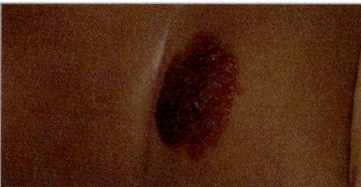

Figure 188A and 188B // Haemangioma

> 💡 Follow-up interval: age in months = follow-up interval in weeks.

> 💡 A haemangioma is a benign proliferation of endothelial tissue and the most common tumour in the neonatal period. A distinction is made between superficial, deep and mixed haemangiomas. Ultrasound, MRI, or CT can help assess lesion depth or differentiate between a haemangioma and vascular malformation.

Diaper dermatitis

- (D) Diaper dermatitis, or diaper rash, is one of the most common skin conditions in infants and toddlers (see Figure 189).
- (E) Prevalence 4-70% in infants, peak incidence 9-12 mo
- (Ae) Form of irritant contact dermatitis caused by skin contact with urine and faeces
- (R) Seborrhoeic dermatitis, infrequent diaper changes, diarrhoea, incontinence
- (Hx) Dermal irritation, red skin, wounds, bumps, and chapped skin
- (PE) (P) Diaper region
  - (A) Symmetrical
  - (S) Variable
  - (S) Variable
  - (O) Moderately to well-demarcated
  - (N) Bright red
  - (E) Erythema, scales, sometimes vesicles and erosions
- (Dx) KOH test or culture ⊖: confirm presence of *Candida albicans*
- (Tx) 💬 Skin care: keep skin dry, increase diaper change frequency, rest without diaper, gentle cleansing with fragrance-free wipes, diaper choice
  - 💊 Zinc oxide ointment, local corticosteroids (class I), or antimycotics for secondary *Candida albicans* infection, ABx for secondary infection
- (P) Common secondary infection with *Candida albicans* (satellite lesions)
- (!) Beware of long-term use of corticosteroids under occlusion (diaper)

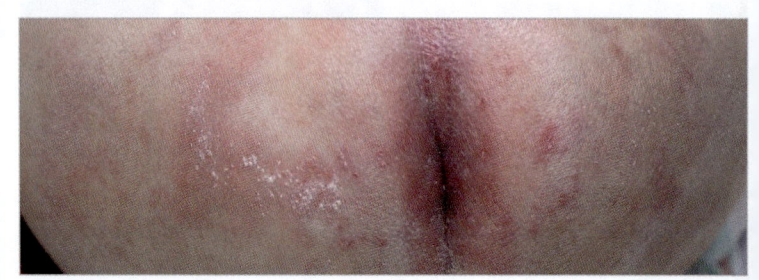

Figure 189 // Diaper dermatitis

Congenital dermal melanocytosis

- D A congenital dermal melanocytosis, or Mongolian spot, is a congenital birthmark (see Figure 190).
- E Prevalence in newborns: 85-100% of Asian descent, <10% of Western European descent, >60% of African descent, 46-70% of Hispanic descent
- Ae Idiopathic, genetic factors involved, colour caused by improper migration of melanocytes from the neural crest to the epidermis during embryonic development
- R Asian descent
- Hx Pale/grey-blue discolouration in the sacral or lumbosacral region, may be accompanied by local excess hair growth
- PE
  - P Sacrum, buttocks, or back
  - A Solitary, sometimes multiple
  - S Lenticular to palm-sized
  - S Variable
  - O Moderately to well-demarcated
  - N Greyish blue, light or dark blue
  - E Macule
- Dx No added value
- Tx Generally no treatment needed, camouflaging possible
  - If persistent: laser therapy
- P Present from birth or from the first weeks of life, regression during childhood, rarely persists into adolescence

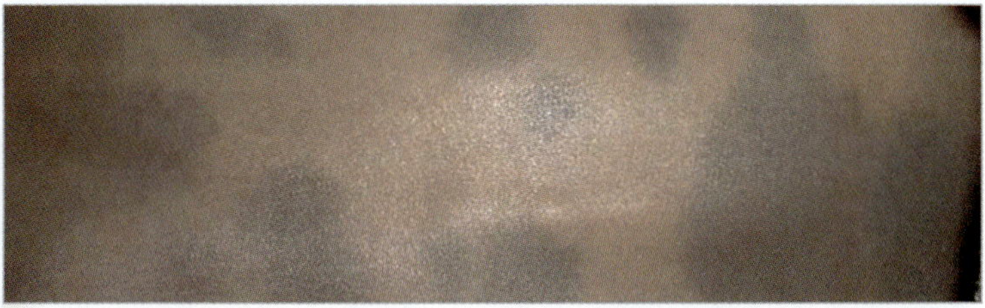

Figure 190 // Congenital dermal melanocytosis

Naevus flammeus

- D A naevus flammeus, also port-wine stain, is a vascular malformation (see Figure 191).
- E Prevalence 0.1-0.2% newborns, incidence in USA 300-500:100,000 newborns per year

- **Ae** Caused by a vascular malformation, capillary dilation in the dermis
- **R** Pale to fair skin
- **Hx** Congenital vascular defect of the skin, initially light red, telangiectatic macule, later wine red
- **PE** **P** Occurs predominantly on the face, followed by the upper part of the torso, unilateral
  - **A** Solitary
  - **S** Few mm to multiple cm, may present with segmental extension e.g. along one of the branches of the trigeminal nerve
  - **S** Variable
  - **O** Unilateral and well-demarcated along the midline
  - **N** Pink or red, darkens with age (dark red to deep purple)
  - **E** Erythematous macule
- **Dx** No added value
- **Tx** 💬 Camouflage if preferred
  - 🔨 • Vascular laser treatment: PDL (first choice), PDT, IPL, argon laser, surgical excision
    - USA: combined Nd:YAG and PDL
- **P** Chronic
- ❗ • Sturge-Weber syndrome is accompanied by a facial naevus flammeus in the ophthalmic nerve region and is associated with vascular malformations of the eye and brain (cause unknown)
  - The port-wine stain is associated with several genetic syndromes (e.g. Klippel-Trenaunay)

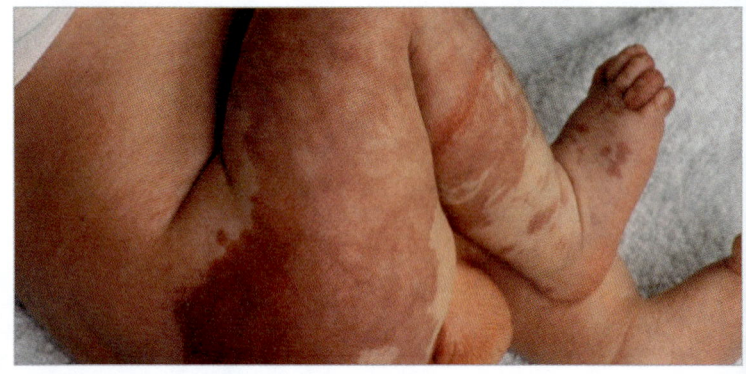

Figure 191 // Naevus flammeus

Seborrhoeic dermatitis of the head (cradle cap)

D Seborrhoeic dermatitis of the head, or cradle cap, is a common form of dermatitis in children, occurring esp. in the first few weeks of life (see Figure 192). For the adult variant, see eczematous dermatoses.

E Prevalence 10% in infants (<1 mo), peak prevalence 3 mo, 7% children (1-2y)

Ae Unclear, presumably associated with sebum overproduction, association with *Malassezia furfur* overgrowth less clear at this age

R Unknown

Hx Thick, yellowish scaling on newborn scalp

PE
- P Scalp
- A Grouped, regional
- S Multiple scales of varying sizes
- S Round or oval
- O Moderately well-demarcated
- N Yellow
- E Scales

Dx Culture or KOH test: to rule out secondary infection

Tx
- Responds well to baths and emollients, remove crusts (e.g. soft brush/fine toothbrush) after softening with oil (e.g. almond, vegetable, baby, white petrolatum), wash hair frequently with baby shampoo
- In more extensive or persistent cases: daily topical corticosteroid (class I), ketoconazole 2% shampoo

P Usually disappears in 3rd to 4th mo of life

! Other variants of childhood seborrhoeic dermatitis occur in flexures, on the torso, or the extremities. Flexural dermatitis is characterised by less scaling and more erythematous, well-demarcated weeping plaques.

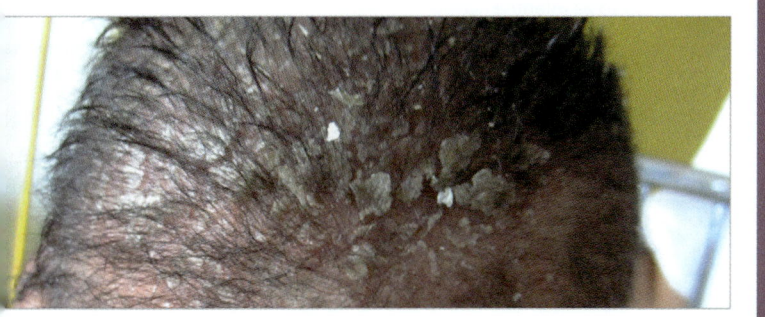

Figure 192 // Seborrhoeic dermatitis

Neonatal acne

- **D** Neonatal acne, or neonatal cephalic pustulosis, is a common acneiform eruption in newborns, typically occurring in the first few weeks of life (see Figure 193).
- **E** Approx. 20% of newborns
- **Ae** Exact mechanism unclear, potential role of circulating androgens (from mother or child) causing a heightened sebaceous gland activity or inflammatory reaction to skin colonisation with *Malassezia* species
- **R** ♂>♀
- **Hx** Development of small papules and pustules, typically within the first 6-12 wk of life
- **PE**
  - **P** Face, esp. cheeks, sometimes scalp
  - **A** Grouped, bound to the sebaceous gland complex
  - **S** Multiple, miliar
  - **S** Round
  - **O** Moderately well-demarcated
  - **N** Red, yellow-white pustules
  - **E** Papules and pustules (often absence of comedones)
- **Dx** No added value
- **Tx** 💬 Daily cleansing with soap and water, avoidance of exogenous oils and lotions

  💊 Pharmacological treatment of neonates is usually not necessary. Low-potency corticosteroids (e.g. hydrocortisone 1% cream), ketoconazole 2% cream, benzoyl peroxide or erythromycin 2% lotions may be used if necessary.
- **P** Eruptions usually resolve spontaneously within four months without scarring
- **!** Acneiform eruptions that develop later on during infancy (from 6-16 mo) are referred to as infantile acne

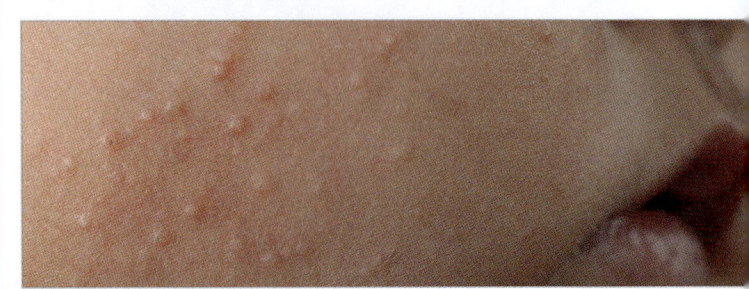

Figure 193 // Neonatal acne (acne neonatorum)

Clinical reasoning

> This section lists several examples of diagnoses to consider for specific complaints.

Allergic reactions

	TYPE I REACTION/ DIRECT HYPERSENSITIVITY	**TYPE IV REACTION/ CELL-MEDIATED HYPERSENSITIVITY**
AETIOLOGY	Inhalant allergens (e.g. pollen), food allergens, medication (e.g. penicillin), wasp and bee stings	Cosmetics, occupational exposure to allergens (e.g. nickel, rubber, glue)
IMMUNE MECHANISM	• IgE-mediated mast cell activation → degranulation mast cell → mediator release • Rapid, minutes to hours	• T helper cell activation → cytokines → tissue damage • Not until 48-72h after contact with allergen
CLINICAL PRESENTATION	• Rash, hives, hay fever, possibly combined with systemic symptoms (e.g. tachycardia, hypotension, or dyspnoea) • Severe reaction: anaphylaxis	• Contact dermatitis • Various skin reactions (ranging from mild to severe)
DIAGNOSTICS	Provocation test (gold standard), percutaneous allergy test (skin prick test), Phadiatop blood test	Epicutaneous testing (patch tests), standard panels are available for common antigens

Table 42 // Allergic reactions

Suspicious skin lesion

```
Suspicious skin lesion
         │
      Coloured
         │
   ┌─────┼─────┐
   ▼     ▼     ▼
Smooth/macula   Scaling/keratotic   Skin-coloured
```

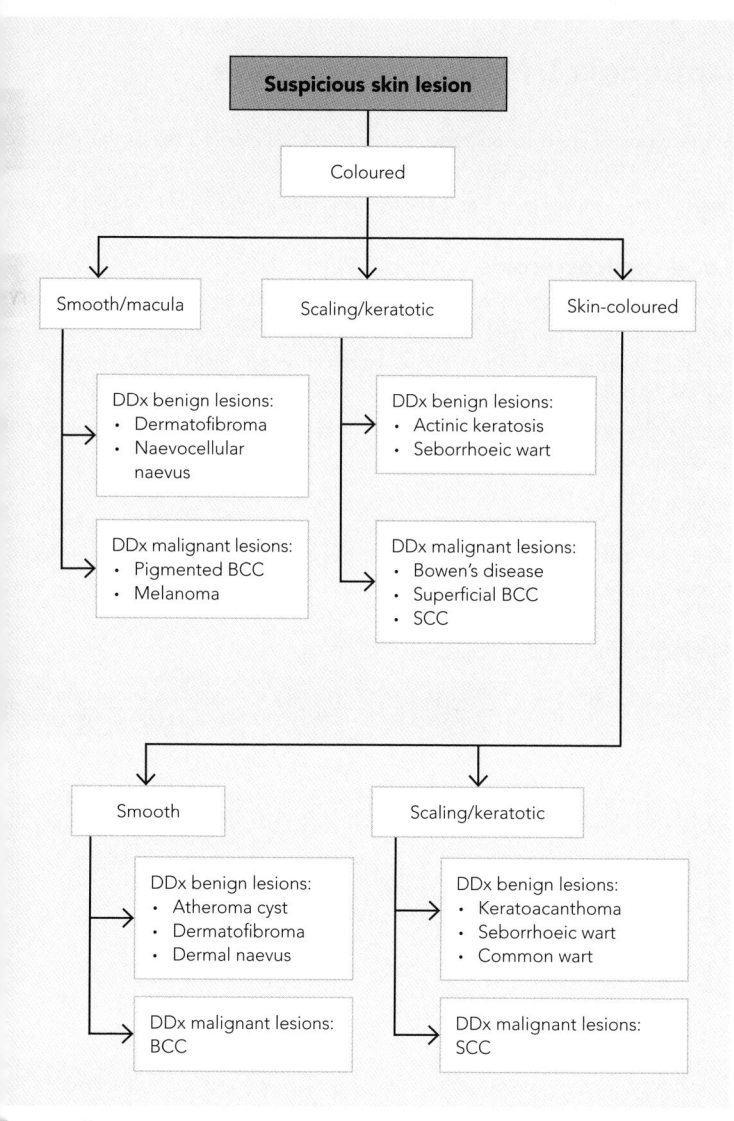

Smooth/macula

→ DDx benign lesions:
- Dermatofibroma
- Naevocellular naevus

→ DDx malignant lesions:
- Pigmented BCC
- Melanoma

Scaling/keratotic

→ DDx benign lesions:
- Actinic keratosis
- Seborrhoeic wart

→ DDx malignant lesions:
- Bowen's disease
- Superficial BCC
- SCC

Skin-coloured

┌─────────────┬─────────────┐
▼   ▼
Smooth   Scaling/keratotic

Smooth

→ DDx benign lesions:
- Atheroma cyst
- Dermatofibroma
- Dermal naevus

→ DDx malignant lesions:
- BCC

Scaling/keratotic

→ DDx benign lesions:
- Keratoacanthoma
- Seborrhoeic wart
- Common wart

→ DDx malignant lesions:
- SCC

Diagram 3 // Suspicious skin lesion, coloured

Appendices

Appendix 1: Medication dosage

Some types of medication require a gradual build-up to reach the effective blood level. This is especially true in medication that is known for toxic effects on heart, kidney, and/or liver. For these medications, a scheme should be followed.

Local corticosteroids

Effective treatment of eczema requires the correct dosage of corticosteroid cream/ointment. However, many patients apply too little, which can delay or reduce improvement. To address this issue, the fingertip unit (FTU) has been adopted. One FTU is the amount of cream or ointment dispensed along the length of the distal segment of the index finger. The required number of FTUs varies per body part and age.

In the event of treatment discontinuation, a tapering (reduction) schedule should be implemented to prevent the rebound of symptoms, as well as adrenal insufficiency in case of oral corticosteroids.

Fingertip Unit (FTU)

AGE	HEAD + NECK	ARM + HAND	LEG + FOOT	CHEST + ABDOMEN	BACK + BUTTOCKS
3-12 mo	1	1	1.5	1	1.5
1-2y	1.5	1.5	2	2	3
3-5y	1.5	2	3	3	3.5
6-10y	2	2.5	4.5	3.5	5
>10y & adults	2.5	3.5	8	7	7

Table 43 // FTU corticosteroids per body part

> A fingertip unit (FTU) weighs approx. 0.5g. A full-body treatment requires around 30g of corticosteroid ointment.

> Do not continue the tapering schedule if there is no improvement. In some cases maintenance treatment of corticosteroids ointments for 3-4x per week is necessary.

WEEK	MONDAY	TUESDAY	WEDNESDAY	THURSDAY	FRIDAY	SATURDAY	SUNDAY
1	X	X	X	X	X	X	X
2	X	X	X	X	X		
3	X	X	X				
4	X	X					
5	X						
6	X						

Table 44 // Example of a tapering schedule for corticosteroids

Prednisone

Prednisone is often used as pulse therapy. It is important to gradually reduce the dosage to avoid a refractory autologous corticosteroid shortage.

For patients undergoing long-term prednisone therapy, it is recommended to monitor urinary glucose levels, weight, and Hb:
- First 3 months of treatment: twice per month
- After 3 months of treatment: once every 1 to 3 months

Indications for proton pump inhibitors in prednisone treatment:
- Use of anticoagulants
- History of duodenal or gastric ulcers
- Concurrent use of NSAIDs
- High-dose corticosteroid therapy
- Older age, heart failure, or diabetes mellitus

DAY	1	2	3	4	5	6	7	8	9	10	11	12	13	14
Dosage (mg)	40	40	35	35	30	30	25	25	20	20	15	15	10	10

Table 45 // Example of a prednisone pulse therapy schedule for 2 weeks

DAY	1	2	3	4	5	6	7	8	9	10	11	12	13	14
Dosage (mg)	40	40	40	35	35	35	30	30	30	25	25	25	20	20

DAY	15	16	17	18	19	20	21
Dosage (mg)	20	15	15	15	10	10	10

Table 46 // Example of a prednisone pulse therapy schedule for 3 weeks

Methotrexate (MTX)

The effective dosage of methotrexate for dermatological conditions varies between individuals and typically ranges between 5-25 mg/week. If treatment is effective, the dose should be tapered to the lowest effective dose. Clinical improvement is expected within 1 to 3 months.

During MTX follow-up, special attention should be given to infections, pregnancy status, and alcohol consumption. Pregnancy and lactation are absolute contraindications.

Dosage

DOSE ADJUSTMENT	DOSAGE
Standard	15 mg/wk
Vulnerable patients*	7.5-10 mg/wk
Dose escalation**	2.5 mg/wk
Maximum dose	25 mg/wk

Table 47 // MTX dosage and adjustment
* Elderly patients or patients with impaired renal function (<50 ml/min)
** Dose escalation should be considered in case of insufficient efficacy, if lab results allow it

Folic acid

Folic acid supplementation is recommended with MTX to reduce toxic effects. Folic acid should be taken once weekly, at least 24 hours after MTX administration.
- For MTX doses <15 mg/week: 5 mg folic acid
- For MTX doses >15 mg/week: 10 mg folic acid

Isotretinoin

In the use of dosages up to 40 mg of isotretinoin, medication should be taken once daily. When dosages are above 40 mg, this should be divided over two to three doses per day. Pregnancy and lactation are absolute contraindications for isotretinoin use.

DOSE TYPE	DOSAGE
Starting dose	0.5 mg/kg/d
Minimum dose	0.1 mg/kg/d
Maximum dose	2.0 mg/kg/d

Table 48 // Starting, minimum, and maximum dosage

CHECK-UP	PRIOR TO TREATMENT	EVERY MONTH	EVERY 3 MONTHS
Pregnancy test (urine/blood)	X	X	X
ALT, ALP, cholesterol, triglycerides	X		X

Table 49 // Check-up during isotretinoin use

> Concerns have been raised about a potential correlation between isotretinoin use and depression or suicide. However, research has since demonstrated that there is no causality between depression and suicide and isotretinoin use.

Fumarates

To reduce the risk of adverse events in fumarate treatment a build-up schedule is used (see Table 50). Additionally, in treatment with fumarates monthly check-ups are performed during the first three months, quarterly until one year after the initial treatment started, and after one year every six months (see Table 51).

> A temporary pause should be considered in case of low WBC (<3 x 109/L, lymphocytes <0.5 x 109/L, eosinophilia (>25%), or acute TB.

WEEK	DOSE	MORNING	AFTERNOON	EVENING
1	30 mg	1	0	0
2			0	1
3			1	1
4	120 mg		0	0
5			0	0
6			1	1
7			1	1
8		2	1	2
9		2	2	2

Table 50 // Build-up schedule fumarates

CHECK-UP	PRIOR TO TREATMENT	DURING TREATMENT
Labs	X	X
ALT, AF	X	X
Creatinin	X	X
Urine	X	X
Pregnancy test (urine)	X	

Table 51 // Check-ups in fumarate treatment

References

💡 You can find the online list of references we used while crafting this pocket by scanning the QR code.

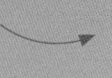

Are you missing a resource or topic? Or is there a new guideline that isn't yet listed here? Let us know! Together we can keep Compendium Medicine up to date.

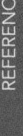

Illustrations & figures

Illustrators

Yente S. Beentjes: *figures 15, 19, and 131*
Dagmar Bouwer: *figure 153*
Susan Deelstra: *figure 10*
Lotte Depuis: *figures 12, 13, 14, and 17*
Gulizar Durak: *figure 154*
Astrid A.H. Feikema: *figures 2, 28, 66, and 148*
Iza Hogenelst: *figures 30, 31, 32, 33, and 34*
Nicky Janssen: *figure 5*
Koen L.C. Ketelaars: *figures 20 and 149*
Rosalie C. Krijl: *figures 3, 4, 6, 7, 9, 18, and 103*
Juliëtte M.E. Linskens: *figure 8*
Delano R. Sanches: *figure 25*
Laura Sanchez: *figures 1, 69, 83, and 160*
Carlijn Sturm: *figure 132*

Sources

01. Photos cover and About us: www.ivarpel.nl
02. Figures 11, 16, 22, 23, 26, 27, 29, 35A, 36, 37, 38, 39, 40B, 41A, 42, 43, 44, 47, 48, 49, 50, 51, 52, 53, 54, 55, 56, 57, 58, 59A, 60A, 60B, 61, 62, 63, 64A, 65, 67C, 68A, 70, 71, 72, 73, 74, 75, 76, 77, 78A, 79, 80, 81, 82, 84, 85, 86, 87, 88, 89, 90, 91, 92, 93, 94A, 95, 96, 97, 98A, 99, 100, 101, 102A, 102B, 104A, 105A, 106, 107, 108, 109, 110, 111, 112, 113, 114, 115, 116, 117, 118, 119, 120, 121, 122C, 123, 124, 125, 126, 127, 128, 129, 130, 133, 134, 135, 136, 137, 138, 139, 140, 141, 142, 143, 144, 145, 146, 147, 150, 155, 156, 157, 159, 161, 162A, 163, 164, 165, 166A, 167, 168, 169A, 170, 171, 172, 173, 174, 175, 176, 177, 178, 179, 180B, 182, 185, 187, 189, 190, 191, 192, and 193: Huidziekten.nl
03. Figure 21: Maas M, Cabri M.M. Normal duplex ultrasound of the left common carotid artery
04. Figure 24: Gram Stain Anthrax / CDC / https://commons.wikimedia.org/wiki/File:Gram_Stain_Anthrax.jpg / Public domain
05. Figures 35B, 41B, 45, 46, 59B, 60C, 64B, 67A, 67B, 68B, 78B, 94B, 98B, 102C, 104B, 105B, 122A, 122B, 158, 162B, 166B, 169B, and 188B: University of New Mexico (z.j.). Photo Gallery of Skin Conditions
06. Figure 40A: Dermatitis of chin from vapors of mustard-1 (NCP 001055) / National Museum of Health and Medicine / https://www.flickr.com/photos/medicalmuseum/ 5243639897 / CC BY 2.0 (https://creativecommons.org/licenses/by/2.0/)

07. Figure 151: Trichomonas pics / isis325 / https://ccsearch.creativecommons.org/photos/ed87697a-3b8a-4253-8df1-754fe454d103 / CC BY 2.0 (https://creativecommons.org/licenses/by/2.0/)
08. Figure 152: Lymphogranuloma venerum - lymph nodes / Herbert L. Fred, MD and Hendrik A. van Dijk / https://commons.wikimedia.org/wiki/File:Lymphogranuloma_venerum_-_lymph_nodes.jpg / CC BY 2.0 (https://creativecommons.org/licenses/by/2.0/)
09. Figure 180A: Morbillivirus measles infection / CDC, Dr. Heinz F. Eichenwald / https://commons.wikimedia.org/wiki/File:Morbillivirus_measles_infection.jpg / Public domain
10. Figure 181: Koplik spots, measles 6111 lores / CDC / https://commons.wikimedia.org/wi-ki/File:Koplik_spots,_measles_6111_lores.jpg / Public domain
11. Figure 183: Rash of rubella on skin of child's back. Distribution is similar to that of measles but the lesions are less intensely red. / CDC / http://phil.cdc.gov/PHIL_Ima-ges/03052002/00002/PHIL_712_lores.jpg / Public domain
12. Figure 184: Fifth disease / Andrew Kerr / https://de.wikipedia.org/wiki/Datei:Fifth_disease.jpg / Public domain
13. Figure 186: Sestamalattia (2) / Emiliano Burzagli / https://commons.wikimedia.org/wiki/File:Sestamalattia_(2).JPG / Public domain
14. Figure 188A: Capillary haemangioma / Zeimusu / https://commons.wikimedia.org/wiki/File:Capillary_haemangioma.jpg / Public domain
15. Figures cover and beginning pages: Traité complet de l'anatomie de l'homme: comprenant la médicine opératoire 1831-1844 / Bourgery, Jean Baptiste Marc; Jacob, Nicolas Henri/ Public domain

Epilogue

Through the collaborative effort of an incredible team consisting of students, illustrators, graphic designers, and medical specialists, with this pocket we have successfully translated our vision into reality. Our goal was to ensure that you, as students and doctors, have access to essential information – literally at your fingertips, regardless of your location.

A heartfelt thank you, Anouk and Dominique, for spearheading the publication of our seventh English pocket! To Otte, Dorina, and Jay Yee – what an incredible journey we have embarked upon together! Your contributions and enthusiasm have been instrumental every step of the way. This has been an intense yet uniquely rewarding process, for which we also want to thank the authors of the previous edition: Linde, Carlijn, Maud, and Gwen.

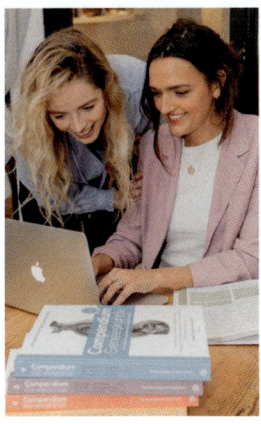

Veerle Smit (L) & Romée Snijders (R)

We are enormously grateful to all the medical professionals who provided valuable feedback and content support, elevating the quality of the text. Your contributions were integral to achieving this result.

This pocket could not have turned out so visually successful without all the illustrators – also mostly medical students – who collaborated on this pocket. Thanks to our team for their exceptional ability to comprehensibly cover the specialty in their graphic work.

We gratefully acknowledge our graphic heroes, Maria and Ivana, whose efforts gave this pocket its recognisable *Compendium Medicine* look. Special thanks also go to Melanie, Pauline, Vera, Laura, and Delano for ensuring the smooth functioning of the entire process.

Last, a sincere thank you to all our colleagues who have *Compendium Medicine* on their bookshelves. Your support has been indispensable in realising our dreams.

We are incredibly proud of this team and hope to see you again soon, in or outside the hospital!

Amsterdam, June 2025

Veerle Smit, MD & Romée Snijders, MD
Doctors and founders of *Compendium Medicine*

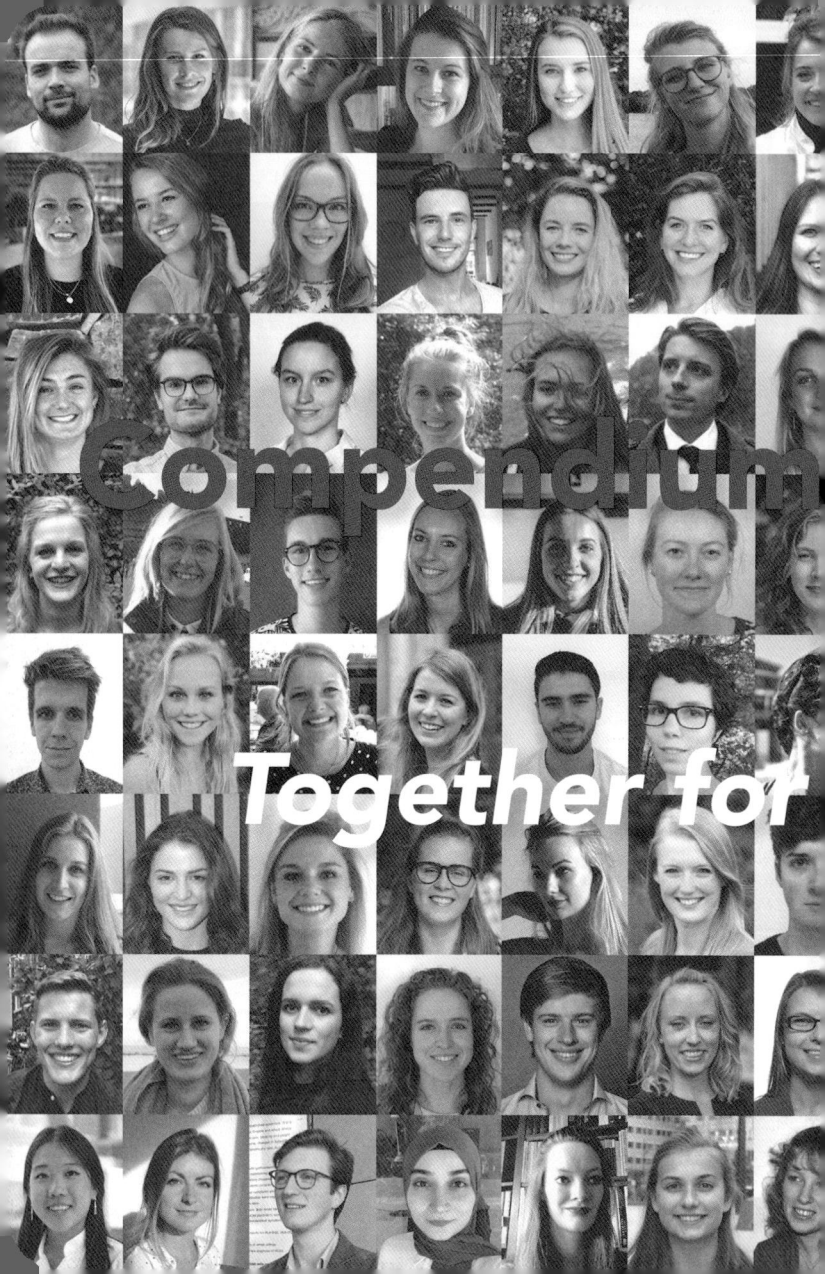

Compendium

Together for

Medicine

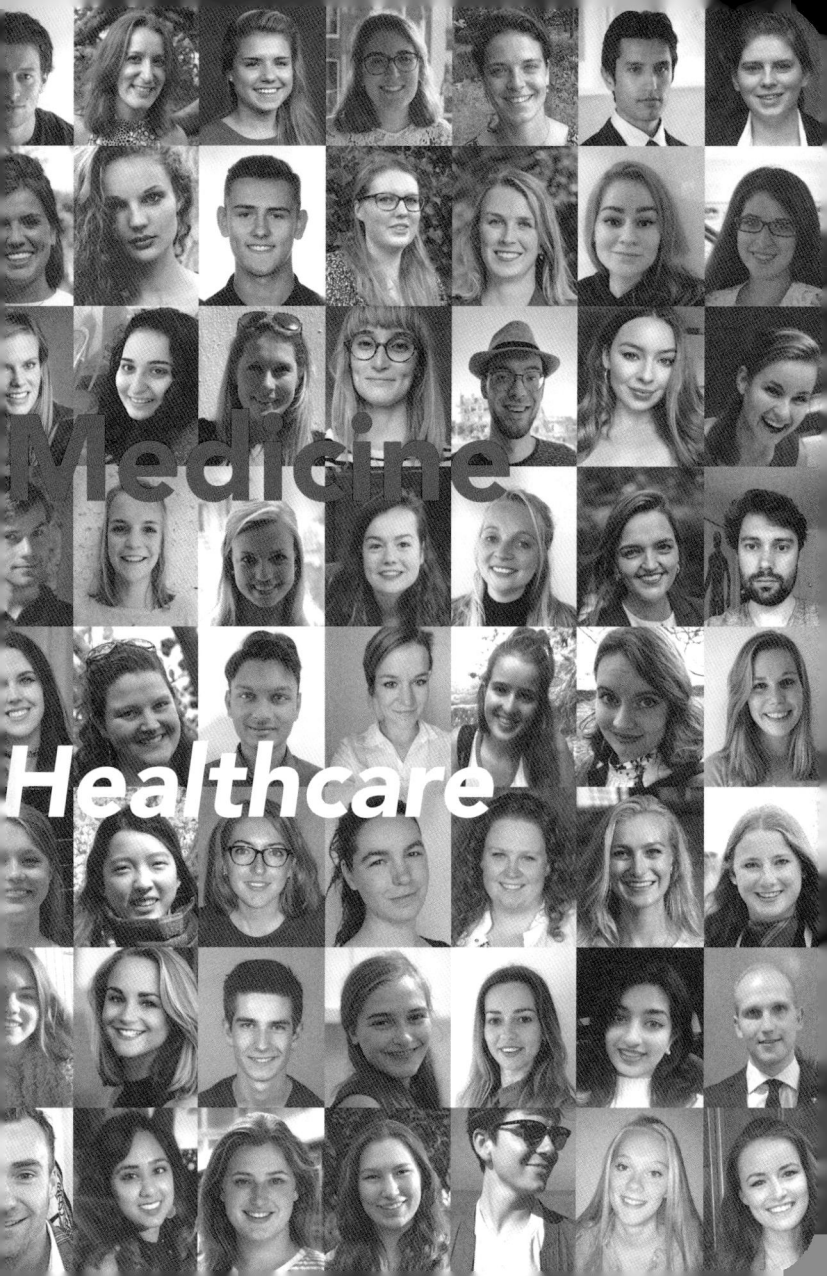

Healthcare

About us

As medical students, we felt overwhelmed by the amount of medical knowledge available. An overview was lacking. Fueled by this need for change, we embarked on a journey that has now brought together over 500 students and doctors to create the entire *Compendium Medicine* book series. Our mission is to help and connect healthcare professionals globally by providing accessible knowledge.

The bigger picture

In 2015, at VU University in Amsterdam, the Netherlands, our paths crossed as we were both pursuing our medical educations. The vast sea of medical knowledge overwhelmed us, highlighting the need for a comprehensive overview. We were surprised by the isolated efforts of every hospital and university, each working on its own 'island', publishing individual books and reference works instead of fostering collaboration.

Motivated to make a difference, we envisioned a solution: a comprehensive guide encompassing all 35 subspecialties, enriched with figures, icons, charts, and mnemonics. Our vision was clear – our books had to be visual, concise, and to the point. With a dedicated team of students and doctors, we started writing an encyclopedia using our unique method. *Compendium Medicine* was born!

Book series

Following almost two years of dedicated effort, the first edition achieved sold-out status even before its official launch: a remarkable start to the ongoing rollercoaster journey. The most rewarding aspect of this experience has been – and still is – the overwhelmingly positive feedback from medical students and specialists. Our narrative caught the attention of prominent Dutch and Belgian newspapers and journals, leading to invitations to feature on popular talk shows on national television.

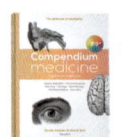

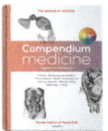

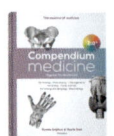

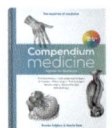

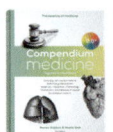

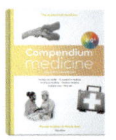

Compendium Medicine book series

Our white-coat pockets

One year later, both of us had started our clinical rotations. We recognized a common challenge faced by many peers: the need for quick and easy access to practical information. In response, we started creating our first series of pockets – concise yet comprehensive pocket-sized booklets designed to provide essential and practical information during a shift.

A period of many milestones followed. Our team expanded every month: from authors to medical specialists, from ambassadors to illustrators. With a growing number of followers on social media, a real community was born. With this team, we worked incredibly hard on new pockets as well as new additions like flashcards and pocket cards. As of now, we have launched a total of 20 different pockets!

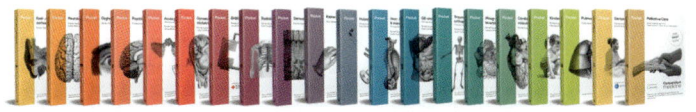

Compendium Medicine pockets

Expanding our mission globally

With the experience gained over the past years, we are committed to making a positive impact on medical students and healthcare professionals worldwide. This new phase kicked off with the distribution of our *Radiology* pocket to all continents. We were amazed to have reached readers from over 92 countries! Their positive feedback was instrumental in propelling us forward, and we are excited to present our seventh pocket in English: *Dermatology*. And this is just the beginning: we are actively working on bringing more pockets to you!

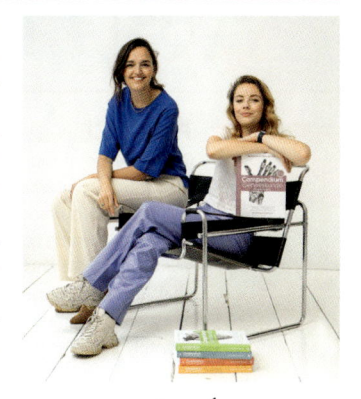

Romée Snijders & Veerle Smit

Doctors and founders of *Compendium Medicine*

Compendium Compass©

We believe that on your journey from medical student to retirement you continuously navigate these five steps. The Compendium Compass© assists you along the way.

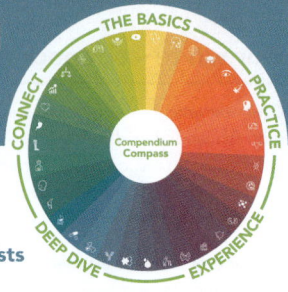

---

1 — THE BASICS

Start at the foundation. Explore all 41 medical specialisms through our comprehensive series, featuring clear diagrams, tables, and illustrations. Visit our website for additional details.

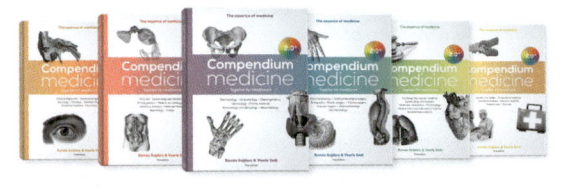

---

2 — PRACTICE

Reinforce your foundational knowledge with our *Compendium Medicine* app and through our social media platforms! The app, which can be downloaded from the Apple and Android app stores, enables you to practice questions on a daily basis and participate in the monthly challenge.

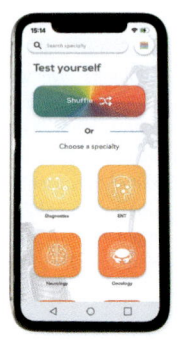

Scan this QR code for more information.

3 **EXPERIENCE**

Learn on-the-go by carrying our pockets and pocket cards with you on the ward, during your shifts and rounds, anytime. Our first pockets are already available worldwide, with many more to come. See below for details!

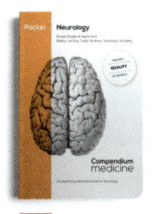

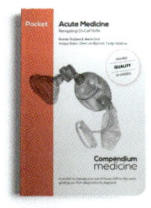

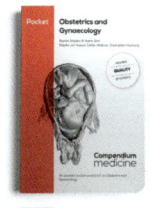

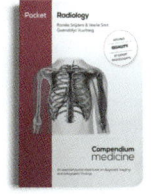

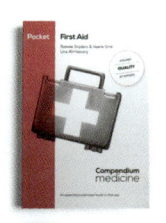

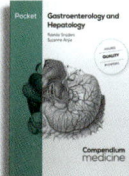

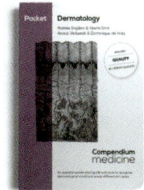

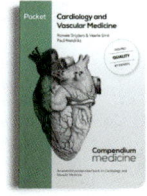

4 **DEEP DIVE**

Explore medical knowledge through extensive reading, immersing yourself in a variety of literature, guidelines, and the latest scientific articles.

5 **CONNECT**

Interested in connecting with individuals in your field? Become a member of our community through our social media platform – a network of students, physicians, specialists, and other healthcare professionals.

Abbreviations

5-FU	5-fluorouacil
ABI	ankle-brachial Index
ABSIS	Autoimmune Bullous Skin Intensity and Severity Score
AB	antibiotics
ABx	antibiotic theraphy
ACE	angiotensin-converting enzyme
ACLE	acute cutaneous lupus erythematosus
ADR	adverse drug reaction
AICAR	5-aminoimidazole-4-carboxamide-1-β-D-ribofuranoside
AIDS	acquired immunodeficiency syndrome
AIN	anal intraepithelial neoplasia
aprox.	approximately
ATZ	anal transition zone
AVN	avascular necrosis
BCC	basal cell carcinoma
BCNS	basal cell naevus syndrome (Gorlin syndrome)
BMI	body mass index
BP	bullous pemphigoid
CADR	cutaneous adverse drug reaction
cAMP	cyclic adenosine monophosphate
cART	antiretroviral combination therapy
CAT	chlamydia antibody titre
CCCA	central centrifugal cicatricial alopecia
CCLE	chronic cutaneous lupus erythematosus
CCR5	C-C chemokine receptor type 5
CI	contraindication
CIN	cervical intraepithelial neoplasia
cm	centimetre
CNS	central nervous system
COPD	chronic obstructive pulmonary disease
COX	cyclooxygenase
CRP	C-reactive protein
CT	computed tomography
CTCL	cutaneous T-cell lymphoma
CVD	cardiovascular disease
CVI	chronic venous insufficiency
CXCR4	C-X-C chemokine receptor type 4
CYP	cytochrome P450
d	day/days
DCS	dissecting cellulitis of the scalp
DDx	differential diagnosis
DFA	direct fluorescent antibody
DHT	dihydrotestosterone
DM	diabetes mellitus
DMF	dimethyl fumarate
DNA	deoxyribonucleic acid
DPCP	diphenylcyclopropenone
DPN	dermatosis papulosa nigra
Dsg1- and 3	desmoglein 1 and 3 (autoantibodies in pemphigus)
DVT	deep vein thrombosis
e.g.	for example
ECG	electrocardiogram
ECM	erythema chronicum migrans
EDP	erythema dyschromicum perstans
EDV	end-diastolic velocity
EIA	enzyme immunoassay
ELISA	enzyme-linked immunosorbent assay
EMm	erythema multiforme minor
EN	erythema nodosum
ENT	ear, nose, and throat
Er:YAG	erbium yttrium aluminium garnet laser
ESBL	extended spectrum beta-lactamase
esp.	especially
ESR	erythrocyte sedimentation rate
EVLT	endovenous laser treatment
FD	folliculitis decalvans
FDG-PET	fluorodeoxyglucose positron emission tomography
FdUMP	fluorodeoxyuridine monophosphate
FFA	frontal fibrosing alopecia
FGFR	fibroblast growth factor receptor
FHx	family history
G6PD	glucose-6-phosphate dehydrogenase
GI	gastrointestinal
GLPLS	Graham-Little-Piccardi-Lassueur syndrome
GNA11	guanine nucleotide-binding protein (G protein), alpha transducing activity polypeptide 11
GNAQ	guanine nucleotide-binding protein (G protein), alpha transducing activity polypeptide Q
GSH	glutathione
GSV	great saphenous vein
h	hour/hours
Hb	hemoglobin
HBS	hepatitis B surface antigen

HCQ	hydroxychloroquine
HGAIN	high-grade intraepithelial neoplasia
HHV	human herpes virus
HIV	human immunodeficiency virus
HLA	human leukocyte antigen
HPV	human papilloma virus
HRA	high-resolution anoscopy
HS	hidradenitis suppurativa
HSIL	high-grade squamous intraepithelial lesion
HSV	herpes simplex virus
Hx	history
IBD	inflammatory bowel disease
ICU	intensive care unit
IF	immunofluorescence
IgA/D/E/G/M	immunoglobulin A/D/E/G/M
IGFR1	insulin-like growth factor-1 receptor
IL	interleukin
IM	intramuscular
incl.	including
IPL	intense pulsed light
IV	intravenous
JAK	Janus kinase
KA	keratoacanthoma
KID	keratitis-ichthyosis-deafness syndrome
KOH	potassium hydroxide (used in fungal microscopy)
KP	keratosis pilaris
KS	Kaposi sarcoma
KSHV	Kaposi sarcoma-associated herpesvirus
L	litre/litres
LEOPARD	a syndrome acronym: lentigines, electrocardiographic abnormalities, ocular hypertelorism, pulmonary stenosis, abnormal genitalia, retarded growth, and deafness
LGAIN	low-grade intraepithelial neoplasia
LGV	lymphogranuloma venereum
LM	lentigo maligna
LMM	lentigo maligna melanoma
LP	lichen planus
LPP	lichen planopilaris
LSIL	low-grade squamous intraepithelial lesion
max.	maximum
MEN 2A	multiple endocrine neoplasia type 2A
mg	milligram
MHC	major histocompatibility complex
min	minute/minutes

min.	minimum
ml	millilitre
MMF	mycophenolate mofetil
MMR	measles, mumps, and rubella
mo	month/months
MPNST	malignant peripheral nerve sheath tumours
MRI	magnetic resonance imaging
MS	multiple sclerosis
NAAT	nucleic acid amplification test
Nd:YAG	neodymium-doped yttrium aluminum garnet (laser treatment)
NF1	neurofibromatosis type 1
NF-κB	nuclear factor kappa B
NNRTI	non-nucleoside reverse transcriptase inhibitor
Nrf2	nuclear factor (erythroid-derived 2)-like 2
NRTIs	nucleoside analogue reverse transcriptase inhibitors
NSAID	non-steroidal anti-inflammatory drug
NYHA	New York heart association
OAC	oral anticoagulation
PAP	Papanicolaou (PAP smear)
PAS	periodic acid-schiff
PCOS	polycystic ovary syndrome
PCR	polymerase chain reaction
PDAI	pemphigus disease area index
PDE4	phosphodiesterase 4
PDL	pulsed dye laser
PDT	photodynamic therapy
PEP	post-exposure prophylaxis
PET	positron emission tomography
PI	pulsatility index
PID	pelvic inflammatory disease
PIH	postinflammatory hyperpigmentation
PLC	pityriasis lichenoides chronica
PLCA	primary localised cutaneous amyloidosis
PLEVA	pityriasis lichenoides et varioliformis acuta
PMHx	past medical history
PMLE	polymorphous light eruption
PPE	personal protective equipment
PPI	proton pump inhibitor
PrEP	pre-exposure prophylaxis
PROM	prelabour rupture of membranes
PRP	platelet-rich-plasma
PSRA	post-streptococcal reactive arthritis
PSV	peak systolic velocity
PTA	percutaneous transluminal angioplasty
PUVA	psoralen and ultraviolet A
PV	pemphigus vulgaris

RA	rheumatoid arthritis
RAS	renin-angiotensin system
RFA	radiofrequency ablation
RNA	ribonucleic acid
RSTL	relaxed skin tension lines
RTI	respiratory tract infection
SCC	squamous cell carcinoma
SCLE	subacute cutaneous lupus erythematosus
SCT	sclerocompression therapy
sec	second/seconds
SEPS	subfascial endoscopic perforator surgery
SIL	squamous intraepithelial lesions
SJS	Stevens-Johnson syndrome
SLE	systemic lupus erythematosus
SNRI	serotonin-norepinephrine reuptake inhibitor
SSPE	subacute sclerosing panencephalitis
SSRI	selective serotonin reuptake inhibitor
SSV	small saphenous vein
STAT	signal transducer and activator of transcription
STI	sexually transmitted infection
t1/2	half-life
TB	tuberculosis
TCA	tricyclic antidepressant
TCC	transitional cell carcinoma
TEC	tyrosine kinase expressed in hepatocellular carcinoma
TEN	toxic epidermal necrolysis
TG2	transglutaminase 2
TG3	transglutaminase 3
Th	T helper
Th2	Th2 – T-helper type 2 cells
TNF	tumor necrosis factor
TPPA	treponema pallidum particle agglutination
USA	United States of America
UV	ultraviolet
UVA	ultraviolet A radiation
UVB	ultraviolet B radiation
VAC	vacuum-assisted closure
VIN	vulvar intraepithelial neoplasia
VZV	varicella zoster virus
WBC	white blood cell
wk	week/weeks
X-ray	radiograph
y	year/years

Index

5th disease	84, 243	Androgenetic alopecia	85, 232
6th disease	84, 243	Angioedema	128, 129
Abx	60	Angioma senilis	195
ABCDE rule	36	Anoscope	47
Abrocitinib	58	Anoscopy	47
Abscess	34	Anterior tibial vein	25
Acanthosis nigricans	178	Antibacterial therapy	60
ACE inhibitors	82	Antibiotic resistance	63
Acne	29, 85	Antibiotics	60
Acne, common subtypes	88	Antihistamines	66
Acne conglobata	85, 89, 90	Anti-inflammatory drugs	52
Acneiform dermatoses	86	Antimycotics	66
Acne keloidalis	85	Antiparasitic therapy	65
Acne keloidalis nuchae	89, 90	Antiviral therapy	65
Acne, neonatal	252	Anus	47
Acne neonatorum	252	Apremilast	54
Acne papulopustular	90	Arrector pili muscle	18
Acne scars	87	Arterial leg ulcer (Fontaine IV)	192
Acne vulgaris	85, 86, 90	Arterial skin conditions	192
Acquired immunodeficiency syndrome (AIDS)	209	Arthropods	45
Acquired melanocytic naevus	166	Asboe-Hansen sign	107
Acrovesicular eczema	116	Athlete's foot	229
Actinic keratosis (AK)	85, 155	Atopic dermatitis	83, 116
Acte cutaneous lupus erythematosus (ACLE)	142	Atrophy	35
Acute urticaria	128	Auramine staining	46
Adalimumab	56	Auspitz's sign	139
Adenocarcinomas	83	Azithromycin	61
Adipose tissue	18	Bacilli, Gram-positive	46
Adnexa	19	Bacterial infections	215
Advancement flap	76	Baricitinib	58
Adverse drug reaction	82	Basal cell carcinoma (BCC)	85, 158
Aesthetic units	21, 22	Becker naevus	167, 169
AIDS	83, 209, 210	Bedsores	183
Allergic contact eczema	118	Benign lichenoid keratosis	153
Allergic reactions	254	Benign skin tumours	146
Allergy testing	44	Bilobed flap	77
Alopecia areata	85, 230	Biologicals	54
Alopecia atrophicans	233	Blister	34
Ambulatory phlebectomy	79	Blushing	84
Amgevita®	56	Bowen's disease	85, 157
Aminoglycosides	62	Braden score	184
Amoxicillin	61	Branches of the facial nerve	24
Anaemia	83	Breast cancer	83
Anaesthetising the skin	41	Broad-spectrum penicillins	61
Anagen effluvium	85	Brodalumab	56
Anagen phase	27	Buccal branch of the facial nerve	24
Analgesics	48	Bulla	34, 35
Anal intraepithelial neoplasia (AIN)	213	Bullous dermatoses	102
Anal swab	47	Bullous impetigo	105
Anatomy	18	Bullous pemphigoid	82, 102, 103
		Bullous pemphigoid (knee)	103
		Buschke-Löwenstein	201

Butterfly erythema secondary to SLE	84
buttonhole sign	155
C2 varicose veins	189
Café-au-lait macule	170
Calcineurin inhibitor	53
Calcium antagonists	82
Campbell de Morgan spots	195
Candle-grease sign	139
Carbapenems	63
Carbuncle	85, 99, 100
Carcinoid syndrome	83
Carcinoma	83
Catagen phase	27
Cauterisation from within the vein	79
CEAP classification: classification of symptoms of chronic venous disorders	188
Cefazolin	61
Cefotaxime	61
Ceftazidime	61
Cefuroxime	61
Celecoxib	48
Cellulitis	84, 215
Cellulitis on the leg	216
Central centrifugal cicatricial alopecia (CCCA)	238
Cephalic pustulosis, neonatal	252
Cephalosporins	61
Cervical branch of the facial nerve	24
Cheeks	22
Cherry angioma	195
Chickenpox	220, 243
Chickenpox, vesicles in	246
Chief complaint	29
Chilblains	194
Childhood diseases	241
Children, generalised erythema in	84
Chin	22
Chlamydia	197
Chronic cutaneous lupus erythematosus (CCLE)	142
Chronic renal insufficiency	83
Chronic venous insufficiency (CVI)	187
Cibinqo	58
Cicatricial alopecia	233, 236
Ciclosporin	53
Ciprofloxacin	63
clarithromycin	61
Classic KS (sporadic)	224
Classic lichen planopilaris	236
Codeine	48
Cold sore	218
Colorimetric scale skin tone classification	38
Colour	31
Comedo	35
Comedonal acne	89
Comedones	87
Common skin pathology	35
Complement binding assay	47
Compound naevus	167
Compression therapy	79
Conditions	86
Condylomata acuminata	200
Congenital dermal melanocytosis	249
Constitutional dermatitis	82, 115, 116
Contact dermatitis	82, 84
Contagious	241
Corticosteroids	51, 52
Corticosteroids, local	256
Cosentyx®	56
Course	29
Course of untreated HIV	212
Coxsackie virus	84
Cradle cap	251
Creams	50
Crossectomy	79
Crust	34
Crusta	34, 35
Crusts	219
Cryotherapy	70
Cushing's syndrome	238
Cutaneous adverse drug reactions (CADR)	136
Cutaneous amyloidosis	181
Cutaneous horn	85
Cutaneous infections, AB used for	60
Cutaneous lupus erythematosus	142
Cutaneous manifestations	62
Cutaneous T-cell lymphoma (CTCL)	164
Cutaneous vascular plexus	18
Cuticle	20, 21
Cutis	21
Cycle of hair growth	27
Cyst	35
Danger zones	23
Dark brown skin	38
Deep femoral vein	25
Delta sign in scabies	204
Dermal naevocellular naevus (compound naevus)	167
Dermal naevus	166
Dermatitis	82, 83
Dermatitis herpetiformis	82, 103
Dermatofibroma	147, 148
Dermatomycoses	226
Dermatomycosis	82
Dermatomyositis	83
Dermatosis papulosa nigra (DPN)	153
Dermis	19
Dermoscopy	36
Dermoscopy: superficial spreading melanoma	36
Dexamethasone	53
Diabetes mellitus (DM)	83
Diagnostics	40
Diaper dermatitis	248

Diaper rash	84, 248
Diclofenac	48
Dimethyl fumarate	68
Dimple sign	148
Dissecting cellulitis of the scalp (DCS)	235
Dissecting folliculitis	236
Distal phalanx	21
DMF	68
Donati suture	74
Dopplers, duplex	43
Doxycycline	62
Dry skin	82
Duhring's disease	103
Dupilumab	58
Dupixent®	58
Duplex ultrasound	43
Dyschromia	35
Dysplastic naevus	85
Ears	22
Eccrine sweat gland	18
ECHO	84
Eczema	29, 115
Eczematous dermatoses	115
Efflorescence	33
Efflorescences, most common	34
Efflorescence, types	35
Electrocoagulation	70
Eliciting factors	29
ELISA	47
Enbrel®	56
Endemic KS (African)	224
Endovenous techniques	79
Enterovirus infections	84
Enzyme-linked immunosorbent assay	47
Epicutaneous test	44
Epidermal/dermal naevocellular naevus (compound naevus)	167
Epidermis	19
Epidermoid cyst	146
Epizoonoses	82
Eponychium	20, 21
Erosion	34, 35
Erysipelas	84
Erysipelas	215
Erythema	35, 83
Erythema chronicum migrans (ECM)	129
Erythema dyschromicum perstans (EDP)	179
Erythema infectiosum	84, 243
Erythema infectiosum, lace-like exanthema in	246
Erythema, local	84
Erythema migrans (Lyme disease)	84
Erythema multiforme	84
Erythema multiforme major (EMM)	131
Erythema multiforme minor (EMm)	130
Erythema nodosum (EN)	84, 109
Erythematosquamous	35

Erythematosquamous dermatoses	137
Erythematosquamous disease	35
Erythematotelangiectatic rosacea	95
Erythematous dermatoses	128
Erythrasma	216
Erythroderma	83
Etanercept	56
Exanthema in exanthema subitum	246
Exanthema in measles	244
Exanthema in rubella	246
Exanthema subitum	84
Exanthema subitum	243
Exanthema subitum, exanthema in	246
Exanthematous childhood diseases	242
Excision	40
Excision biopsy melanoma	70
Excision margins	71
Exclamation mark hair	232
Excoriation	34, 35
Excoriations	83
Exicional biopsy	41
External iliac vein	25
Face	21
Facial erythema	84
Facial nerve	24
Facial pustules	85
Fair skin	38
Fall out/return to anagen phase	27
Febrile erythema of unknown origin	84
Femoral vein	25
Fentanyl	48
Fibular veins	25
Fingertip Unit (FTU)	256
Fissure	35
Fitzpatrick skin type classification	36
Flaps, local, most commonly used	76
Flat skin lesions	33
Flixabi®	56
Flucloxacillin	61
Fluorescence and corresponding pathogens	37
Fluorescence microscope	42
Fluorouracil 5% (5-FU)	68
Flushes secondary to carcinoid syndrome/pheochromocytoma	83
Folic acid	258
Folliculitis	82, 85, 96, 97
Folliculitis barbae	85
Folliculitis decalvans (FD)	235
Fontaine	192
Forehead	22
Frontal bossing alopecia	236
Frontal fibrosing alocepia (FFA)	235
FTU	256
Fumarates	259
Furuncle	85, 99, 100
Gastric cancer	83

INDEX // 277

Generalised erythema	83
Generalised erythema in children	84
Genital herpes	199
Gentamicin (IV)	62
German measles	243
Giant condylomata acuminata	201
Gonorrhoea	198
Gorlin syndrome	159
Gout	83
Gram-negative	61
Gram-negative bacteria	46
Gram-positive	61
Gram-positive bacteria	46
Gram staining	46
Granulocytes	46
Granuloma annulare	111
Grawitz tumour	83
Greater auricular nerve	24
Great saphenous vein	25
Groups of antibiotics	60
Guselkumab	56
Guttate psoriasis	141
Haemangioma	246
Haematoma	35
haematoxylin eosin staining	42
Hair follicle	18
Hair follicle receptor	18
Hair growth	27
Hair growth, cycle of	27
Hair loss	85
Hair root	18
Hairs	19
Hair shaft	18
HALO naevus	169
Halo naevus	167
Handling of needle and needle holder	73
HCQ	66
Herpes, genital	199
Herpes labialis	218
Herpes, oral	218
Herpes simplex	85
Herpes virus	85
Herpes zoster	85, 219, 220
H&E staining	42
Hidradenitis suppurativa (HS)	92
Hidradenitis suppurativa with fistulas	93
High-grade intraepithelial neoplasia (HGAIN)	214
High-resolution anoscopy (HRA)	47
Hirsutism	237
Histopathological testing	42
History-taking for dermatological symptoms	29
HIV	209
Hive	34, 35
Hives	82, 83, 84
HIV replication and targets of antiretroviral drugs	211
HIV, untreated, course of	212
Hodgkin	83
H plasty	76
HRA	47
HSV	85
Hulio®	56
Human immunodeficiency virus (HIV) infection	209
Human papilloma virus (HPV) induced malignancies/premalignancies	212
Humira®	56
Hurley-stage disease severity	93
Hutchinson's sign	163
Hydrochlorothiazide	82
Hydroxychloroquine	66, 68
Hyperhidrosis	240
Hyperkeratosis	35
Hyperparathyroidism	83
Hyperthyroidism	83
Hypodermis	18
Hyponychium	20, 21
Hypothyroidism	83
Hyrimoz®	56
H zone	160
Iatrogenic KS (immunocompromised)	224
Ibuprofen	48
Ice-pick scars	87, 90
Ichthyosis	84
Idiopathic (red man syndrome)	84
IgE immunoglobulins, inceased levels	45
IL inhibitors	55
Ilumya®	56
Immunofluorescence	47
Immunofluorescence (IF) biopsy	42
Immunohistochemical testing	42
Immunological function, skin	26
Immunosuppressive drugs	51, 52
Immunosuppressive drugs, other	54
Impetiginisation	101
Impetigo	85
Impetigo vulgaris	100
Imraldi®	56
Infantile haemangioma	246
Infections	45
Infectious diseases	84
Infectious exanthem	135
Infiltrative BCC	159
Inflectra®	56
Infliximab	56
Infraorbital nerve of the trigeminal nerve	24
Injecting varicose veins	79
Insect bite	82, 84
Interleukin (IL) inhibitors	55
Interrupted, mattress suture	74
Intertriginous eczema	121

Intertrigo	84
Intralesional corticosteroids	51
Invasive, non-pharmacological treatment	70
Iron deficiency	83
Irritant contact dermatitis	119
Isotretinoin	87, 259
Itching	82
Ixekizumab	56
Jakavi®	58
JAK inhibitors	58
Janus kinase (JAK) inhibitors	58
Junctional naevus	167
Kahler's disease	45
Kaposi sarcoma (KS)	223
Kaposi sarcoma subtypes	224
Keloid	148
Keratoacanthoma	85, 150
Keratoacanthoma (KA)	149
Keratolytics	66
Keratosis pilaris	85
Keratosis pilaris (KP)	114
Kiss of death	200
Knot-tying	73, 78
Koplik spots	245
Lace-like exanthema in erythema infectiosum	246
Large lump	34
Large nodule	34, 35
Laser therapy	80
laxative	48
Lentigo maligna (LM)	85, 163
Lentigo simplex	172
LEOPARD syndrome	173
Leukaemia	83
levofloxacin	63
Lichen amyloidosis	182
Lichenification	35, 83
Lichen planopilaris (LPP)	235
Lichen planus (LP)	83, 112
Lichen ruber planus	82
Lichen sclerosus	134
Lichen simplex chronicus	82, 125
Light brown skin	38
Limberg flap	77
Lipoma	151
Lipoma excision, therapeutic	72
Lipoma, removed	72
Liver disease with cholestasis	83
Local corticosteroids	51, 256
Local erythema	84
Local flaps, most commonly used	76
Loss of the epidermis	34
Lower extremities, venous system	25
Lower lip	22
Low-grade intraepithelial neoplasia/LGAIN	214
Lump	34

Lunula	20
Lyme disease	84
Lymphoedema	186
Lymphoedema legs	186
Lymphogranuloma venereum (LGV)	208
Lymphology	186
Lymphomas	83
Macrolides	61
Macular cutaneous amyloidosis	182
Macule	34, 35
Malignancy	83
Malignancy risk factors	28
Malignant reticulosis	84
Malignant skin tumours	158
Marginal mandibular branch of the facial nerve	24
Martorell's ulcer	193
Measles	84, 241
Measles, exanthema in	244
Medication dosage	256
Medication, hair loss	85
Medium brown skin	38
Melanoma	85, 161
Melanoma excision	71
Melanoma, excision biopsy	70
Melasma	173
MEN 2A syndrome	182
Mental nerve of the trigeminal nerve	24
Meropenem	63
Methotrexate (MTX)	54, 258
Methylene blue staining	45
Microbiological testing	45
Micronodular BCC	159
Microscopy	45
Mohs micrographic surgery	78
Molluscum contagiosum	220
Mongolian spot	249
Mononucleosis infectiosa	84
Morbilli	84, 243
Morpheaform BCC	159
Morphine	48
Most common efflorescences	34
Motor nerve branch	23
MTX	258
Muller procedure	79
Multiple myeloma	45, 83
Multiple sclerosis (MS)	82
Mycological test	45
Naevi	166, 168
Naevocellular naevus	166, 167
Naevus flammeus	249
Naevus flammeus (port-wine stain)	84
Naevus sebaceous	169
Naevus spilus	169
Nail bed	21
Nail defects, psoriasis vulgaris	140
Nail external	8, 20

Nail fold	21
Nail internal	21
Nail matrix	21
Nail plate	20, 21
Nail root	21
Nails	20
Naproxen	48
Nasolabial flap	77
Necrotising fasciitis	217
Neonatal acne	252
Neonatal cephalic pustulosis	252
Nerve branch	23
Nerve palsy, symptoms of	23
Neurofibroma	154
Nikolsky sign	107
Nikolsky-II sign	107
Nodular BCC	159
Nodular dermatoses	109
Nodule	34, 35
Non-bullous, pemphigoid	82
Non-Hodgkin	83
Non-medicated therapy	50
Nonspecific viral exanthems	84
Noonan syndrome	173
Normal duplex ultrasound of the left common carotid artery	43
Nose	22
Notalgia paresthetica	127
NSAIDs	48
Nummular dermatitis	82, 122
Oedema	35
Ointments	50
Olumiant®	58
Omalizumab	58
Onychomycosis	226
Onychomycosis of the toenail	227
Opioids	48
Oral herpes	218
Oral retinoids	67
Otezla®	54
Oxycodone	48
Pacinian corpuscle	18
Paediatrics	241
Pale skin	38
Palmar erythema	84
Palmoplantar pustulosis (PPP)	101
Papillomatous naevus	167
Papula	35
Papule	34
Papules	83
Papulomatous dermatoses	111
Papulopustular acne	89
Papulopustular rosacea	87, 95
Paracetamol	48
Parakeratosis	35
Paraneoplastic	83
Parasitic diagnostics	45
Parasitic infections	83
Paronychium	20
PASS ONE©	30
PASS ONE© arrangement	32
Past dermatological history	29
Patch test	44
Patient history	28
PDE4 inhibitor	54
PDT	80
Pediculosis capitis	201
Pediculosis pubis	202
Pemphigoid	82
Pemphigus vulgaris	106
Penicillinase-resistant penicillins	61
Penicillins	61
Perifolliculitis capitis abscedens et suffodiens (dissecting folliculitis)	236
Periocular dermatitis	85
Perioral dermatitis	85, 91, 92
Periorbital	22
Pernio	193
Peutz-Jeghers syndrome	173
Pfeiffer's disease	84
Phadiatop test	45
Pharmacological treatment	48
Pheochromocytoma	83
Photodynamic therapy (PDT)	80
Phthiriasis pubis	202
Physical examination	30
Pigmentation disorders	170
Pimples	85
Piperacillin	61
Pityriasis alba	177
Pityriasis lichenoides	144
Pityriasis lichenoides chronica (PLC)	146
Pityriasis lichenoides chronicus	144
Pityriasis lichenoides et varioliformis acuta	144
Pityriasis lichenoides et varioliformis acuta (PLEVA)	146
Pityriasis rosea	137, 138
Pityriasis rosea mother lesion	138
Pityriasis versicolor	174
Plaque	34, 35
Plaquenil®	68
PMNLs	46
Polycystic ovarian syndrome	238
Polycythaemia vera	83
Polymorphonuclear leukocytes	46
Polymorphous light eruption (PMLE)	132
Popliteal vein	25
Pore of sweat gland duct	18
Port-wine stain	84, 249
Posterior tibial vein	25
Postinflammatory hyperpigmentation (PIH)	176
Postmenopausal	83
Post-pregnancy hair loss	85
Prednisolone	53

Prednisone	53, 257
Pregnancy	83
Premalignant skin lesions	155
Presentation of psoriasis in different skin types	32
Pressure ulcer grading system	185
Pressure ulcers	183
Primary hyperhidrosis	241
Proctological examination	47
Proctoscope	47
Progressive macular hypomelanosis (PMH)	180
Protective functions, skin	26
Prurigo	126
Prurigo nodularis (PN)	110
Pruritus	82
Pseudofolliculitis barbae	97, 98
Psoriasis	29, 82, 83
Psoriasis inversa	141, 142
Psoriasis vulgaris	138
Punch biopsy	41
Purpura	35
Pursestring suture	77
Pustular dermatoses	86
Pustule	34, 35
Pustules, facial	85
PUVA	79
Pyodermas	96
Pyogenic granuloma	195
Quinolones	63
Radioallergosorbent test (RAST)	44
Raspberry tongue	245
RAST	44
Raynaud's phenomenon	84
Rectum	47
Red man syndrome	84
Relaxed skin tension lines (RSTL)	22
Remicade®	56
Removal, suture	78
Remsima®	56
Retinoids	67
Rhagade	35
Rhinophyma	96
Rhomboid flap	77
Ringworm	228
Rinvoq®	58
Risankizumab	56
Rosacea	84, 85, 94, 96
Rosacea papulopustulosa	96
Rosacea subtypes	95
Rosacea telangiectasia	96
Roseola infantum	243
Rotation flap	76
Rubella	84, 241, 243, 246
Running intracutaneous suture	75
Running mattress suture	75
Ruxolitinib	58
Scabies	82, 203

Scale	34
Scalp	22
Scalp psoriasis	141, 142
Scarlatina	243
Scarlet fever	84, 243
Scarring alopecia	233
Sclerosis	35
Sclerotherapy	79
Scratch mark	34
Sebaceous glands	19
Sebaceous naevus	167
Sebaceous (oil) gland	18
Seborrhoeic dermatitis	83, 123
Seborrhoeic dermatitis of the head	251
Seborrhoeic keratosis	152
Secondary hyperhidrosis	241
Secondary impetigo	101
Secondary syphilis	84
Secukinumab	56
Senile comedones	85
Sensitive nerve branch	23
Sensory function, skin	27
Sensory nerve fiber	18
Serological testing	46
Serology	44
Sexually transmitted infections (STIs)	29, 197
Sezary syndrome	84
Shave biopsy	41
Shingles	85, 219
Siliq®	56
Sipple syndrome	182
Skin	18
Skin biopsy and excision	40
Skin cancer	29
Skin colour	38
Skin excision	40
Skin layer	19
Skin lesions, suspicious	85
Skin lesion, suspicious	255
Skin pathology, common	35
Skin prick test	44
Skin tone classification, colorimetric scale	38
Skin tumours	146
Skin type	36
Skin type classification, Fitzpatrick	36
Skin types and names	38
Skyrizi®	56
Slapped cheeks	246
SLE	84
Small lump	34
Small saphenous vein	25
Solar erythema	83
Solar erythema (sunburn)	84
Solar lentigo	171
Soluble sutures	73
Spilus naevus	167
Spitz naevus	167, 169

Squama	34, 35
Squamous cell carcinoma (SCC)	85, 160
Staphylococcal scalded skin syndrome (SSSS)	84
Statis dermatitis	82
Stelara®	56
Steroid acne	85
STIs	197
Stolz's ABCDE rule	36
Strawberry naevus	246
Stretch test	175
Stripping	79
Subacute cutaneous lupus erythematosus (SCLE)	142
Sub-branch of the facial nerve	24
Subcutis	19
Sunburn	84
Superficial BCC	159
Supraorbital nerve of the trigeminal nerve	24
Supratrochlear nerve of the trigeminal nerve	24
Surgery, Mohs micrographic	78
Suspicious skin lesion	255
Suspicious skin lesion, coloured	255
Suspicious skin lesions	85
Sutton-naevus	167
Suture removal	78
Suturing	73
Suturing techniques	73, 74
Sweat glands	19
Switch therapy	63
Syphilis	204
Syphilis, stages	206
Tacrolimus	53
Taltz®	56
Telangiectasias	35
Telogen effluvium	85, 236
Telogen phase	27
Temporal branch of the facial nerve	24
Tetracyclines	62
The clap	198
The great pretender	205
Therapeutic lipoma excision	72
Thermoregulation	26
Three-day measles	243
Tildrakizumab	56
Tinea capitis	227
Tinea corporis	228
Tinea pedis	229
Tinea unguium	226
TNF-alpha blockers	54, 56
Tofacitinib	58
Topical antibiotics	65
Topical fluorouracil	68
Topical retinoids	67
Toxic epidermal necrolysis (TEN)	107
Toxicoderma	62, 83
Traction alopecia	239, 240
Tramadol	48
Transposition flap	76
Trauma hairloss	85
Treatment of varicose veins	79
Treatment, wound	78
Tremfya®	56
Trichomonas vaginalis	208
Trichomoniasis	207
Trichomycosis	227
Trichosis	230
Trichotillomania	85
Trigeminal nerve	24
Tumours	35, 83
Tumours, skin	146
Type and name, skin	38
Ulcer	34, 35
Ulceration in syphilis	207
Upadacitinib	58
Upper lip	22
Urtica	34
Urticaria	129
Ustekinumab	56
UVA	79
UVB	79
Varicella	82, 220, 243
Varicose veins, injecting	79
Varicose veins, treatment of	79
Vascular conditions	187
Veins, varicose	79
Venous insufficiency	190
Venous leg ulcer	190, 191
Venous skin conditions	187
Venous system of the lower extremities	25
Verruca plantaris	222
Verruca vulgaris	221
Very dark brown skin	38
Very light beige skin	38
Vesicle	34, 35
Vesicles in chickenpox	246
Viral infections	218
Vitamin D3 production	27
Vitiligo	175
V-Y plasty	76
Wart	221
Wheal	34
Window phase	210, 214
Wood's lamp	36
Wool wax allergies	51
Wound	34
Wound treatment	78
Xeljanz®	58
Xerosis cutis	82, 83, 126
Xolair®	58
Zessly®	56
Ziehl-Neelsen staining	46
Z plasty	77
Zygomatic branch of the facial nerve	24